Atlas of Oral and Maxillofacial Rehabilitation

Edited by
Kan-ichi Seto, D.D.S., Ph.D.
Professor and Chairman
1st Dept. of Oral and Maxillofacial Surgery
School of Dental Medicine, Tsurumi University, Japan

With contribution by
Masaro Matsuura, D.D.S., Ph.D.
Professor and Chiarman
Section of Oral Implantology, Department of Oral Rehabilitation
Fukuoka Dental College, Japan

Kazuo Shimozato, D.D.S., Ph.D.
Professor and Chairman
Dept. of Oral and Maxillofacial Surgery-II
School of Dentistry, Aichi-Gakuin University,Japan

Masaaki Goto, D.D.S., Ph.D.
Professor and Chairman
Dept.of Oral and Maxillofacial Surgery
Saga Medical School, Japan

Takayoshi Nomura, D.D.S., Ph.D.
Assistant Professor
1st Dept. of Oral and Maxillofacial Surgery
School of Dental Medicine, Tsurumi University, Japan

Quintessence Publishing Co.,Ltd.
Tokyo ,Berlin, Chicago, London, Paris, Barcelona, São Paulo, New Delhi, Moscow, Prague,Warsaw, and Istanbul

Printing and Binding: Sun Art Printing Co., Ltd. Osaka
Printing in Japan
ISBN 4-87417-796-4　C 3047

Preface

Oral and maxillofacial rehabilitation means that where any function or physical structure in the oral-maxillofacial region has been lost, restoration is made to the extent that patients can return to a normal social life. Even though it might be assumed that defects in the oral and maxillofacial region most commonly have their origin in congenital malformation, injury or inflammation, defects resulting from surgical treatment for malignancy are, in fact, currently much more frequent. Recent enormous advances in reconstructive surgery have allowed the range of curable cancers to be greatly expanded, therefore the cure rate for malignancies of the oral cavity has increased dramatically. However, under present circumstances, full use of various techniques such as pedicles or free flaps has not always led to a complete reconstruction of function. Furthermore, defect reconstruction of the hard palate or of the alveolus with dentition covered by masticatory mucosa or sites presenting complex forms, such as those involving the orbit or auricle, is difficult. Maxillofacial prosthetic techniques employing artificial forms or appliances based upon dental practice are required for such defects. Within the academic system, as reconstructive surgery and maxillofacial prosthetics developed independently, mutual exchange of information was notably minimal. However, at present when a defect involving a large field is encountered, affected areas are spread across several zones, owing to the expansion of the curable cancerous region. The simultaneous use of both surgical and dental prosthetic techniques has compelled their fusion and integration within the treatment system.

Incidentally, the Japanese Academy of Maxillofacial Prosthetics has a history of special development, having initiated a multidisciplinary dental academy based upon the initiative of oral and maxillofacial surgeons and prosthodontists. This undertaking has continued into the present era and is proving its worth in current practice. In future, we intend to pursue our development as an Academy of Maxillofacial Rehabilitation in response to changing patient needs. This will include all dental and relevant medical fields as well as reconstructive surgery. Since oral and maxillofacial functionality is of fundamental importance and of a complexity far beyond ordinary considerations, the rehabilitation of patients suffering defects of the parenchyma can never be easy.

Although a dedicated technological work on oral and maxillofacial rehabilitation has long been desired, particularly in Southeast Asia which has a high incidence of oral cavity cancer, in practical terms none has been available. We, frankly speaking, feel some anxiety as to whether the present volume can fully meet this need. However, we consider that, at least, we can supply documented and illustrated information regarding current technological standards based upon the establishment of a concept of maxillofacial rehabilitation in Japan. We will be quite satisfied if this volume serves as a foundation for future international development in this field.

To provide the most widespread help to people who lose oral and maxillofacial functions and forms, who suffer due to the exigencies of war, or from diseases such as oral cancer, we would be extraordinarily happy if the present volume were to pass into the hands of the surgical team in an underprivileged hospital, an under financed dental college, a rural clinic, or a remote tropical dental laboratory.

It is brought to notice that the present volume was published with considerable support from a Non-Profit Organization, Asia Fight against Oral Cancer (AFOC).

Winter, 2003
Kan-ichi Seto

Contributors

Hideharu Usui,D.D.S.,Ph.D.
Assistant Professor
Dept. of Oral and Maxillofacial Surgery-II
School of Dentistry, Aichi-Gakuin University, Japan
Chief, Section of Maxillofacial Prosthetics
Usui Dental Clinic, Japan

Hideki Sekiya, D.D.S.
Instructor and Reserch Associate
1st Dept. of Oral and Maxillofacial Surgery
School of Dental Medicine, Tsurumi University, Japan

Hirohumi Kido, D.D.S., Ph.D.
Associate Professor
Section of Oral Implantology
Department of Oral Rehabilitation
Fukuoka Dental College, Japan

Kan-ichi Seto, D.D.S., Ph.D.
Professor and Chairman
1st Dept. of Oral and Maxillofacial Surgery
School of Dental Medicine, Tsurumi University, Japan

Kazuo Shimozato, D.D.S., Ph.D.
Professor and Chairman
Dept. of Oral and Maxillofacial Surgery-II
School of Dentistry, Aichi-Gakuin University, Japan

Koichiro Ihara, D.D.S., Ph.D.
Assistant Professor
Dept. of Oral and Maxillofacial Surgery
Saga Medical School, Japan

Koji Kawaguchi, D.M.D., Ph.D.
Assistant Professor
1st Dept. of Oral and Maxillofacial Surgery
School of Dental Medicine, Tsurumi University, Japan

Masaaki Goto, D.D.S., Ph.d.
Professor and Chairman
Dept. of Oral and Maxillofacial Surgery
Saga Medical School, Japan

Masaro Matsuura, D.D.S., Ph.D.
Professor and Chiarman
Section of Oral Implantology
Department of Oral Rehabilitation
Fukuoka Dental College, Japan

Michio Shikimori, D.D.S., Ph.D.
Associate Professor
Dept. of Oral and Maxillofacial Surgery
Saga Medical School, Japan

Motoo Yokoi, D.D.S., Ph.D.
Chief, Dept. of Oral and Maxillofacial Surgery
Nagoya City University Hospital,Japan

Nobuhiro Noguchi, D.D.S.
Instructor and Reserch Associate
Dept. of Oral and Maxillofacial Surgery
Saga Medical School, Japan

Takayoshi Nomura, D.D.S., Ph.D.
Assistant Professor
1st Dept. of Oral and Maxillofacial Surgery
School of Dental Medicine, Tsurumi University, Japan

Yoshimasa Yamaguchi
Dental technician
Dept. of Oral and Maxillofacial Surgery
Saga Medical School, Japan

Yoshio Yamashita, DY.D.S., Ph.D.
Assistant Professor
Dept. of Oral and Maxillofacial Surgery
Saga Medical School, Japan

Yukinobu Satoh
Dental technician
Division of Maxillo-Facial Prosthetics
Usui Dental Clinic, Japan

Contents

SECTION 1

Foundations of Maxillofacial Prosthetics

CHAPTER 1

Classification of maxillofacial prostheses

Maxillofacial prosthetics is the restoration of maxillofacial defects using prostheses. The defect sites to be restored by maxillofacial prosthetics include the maxilla, soft palate, mandible, facial skin, eye, nose, and ear.

1. Prostheses for maxillary defects

Any maxillary defect may have an effect on the bone of the jaw, including the dental alveoli and the hard palate. Prostheses for maxillary defects including those of the dental alveoli are referred to as "maxillodental prosthesis (or jaw prosthesis)". With this type of prosthesis the healthy region is covered by a denture plate, the defective region is sealed by an obturator, and the posterior margin of the maxillodental prosthesis (or jaw prosthesis) is extended to cover the defect region of the soft palate.

- Immediate maxillary prostheses and permanent maxillary prostheses :

With maxillary resection, maxillodental prosthesis that are produced preoperatively and are inserted on the completion of surgery are referred to as "immediate maxillary prostheses" or "resection prostheses". Insertion of the immediate maxillary prosthesis has the effects of minimizing postoperative dysfunction and preventing patients from feeling the loss of maxillary parenchyma. Later, after the wound has stabilized, a permanent maxillary prosthesis is produced. However, the permanent maxillary prosthesis cannot be used permanently as-is because the form of the resected wound gradually changes, making reproduction or repair necessary.

- Palatal prostheses :

When surgery causes a palatal bone defect, it is essential to prepare an artificial palatal plate for insertion at the completion of the surgery. Another objective of preparing a palatal plate is to assist with tongue functions by producing a plate with appropriate thickness to lower the palate for cases in which there is insufficient tongue lift because of a tongue defect or tongue dysfunction.

2. Prostheses for defects of soft palate

Although most soft palate defects are incidental to maxillary defects, limited defects of the soft palate may occur as a result of excision of soft palatal and oropharyngeal tumors. In such cases, when recovery of the articulatory function is the principal purpose, a valve or extended valve is attached to the palatal plate to assist in the restoration of the defect and in phonation.

The case ($H_5S_3D_0T_3$) shown in Figs. 1 to 3, with a defect exceeding half of the maxilla and an extensive defect extending to the posterior margin of the soft palate, was reconstructed using a forearm flap with bone from the radius, followed by insertion of a maxillodental prosthesis with open-type obturator.

- Speech aid :

An appliance to assist phonation is applied to the soft palatal defect to alleviate shortening due to scarring or dyskinesia due to denervation. A speech aid should be used to alleviate velopharyngeal failure, a palatal lift should be made for alleviation of dyskinesia, and the posterior margin of the maxillodental prosthesis should be extended to alleviate a soft palatal defect.

3. Prostheses for mandibular defects

Mandibular defects require reconstruction of the jaw. In particular, when the continuity of the mandible has been lost, prosthetic treatment is almost impossible without reconstruction. Since mandibular reconstruction involves repair of the bone in the defective region, ordinary dentures can be inserted rather than maxillodental prostheses in cases in which reconstruction is excellent. On the contrary, with extensive surrounding soft-tissue defect and poor tongue function, or if the oral cavity is filled with a large flap, or the intermaxillary relationship is poor, inserting dentures can be difficult, or it may be impossible to achieve functional recovery even if prosthetic treatment is performed.

In some cases involving debridement for a minimum soft tissue defect, the production of a denture might be possible even if no mandibular reconstruction has been performed (Figs. 4 and 5).

- Preprosthetic surgery :

In the production of maxillary prostheses, it is essential to achieve conditions that make it possible to insert those prostheses. In many cases of reconstruction, it is impossible to insert prostheses due to the occupation by flaps.

- Vestibuloplasty :

There are two main types of cases in which dentures cannot be inserted on the mandible.

The first type are cases in which there is no immov-

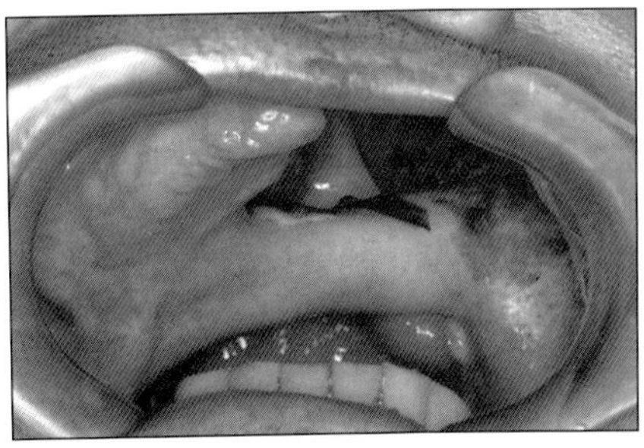

Fig. 1 Case in which reconstruction was done using forearm flap and with bone from the radius following the resection of squamous cell carcinoma on the soft palate region. This defect is described as $H_5S_3D_0T_3$ according to HS classification.

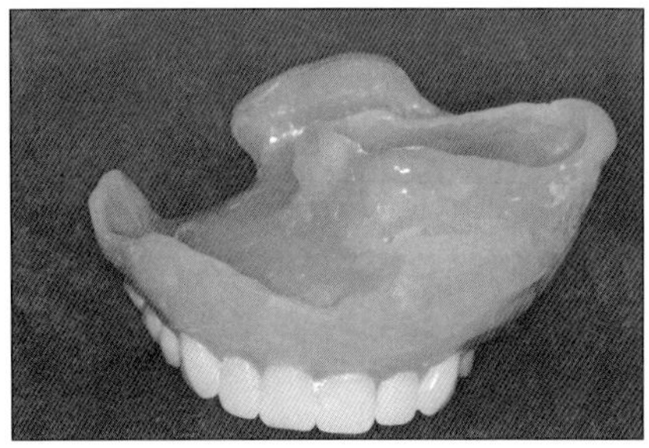

Fig. 2 Maxillodental prosthesis.

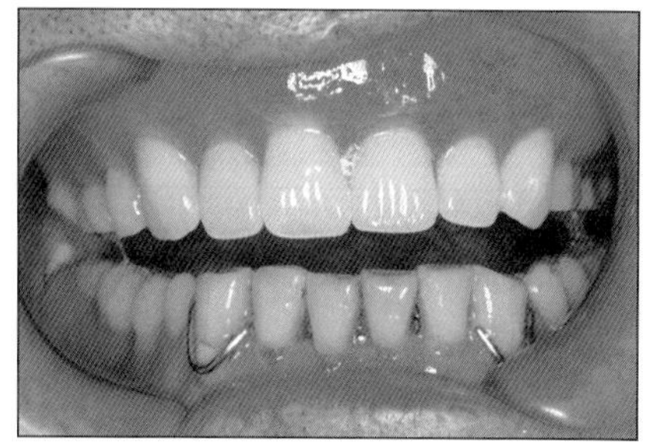

Fig. 3 With Maxillodental prosthesis inserted for the case shown in Fig. 1.

Fig. 4 *(left)* Denture for case in which marginal mandibulectomy was done due to ameloblastoma.
Fig. 5 *(right)* Intraoral view of the same case with denture inserted. In this case, it was possible to produce dentures without doing preprosthetic treatment.

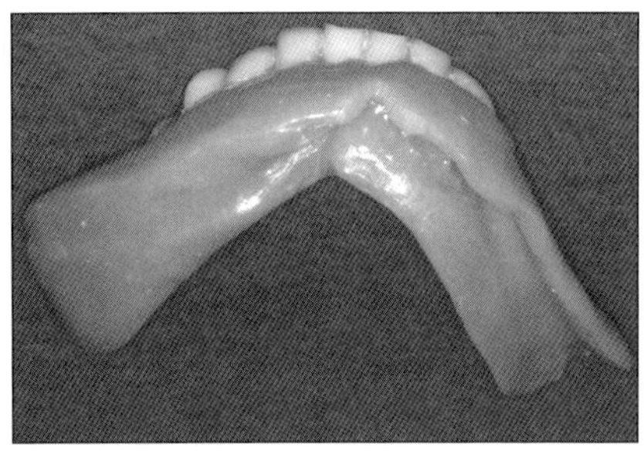

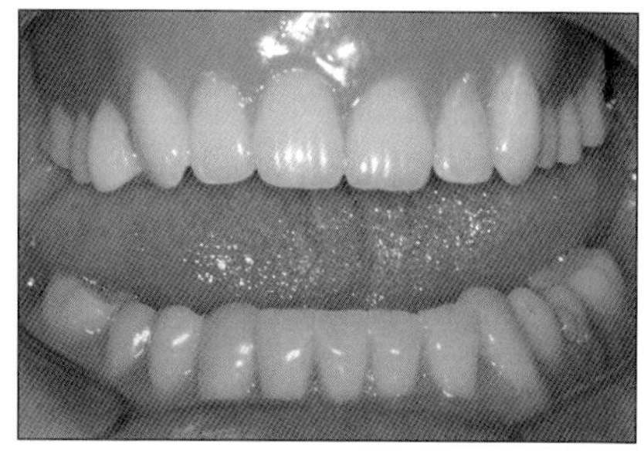

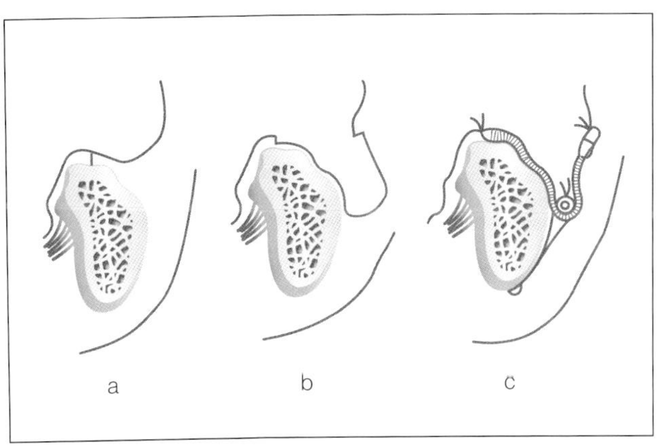

Fig. 6 Schema showing procedure for vestibuloplasty for cases in which the immovable region has been lost because of reefing of the mucosal wound after the resection of tumors:
a: Incision line. **b:** The mucosa is excluded buccally to form the grafting space without bone exposure. **c:** Traction suturing is done following suturing of the split-thickness skin graft.

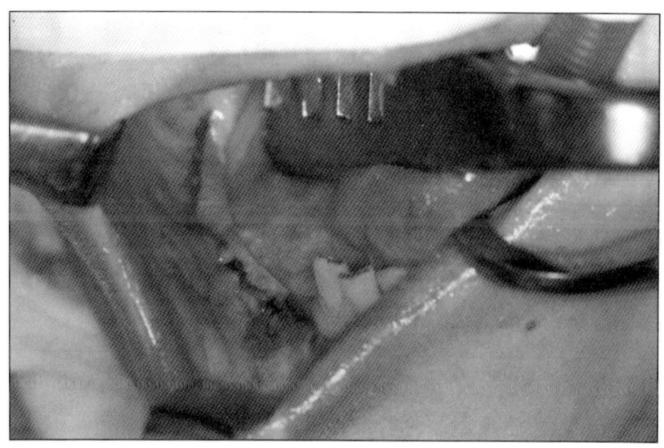

Fig. 7 Case in which reconstruction was done using a free iliac bone transplant after excision of mandibular ameloblastoma. Because of shrinkage of the wound after suturing, there was no immovable mucous membrane. Therefore vestibuloplasty was performed using a split-thickness skin graft.

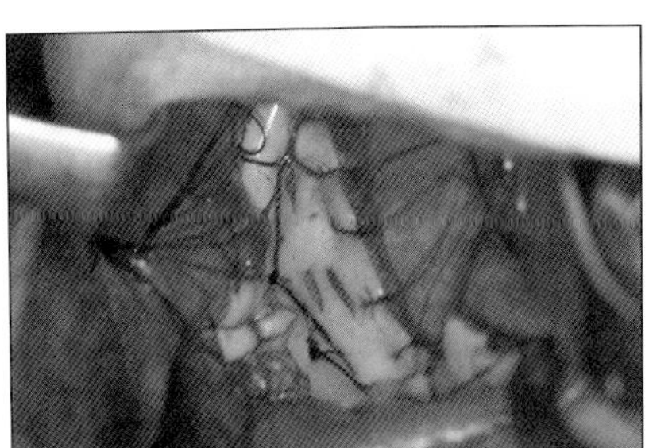

Fig. 8 The mucosa was moved to the buccal side to prepare the grafting space. The skin harvested from the femoral region was grafted, and a tie-over dressing was done following traction suturing.

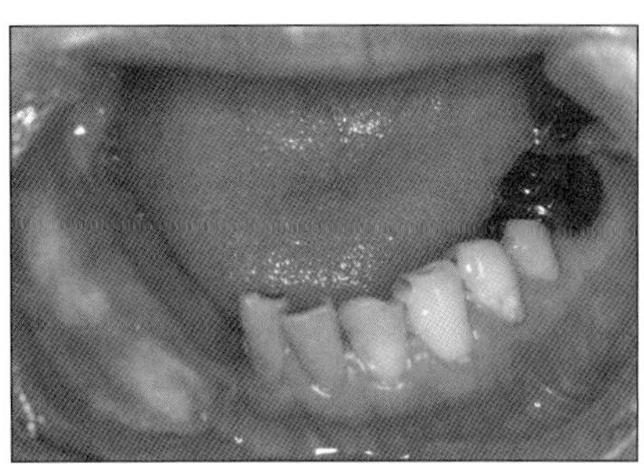

Fig. 9 Postoperative intraoral view. Vestibule has been sufficiently prepared.

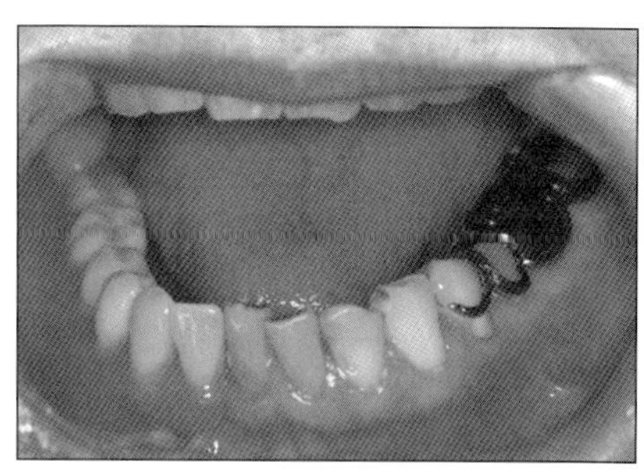

Fig. 10 Intraoral view of the same case with denture inserted.

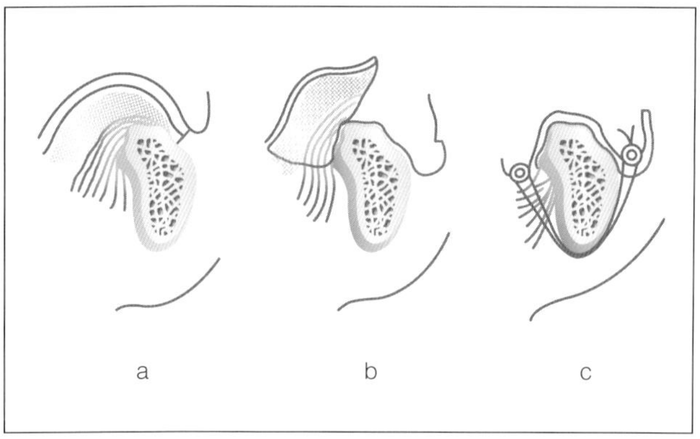

Fig. 11 Schema for vestibuloplasty for case in which the alveolar crest is covered by a myocutaneous flap:
a: Incision line. **b:** A flap is peeled back from the alveolar crest, then the hypodermis and muscular body are resected. **c:** Traction suturing is done following suturing of the thinned skin.

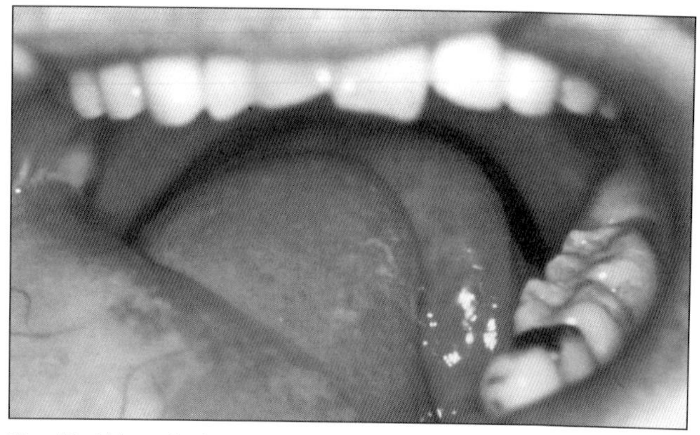

Fig. 12 Although the oral floor was reconstructed with a rectus abdominal flap after resection of carcinoma of the oral floor, displacement of the tongue to the left because of excessive volume of the flap resulted in dysmasesis and dysphagia.

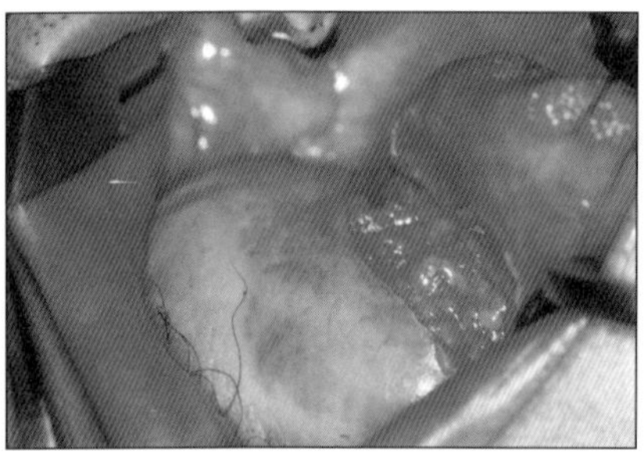

Fig. 13 A diamond-shaped incision was made in the left half of the flap skin and drastic resection of the hypodermis was done.

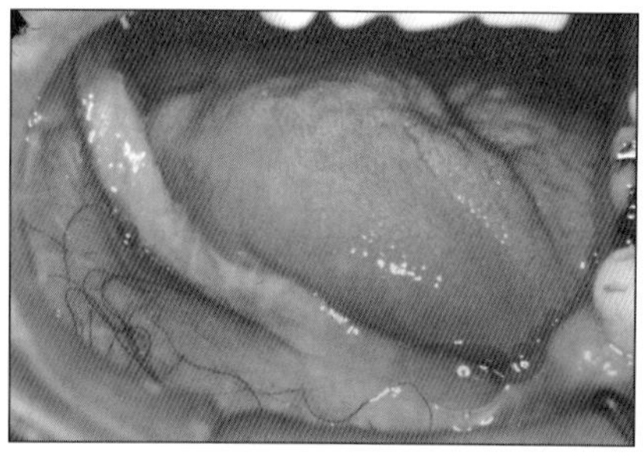

Fig. 14 The thinned skin was tightly adhered to the alveolar crest by traction suturing, to form an immovable region. The tongue position also returned almost to normal.

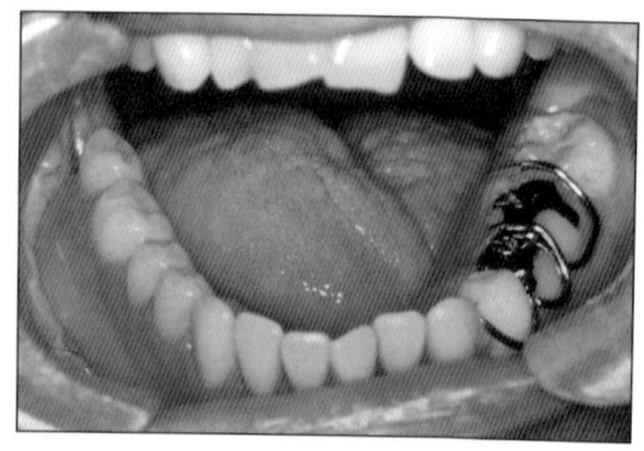

Fig. 15 Intraoral view of the same case with denture inserted.

able region for the insertion of dentures, due to the gingival resection following the excision of tumors and reefing of the buccal mucosa with the oral-floor mucosa. In this type of case, the crest of the alveolar bone is incised and a graft floor is prepared by moving the mucosa to the buccal side, followed by the grafting of skin or mucosa (Figs. 6 to 10).

In the other type of case, resection of the thick flap over the alveolar ridge is done, leaving only the epidermis. The epidermis is then attached to the alveolar ridge to form an immovable region (Figs. 11 to 15).

• Jaw prostheses using implants :

The achievement of prosthesis retention and stability is often difficult in patients with jaw defects, although the retention of prostheses with implants in the maxilla and mandible is an effective method. In cases of extensive defects and complex reconstruction, however, special preparation of the denture placement region is necessary since simply inserting implants alone is insufficient to ensure successful placement of the prosthesis. Mucosa in particular is needed around the implants, so mucous membrane grafting, from the palate or elsewhere, is necessary. In both of the cases shown in Figs. 16 to 23, the mucous membrane graft was performed in the second surgery.

Even for a facial prosthesis, implants are used as secure retentive sources for the "Epithese".

4. Facial prostheses

The prosthesis for a facial defect is referred to in Japan as an "Epithese". Since there is no adequate term in Japanese to describe a prosthesis for a facial defect, the German word, "Epithese", is commonly used. The most frequent defects (in Japan) are midface defects centering on the orbit, followed in frequency by defects of the external ear and auricle, although these are relatively rare among the Japanese, who have a comparatively low incidence of skin cancer.

A major role of the "Epithese" is the esthetic restoration of defects around the orbit; other roles include the restoring of dysfunctions involved in articulation, swallowing, and mastication, functioning to separate the nasal and oral cavities in defects extending through the buccal area to the lip. However, a perfect closure between the nose and the oral cavity is difficult to achieve in practice, and it is more desirable to use skin flaps to reconstruct skin defects other than those involving the orbit, and to have only the orbit covered by an "Epithese".

The most extreme challenge is to keep the "Epithese" from ever becoming displaced on the expressive face. With today's developments in electronic engineering, we can expect the completion of various types of "Epithese" that will allow movement and will adapt to facial expressions (Fig. 24).

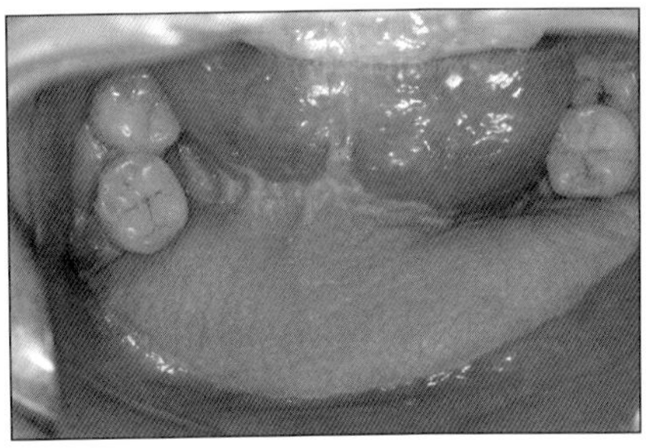

Fig. 16 The alveolar crest was reconstructed using a scapular flap after the resection of mandibular gingival cancer. An implant prosthesis was used since it was too difficult to insert an ordinary denture.

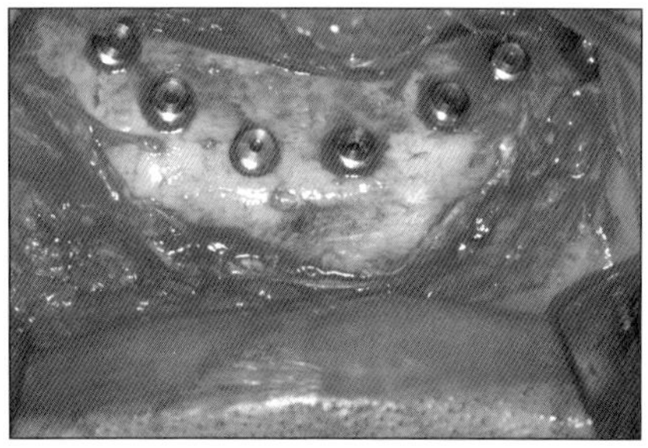

Fig. 17 The border between the flap and the mucosa was cut to expose the scapular, into which 6 implants were placed.

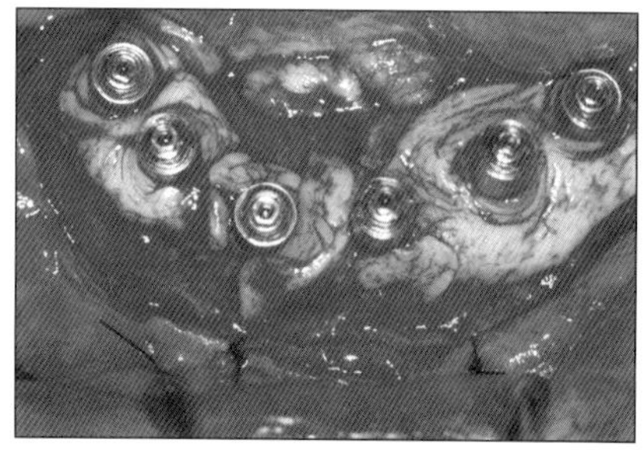

Fig. 18 In the second surgery, performed 3 months later, the hypodermis was drastically reduced, the oral mucosa was grafted around the implants, part of the skin was resected, and the graft was fixed in position by the use of a stent on the implants.

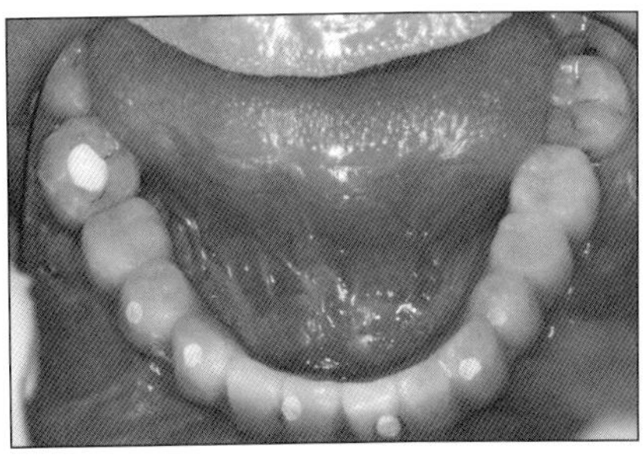

Fig. 19 A superstructure was created after about 3 months. This photograph shows the intraoral view with the provisional restoration inserted.

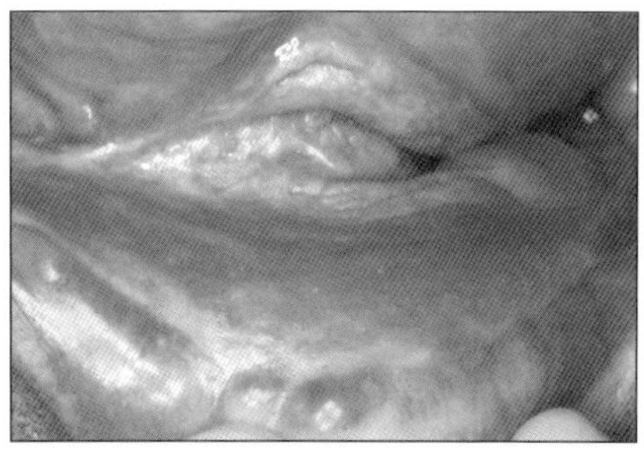

Fig. 20 Case in which reconstruction was done using a cervical skin flap following the resection of mandibular-mucosal squamous cell carcinoma. It was impossible to insert a denture because the mandible was located within the flap.

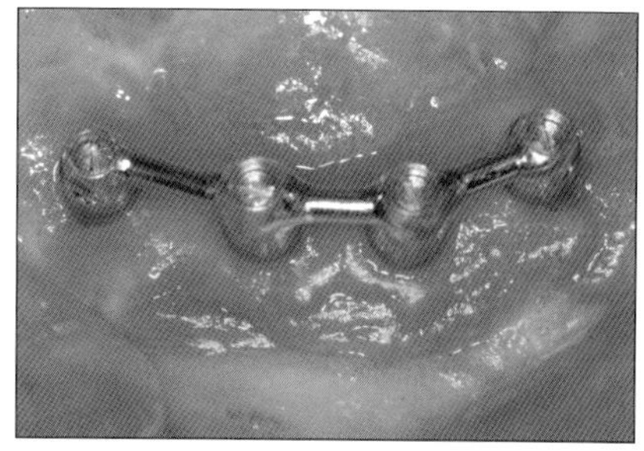

Fig. 21 During the second surgery, following the placement of 4 implants, the oral mucosa was grafted to form the oral vestibule. An over denture with bar attachment was produced.

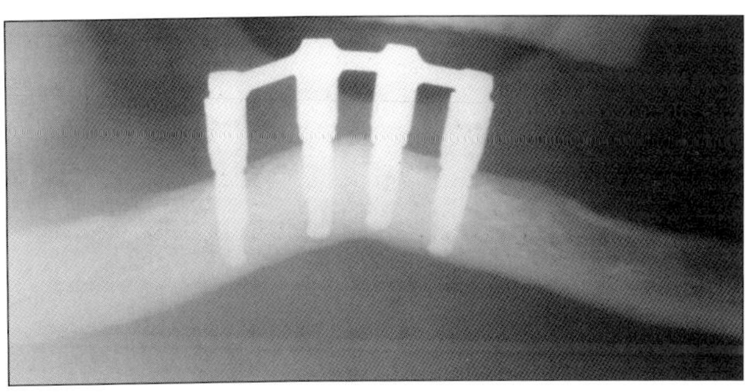

Fig. 22 Postoperative radiograph.

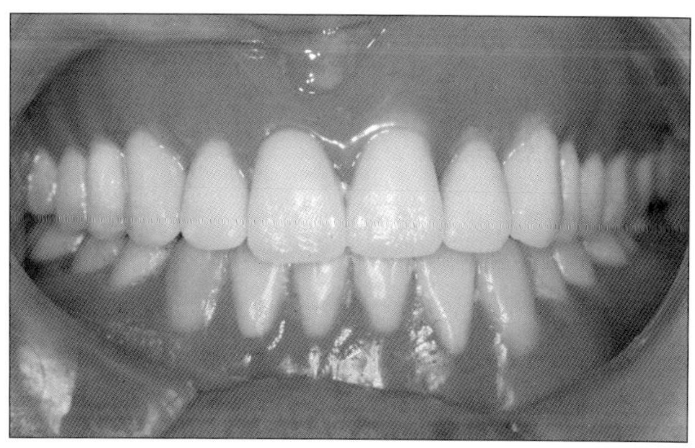

Fig. 23 Intraoral view with denture inserted.

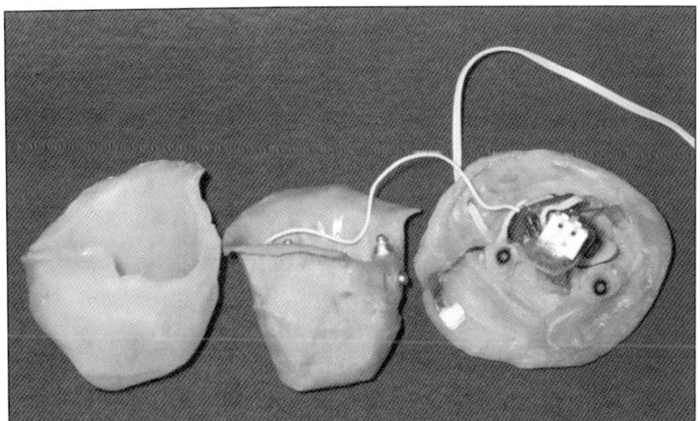

Fig. 24 Prototype model of blinking "Epithese".

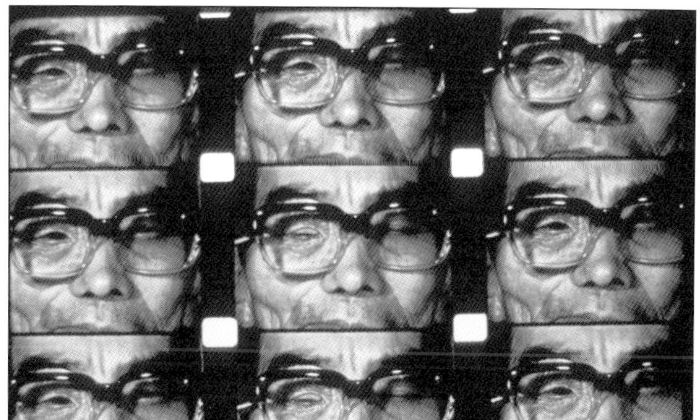

Fig. 25 Blinking "Epithese".

CHAPTER 2

Surgical simulation for maxillofacial prosthesis

In maxillofacial rehabilitation, it is of value before surgery to predict the postoperative defective status and the reconstructed contour of the jaw bone, and the final contours of maxillodental prostheses and of facial prostheses.

With the development of computers and the popularization of such diagnostic imaging apparatus as CT and MRI, surgical simulations on computers have been becoming possible. However, there are inconveniences including the need to install computers, the necessity for skilled operators, and the fact that actual surgical instruments cannot be used. The actual skull model created by means of the stereo lithography technique is capable of providing simulations for which surgical instruments can actually be used, as well as "hands-on" observation. In this chapter, an actual craniofacial skull model is used to describe surgical simulations.

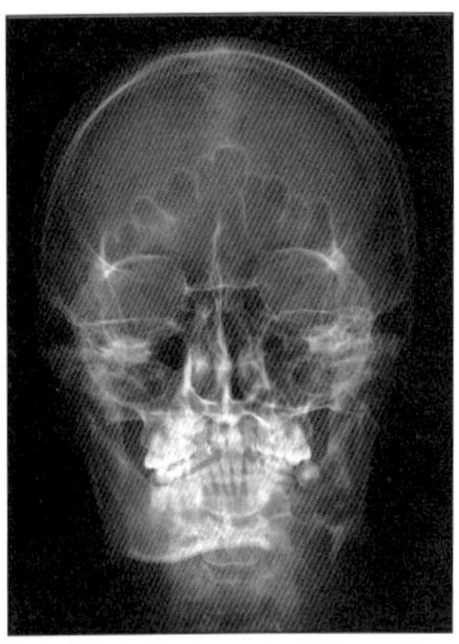

Fig. 1 Ameloblastoma developed on the left side of the mandible.

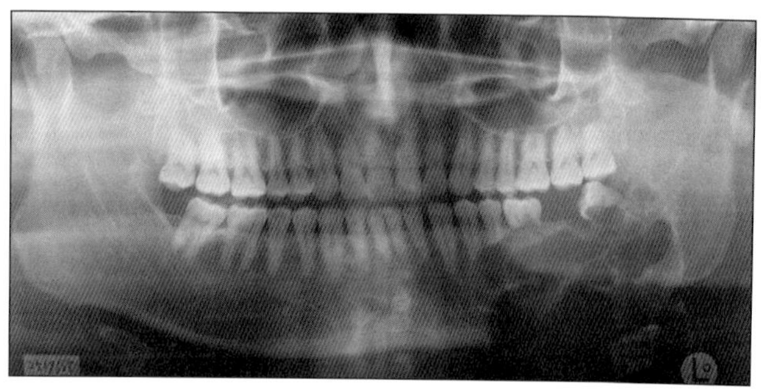

Fig. 2 On the panoramic radiograph, a multilocular radiolucent area is observed from the mandibular left premolar region to the ramus.

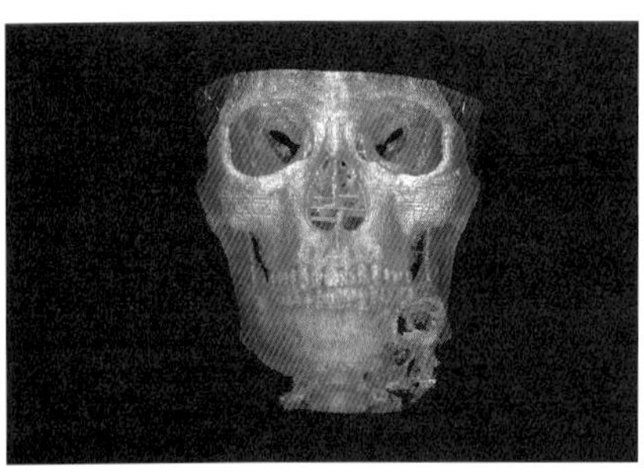

Fig. 3 The craniofacial skull model fabricated by means of the stereo lithography technique on the basis of CT data.

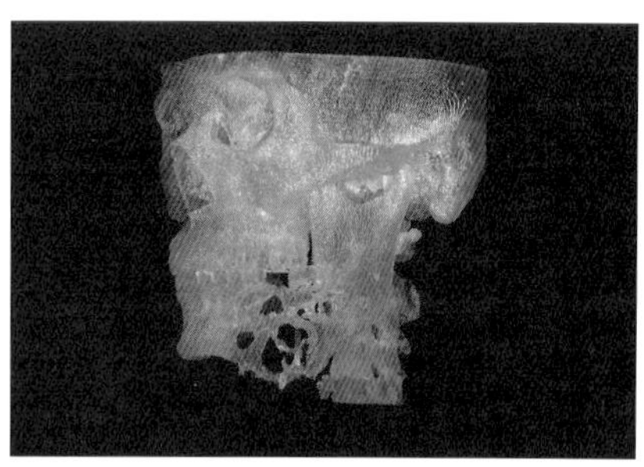

Fig. 4 The left side of the mandible is swollen due to tumors, and the cortical bone appears as reticular structure.

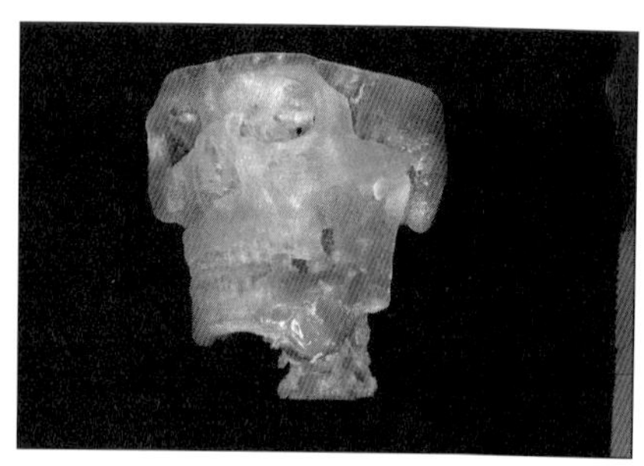

Fig. 5 The mandible must be separated for surgical simulation, so the swollen region is filled with paraffin wax to protect the reticular structure from breakage.

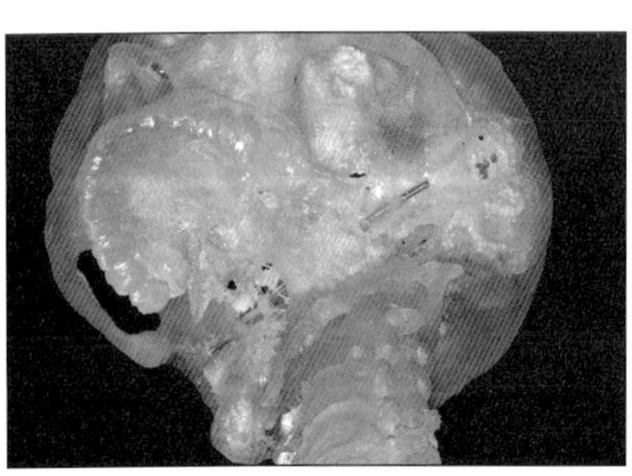

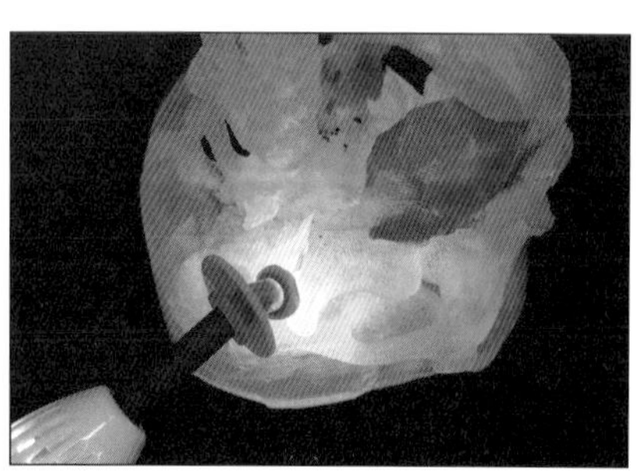

Fig. 6 *(left)* A pin has been inserted into the mandibular fossa both sides so that the mandible can do hinge movement following separation from the skull.

Fig. 7 *(right)* After separation a hole is made in the condylar head in the mandibular model on both sides, and the pins are inserted into these holes, which makes it possible to reposition the mandible to the skull accurately and return it to the original position for setting with a light-curing resin. The mandibular model allows hinge movement on the cranial bone.

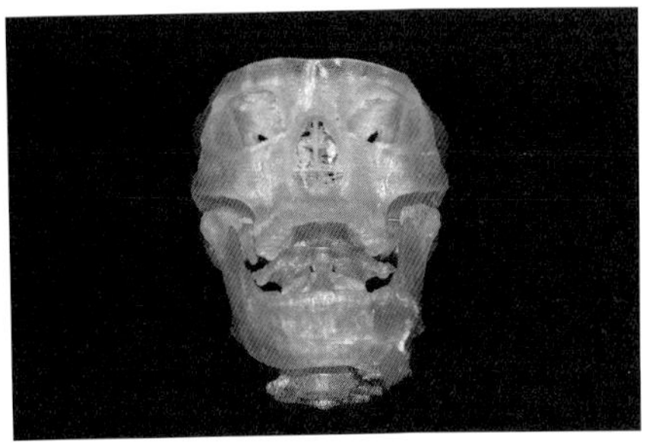

Fig. 8 The state in which hinge movement of the mandible has become possible through insertion of a metal pin into the separated head of the mandibular condyle.

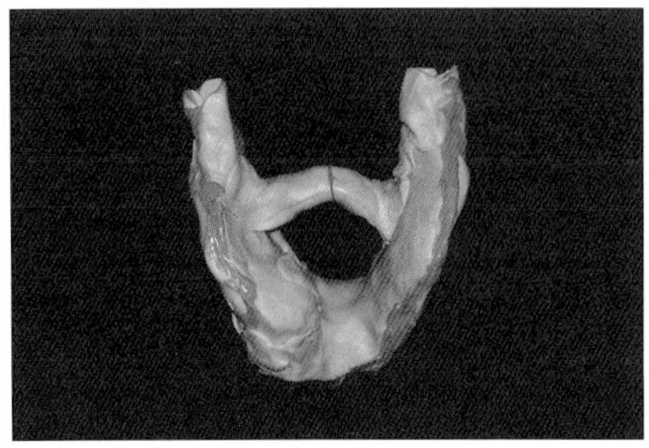

Fig. 9 Duplication of the mandibular model. For fabricating the duplication of the mandibular original model, an impression is made with dental impression material. The opening for the pouring of fluid resin should be prepared.

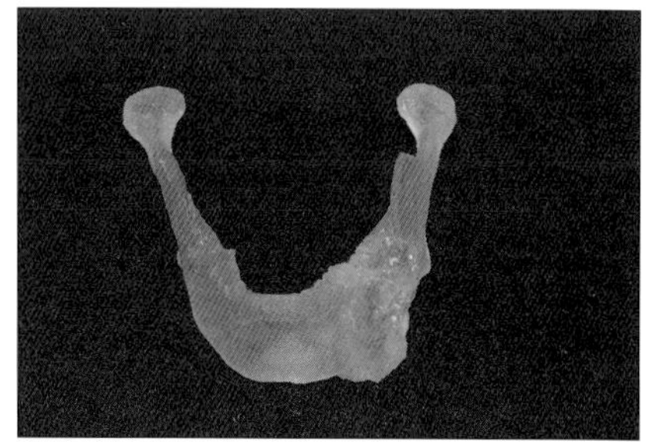

Fig. 10 The duplicated mandibular model fabricated using transparent liquid resin.

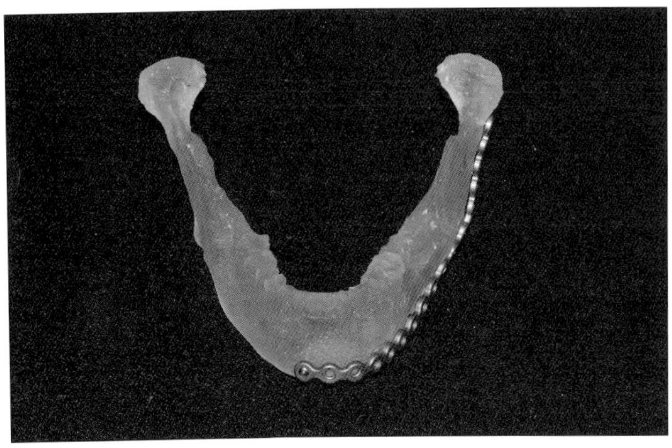

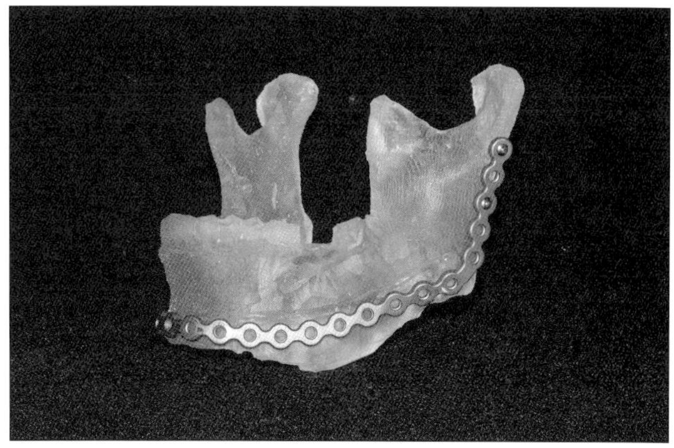

Figs. 11 and 12 The reconstruction plate should be bent to fit the mandible after removal of the swollen region taking into consideration the symmetry of the mandible.

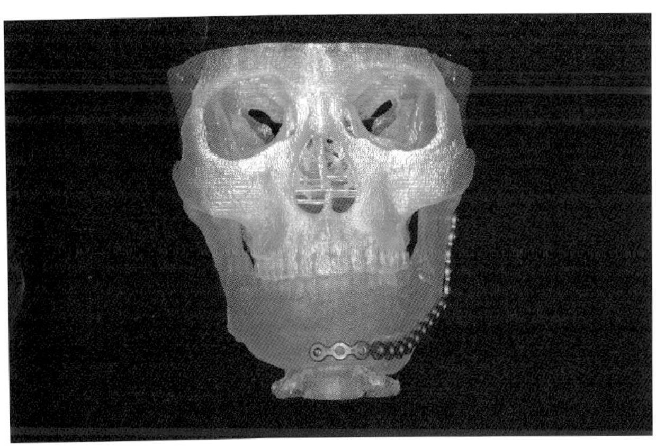

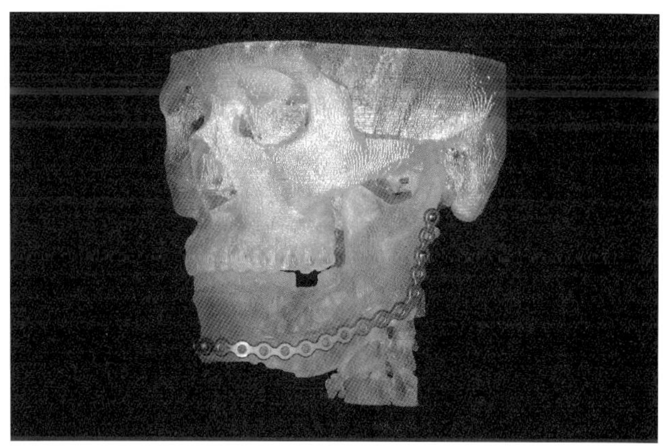

Figs. 13 and 14 The duplicated mandibular model is repositioned at the mandibular fossa.

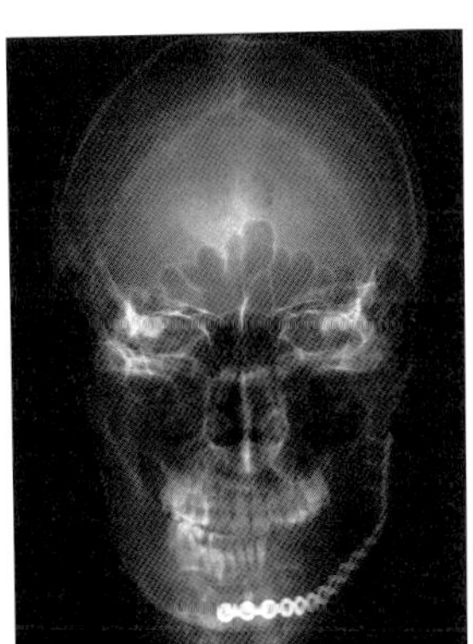

Fig. 15 Postoperative radiograph, frontal view.

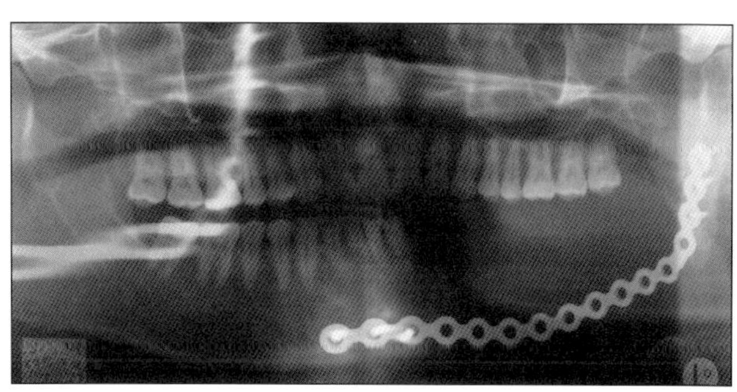

Fig. 16 Postoperative panoramic radiograph. If the bone grafting can be performed along this plate, good facial symmetry and good occlusal relationship will be maintained.

CHAPTER 3

Conversation, mastication and deglutition

The oral cavity, pharynx, and larynx have undergone drastic changes since humans began to walk upright. Although the distal position of the larynx was convenient for language function, a complex "larynx-up" motion became necessary for deglutition. Because of the distal position of the larynx, it is difficult to treat dysphagia in humans, for whom the language function as a communication tool has developed through a diminution of eating function.

This chapter discusses the changes in conversational and eating functions in conjunction with descriptions of their normal mechanisms and their evaluations when defects have resulted from intraoral tumor surgery. The evaluations of conversational and eating functions after resection of tumors contribute to the development of surgical techniques as well as to improvements in issues of tumor resection and reconstructive surgery.

The relationships between postoperative oral functions, the resected range of the tongue, the oral floor or mandible, and the flaps used for reconstruction have already become clear. Seto et al.[1)] stated that the articulatory function was unaffected by any type of flap while postoperative oral function decreased with increase of the resected range of the tongue, oral floor, or mandible, and that a relatively massive flap for reconstruction allowed the restoration of the articulatory function. They also reported that eating and deglutitive functions decreased with increase of the resected range of the tongue, oral floor, or mandible, and was also unaffected by any type of flap. However, the type of flap employed for reconstruction is largely determined by the extent of the defect and the function varies widely according to the method used for suturing. Excellent deglutitive function has been shown in cases making use of the mobility of the residual tongue by reconstruction with a forearm flap for hemiglossectimized cases, and it was shown that stronger contact between the maxilla and the reconstructed tongue provided excellent function in subtotal-excision cases. Therefore, it has become clear that more precise reconstruction is required for restoration of the deglutitive function than for that of the articulatory function.

In maxillary defects, the important factors are the extent of the soft palate defect and the number of teeth available for retention of dentures/prostheses for the defective maxilla or mandible. A defect of the soft palate gives rise to velopharyngeal failure, and by extension, causes hypernasality and dysphasia or swallowing disorder. The functional evaluations listed below are important for adaptive evaluation of speech aids (speech bulb, palatal lift prostheses).

Conversational function

Oropharyngeal functions are classified into the velopharyngeal function (VP function) for control of the voice and the narrow articulatory function for controlling the voice with such oral organs as the tongue, teeth, and lips, using air flowing into the oral cavity, with the air stream divided into the oral and nasal cavities.

Velopharyngeal function :
Hypernasality is caused by the stream of air into the oral cavity flowing into the nasal cavity instead due to defects of the hard and/or soft palate. While hard palatal defects are addressed by prostheses and implantation, the functional restoration of soft palatal defects is difficult because of the moving site. Anatomically, the muscle sling formed in the soft palate is lifted by the levator muscle of the velum palatini to close the rhinopharynx (valvular closure). In addition, the velopharyngeal function may be compensated for by the contraction of the muscle that forms the posterior pharyngeal wall and lateral pharyngeal wall to narrow the pathway to the nasal cavity (sphincteral closure). This muscular contraction and narrowing of the pathway occur during swallowing or during speech in cleft-palate patients (Fig. 1).

Articulatory function:
Articulatory disorders that develop after resection of the tongue, oral floor and mandible, are particularly likely to be caused by disorders of tongue movement. Therefore, when some contact with the palate is provided by soft-tissue reconstruction, it becomes possible to create similar articulation by compensation for the articulatory point, with restoration of conversational function (Fig. 2). Particularly, in the case of total or subtotal extirpation of the tongue, anterior augmentation and a slight parapharyngeal decrease are effective in the reconstruction. Also, consequent upon the compensatory articulation of the glottis (glottal stop and glottal fricative), speech intelligibility may be restored

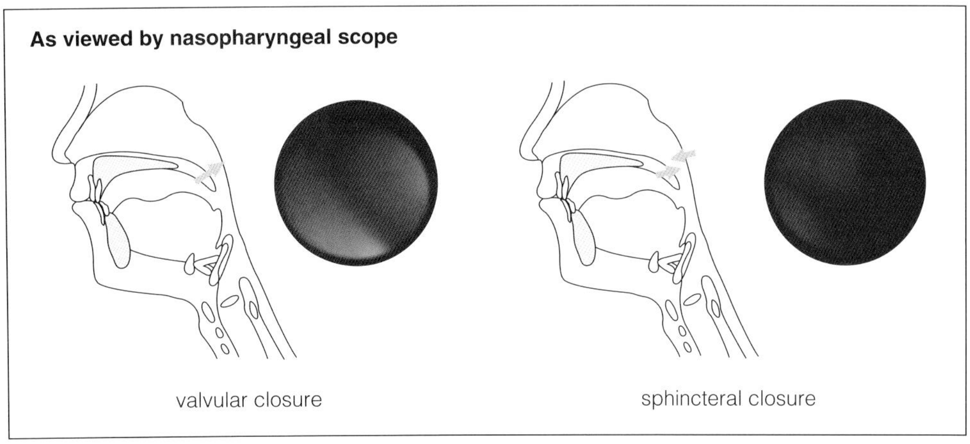

Fig. 1 Types of velopharyngeal closure. (left; valvular closure, right; sphincteral closure).

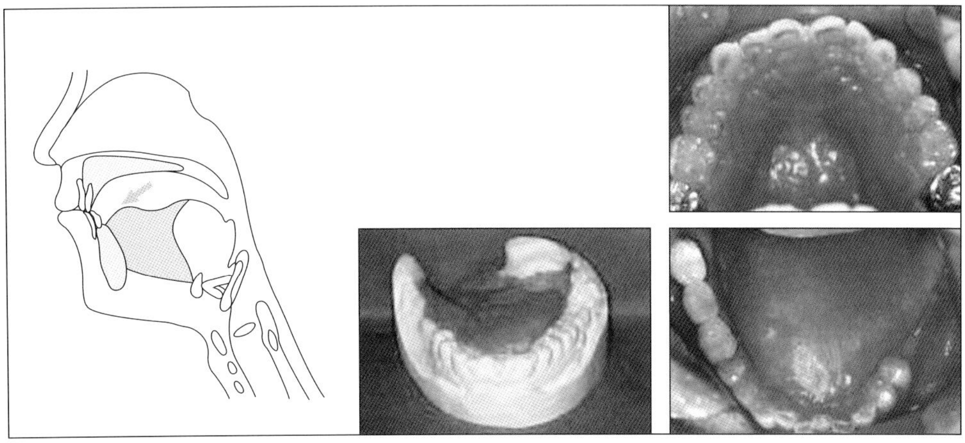

Fig. 2 Compensational articulation. The reconstructed tongue (flap of rectus abdominis muscle) comes in contact with the palate. Mandibular anterior-and-posterior motion changes the articulatory point for compensational pronunciation.

Fig. 3 Soft blowing test.

The patient blows through a straw to make bubbles in a container, such as a cup, filled 1/3 full of water. The duration ratio (blowing ratio) of blowing duration in nasal breathing relative to blowing duration in oral breathing is determined. Breath leakage from the nasal cavity is observed with a mirror during this procedure.

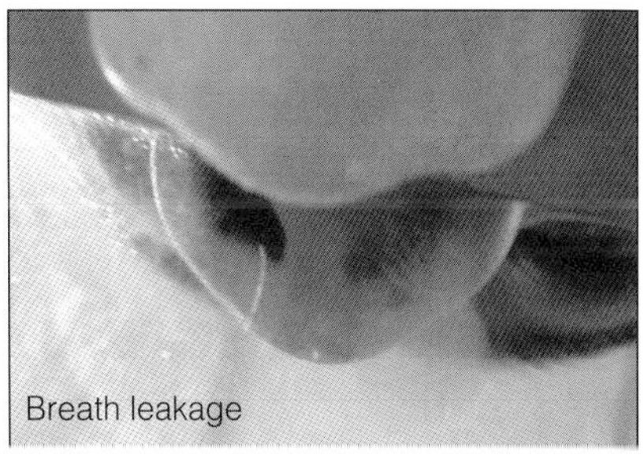

$$\frac{\text{Expiratory duration in nasal breathing}}{\text{Expiratory duration in oral breathing}} \begin{array}{l} = 1.0 \text{ (normal)} \\ < 1.0 \text{ (closing failure)} \end{array}$$

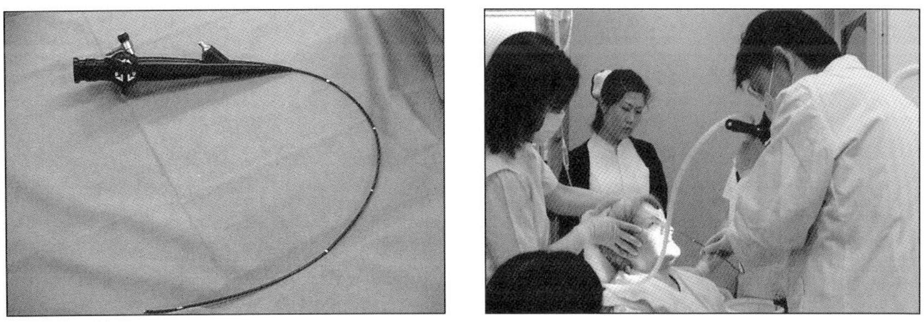

Fig. 4 Nasopharyngeal (rhinopharyngeal) fiberscope. Direct observation of actual condition of closed rhinopharynx, laryngeal periphery, and glottis.

to some extent.

Functional evaluations (Objective evaluations) :

1) Velopharyngeal closure function

When both hard and soft palatal defects are present, it is necessary to do clinical determination of whether the cause is velopharyngeal deficiency or nasooral fistula.

• **Soft blowing examination** (Fig. 3):

When the expiratory duration ratio (blowing ratio) between blowing duration with nostrils open and blowing duration with nostrils closed is below the standard reference value of 100%, closing failure should be suspected. Breath leakage should be ascertained by applying a mirror to the nose.

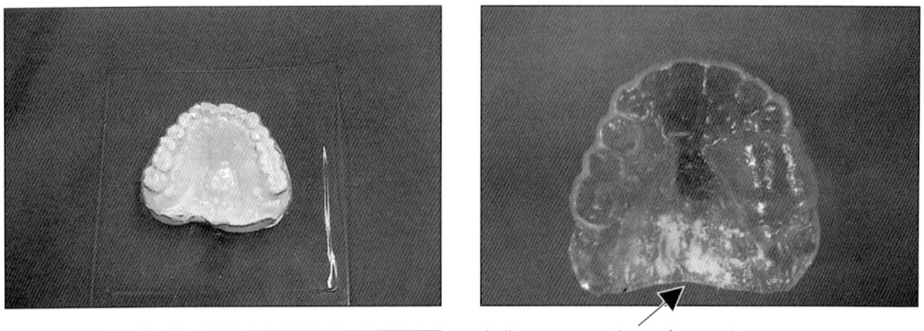

Fig. 5 Static palatography (upper photo) and measurement of palatal pressure (lower photo). Maxillary simple impression and palatal base (upper left), Palatogram (upper right).

Adherent portion of powder = tongue-contact site.

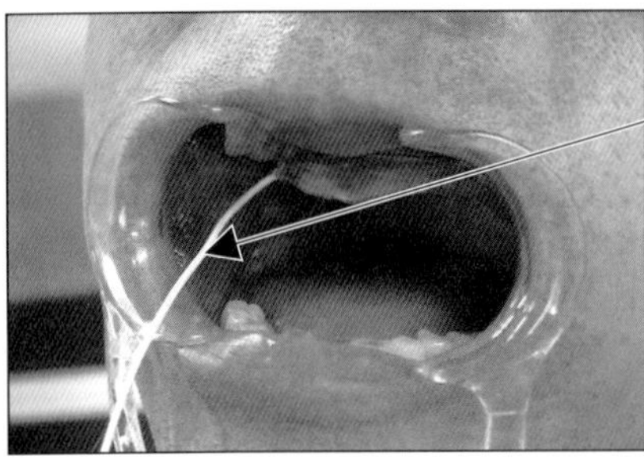

A pressure sensor is provided.

Table 1 Hearing impression of resonance and consonantal strain.

- syllable /ma/changes in hypernasality.
- vowels /a/ and /i/, and syllables change in hypernasality /pa/, /ta/, /ka/, /sa/, /ba/, /da/, and /ga/.

Table 2 English consonant chart and vowel diagram.

Manner of articulation	*Place of articulation*						
	Bilabial	*Labio-dentel*	*Lingual dentel*	*Lingual alveolar*	*Lingual palatal*	*Lingual velar*	*Glottal*
Plosive	p (pipe)			t (toe)		k (cat)	
	b (baby)			d (dad)		g (goat)	
Fricative	hw (what)	f (fat)	θ (thin)	s (sack)	ʃ (shoe)		h (hat)
	w (watt)	v (vat)	ð (than)	z (zoo)	ʒ (rouge)		
Affricate					tʃ (church)		
					dʒ (judge)		
Nasals	m (man)			n (no)		ŋ (sing)	
Glide				l (lake)	r (rat)		
					j (yet)		
Vowels		*Front*				*Back*	
		i (eat)				u (food)	
		ɪ (it)		ɜ˞ɚ (further)		ʊ (book)	
		e (ate)		ə (above)		o (omit)	
		ɛ (bed)		ʌ (above)		ɔ (jam)	
		æ (at)				ɒ (watch)	
		a (bath)				ɑ (father)	

Table 3 Speech Intelligibility.

Normal, Intelligible (80% understood)
Moderately intelligible (50-80% understood)
Partially intelligible (50% understood)
Not intelligible or no speech

• **Hearing impression for resonance and consonantal strain** (Table. 1): Have the patient actually pronounce various vowels, consonants, and syllables.

• **Nasopharyngeal fiberscope** (Fig. 4): Direct-vision observation using a fiberscope

2) Articulatory function

• Static palatography : Contact between the tongue and the palate is observed as shown by the adhesion to the palatal plate of a powder coating first applied to the tongue (Fig. 5). Vaseline is applied to the palatal plate.

3) Integrated speech examinations (Objective evaluations)

Method of evaluation by having patients actually pronounce various vowels, consonants, and syllables while an evaluator listens to the actual pronunciation

• **Speech ability for single consonant-vowel syllables**[2] (Table. 2): is assessed by the number of audible syllables.

• **Speech intelligibility**[3] (Table. 3): is a graded evaluation of the extent to which daily conversation can be clearly understood.

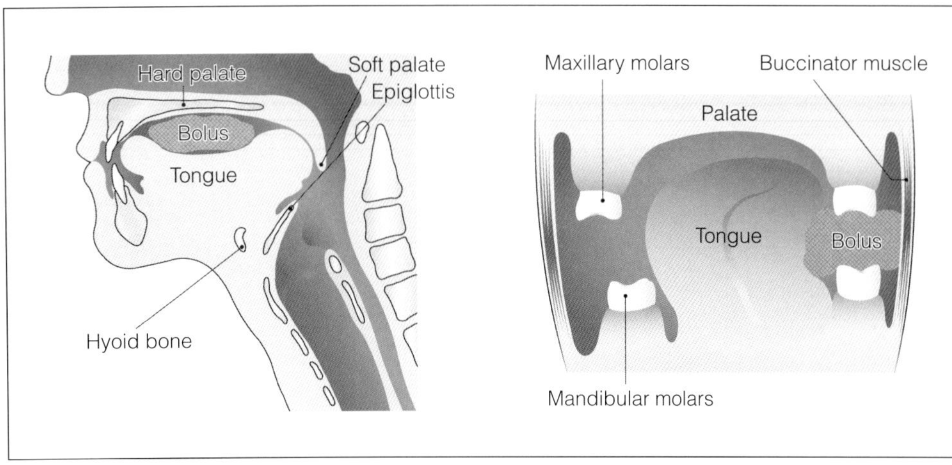

Fig. 6 Preparative stage.

Eating function (Mastication)

Masticatory function (Preparation for deglutition): Mastication is the preliminary stage prior to the oral stage of swallowing, and is referred to as the preparatory phase. The work of altering foods through mastication, so that they have the size and physical properties that make swallowing possible, is integral to deglutition (Fig. 6).

Tongue function (movement): During mastication, the tongue transfers food to the tooth, then it transfers the prepared food to the pharyngeal cavity for deglutition. The only difference between this and the oral stage of deglutition is the transit direction. Tongue function is important for mastication. In jawbone defects, mastication cannot be restored without the restoration of affected-sided tongue movement even if occlusion itself is restored with dentures and implants (Fig. 6). When the masticatory function is evaluated as being poor, it is necessary to include functional examinations of the tongue or oral stage of deglutition.

Functional evaluations (Objective evaluations) :

- **"Nuts mastication" method:** Screening is a traditionally-used method of determining masticatory efficiency according to the residue on a sieve of specimens such as nuts. Have the patient masticate a specimen such as nuts, and then spit it out. Pass the spat-out sample through a fixed-mesh sifter. The quantity remaining on the sieve determines masticatory efficacy. However, mesh size settings vary.[4]
- **Elution examination from specimens:** Masticatory efficiency is determined by measuring the elution of glucose and gelatin from a "gummi" candy, the elution of sugar from gum, the elution of starch from rice, and the elution of ATP from ATP granules. Allowed time and other criteria must be established in each case.
- **"Gummi" breaking method** (Fig. 7)**:** This method examines the number of pieces into which a "gummi" candy of fixed hardness is broken.
- **Gum color-change method:** Alteration of the color of gum by chewing is measured using a colorimeter.[5]

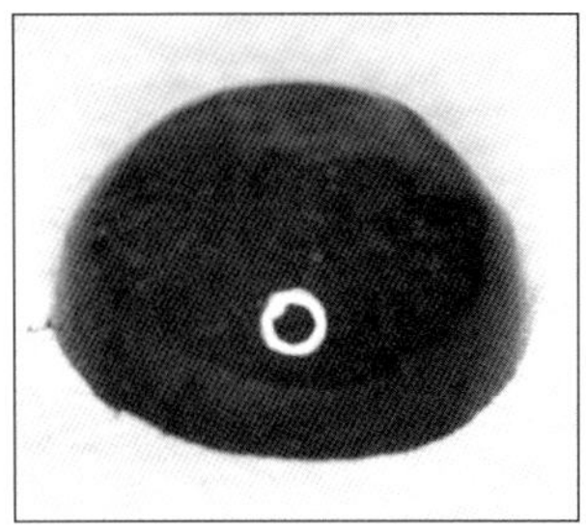

Fig. 7 "Gummi" Points. We assess function according to this chart after 30 seconds of chewing a "gummi" candy.
5: Broken into over three pieces
4: Broken into two pieces
3: Shape is changed
2: Shows marks
1: No change

Eating function (Deglutition)

The oral stage refers to the stage of transferring to the pharyngeal cavity the bolus held in the palate following mastication in the preparative stage, and the pharyngeal stage refers to the stage in which the bolus is moved to the esophagus, and "larynx-up" (swallowing reflex) occurs to prevent intrusion into the trachea.

"Misdeglutition aspiration" refers to the intrusion of the bolus into the trachea.

In the case of mandibular defect of the tongue and oral floor, the contact pressure of the reconstructed or residual tongue upon the palate and also the presence or absence of resection of the suprahyoid muscles or mandibular anterior arch have an influence upon functional restoration. Particularly, in soft palatal defect, movements of the lateral and posterior pharyngeal wall have an effect on the prognosis for deglutitive functional restoration in the case of insertion of soft-palatal prostheses.

1) Deglutitive function (Oral stage) (Fig. 8)

2) Deglutitive function (Pharyngeal stage) (Fig. 9)

Relationships with the respiratory tract are also illustrated.

3) Functional evaluations (Objective evaluations)

It is important to begin with accurate screening of misdeglutition and to evaluate what disorder of misdeglutition is occurring and in which stage of deglutition it occurs.

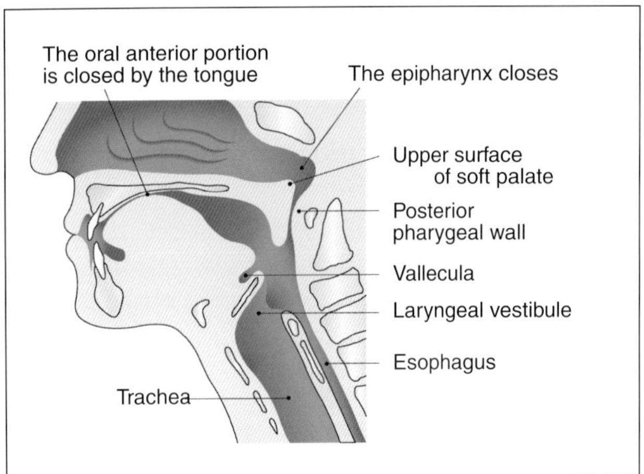

Fig. 8 Oral stage.

Table 4 Modified water drinking test.

- Have patient hold, in the dominant hand, a cup containing 30ml, or as little as 3ml of water at room temperature, then drink the water in an ordinary way. Observe the following profiles and episodes. (Repeat several times.)
- Profiles
  1. Patient can drink all the water in a single swallow without choking.
  2. Patient can drink all the water in two or more swallows without choking.
  3. Patient can drink all the water in a single swallow each time but chokes occasionally.
  4. Patient chokes occasionally in spite of drinking water in two or more swallows.
  5. Patient chokes frequently and cannot drink the entire quantity of water.

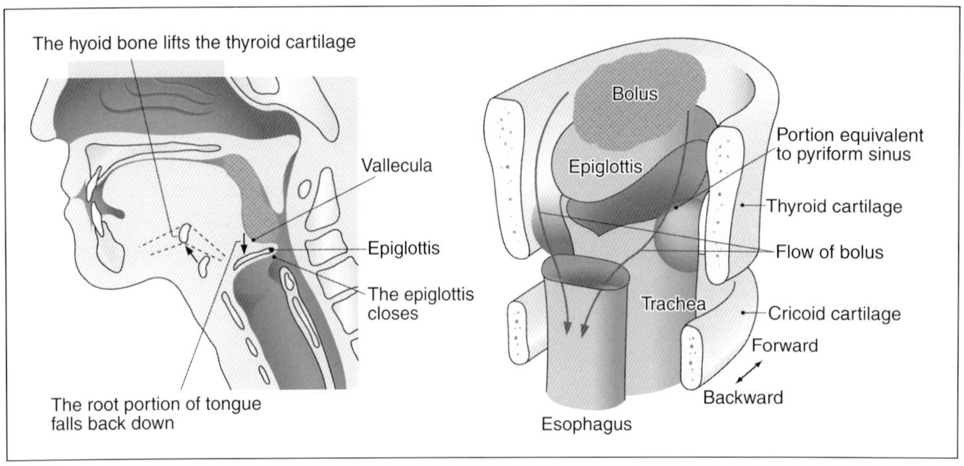

Fig. 9 Pharyngeal stage.

• **Modified drinking test:** This is a test for evaluating the presence or absence of misdeglutition in the early postoperative stage (Table 4). Episodes should be recorded except for the profiles shown in the table. Inhaling of air with water and occurrences such as leakage from the lips are important. Assessment criteria are as follows: "normal" is when it is possible for the patient to drink the water in 5 seconds or less and the way of drinking fits Profile 1; the borderline between normal and abnormal is when it takes 5 seconds or more to drink the water and the way of drinking is inferior to Profile 2, which is the borderline (suspected); abnormal is when the way of drinking fits Profiles 3 to 5. Additional deglutitive contrastradiogram and fiberscope examinations are required.

• **RSST (Repetitive Saliva Swallowing Test):** The extent of the swallowing reflex is determined by measuring the amount and the number of times that the thyroid cartilage lifts (Fig. 10).

• **Auscultation of neck:** Auscultation of the lateral skin of trachea immediately below the cricoid cartilage. Misdeglutition is confirmed by expiration after swallowing water plus subsequent bubbling sounds during inspiration (Fig. 11).[6]

• **Static palatography and the measurement of palatal-pressure:** Examination with a pressure probe is added to the examination of whether the tongue makes contact with the palate or not, as for articulation (Fig. 5).

• **Videofluorography (VF):** A contrast radiogram is performed with a fluoroscopic apparatus following injection of a contrast medium into water, jelly, and paste foods. Duration of passage through the oral cavity and how long each item remains in the pharyngeal cavity are observed and recorded. The misdeglutition is classified into two types. In cases of misdeglutition at the moment of "larynx-up", insufficient laryngeal atresia due to limited raising of the larynx results in the direct inflow of the bolus into the respiratory tract (Fig. 12, left). In cases of misdeglutition at the moment of "larynx-down", the accumulation and overflow of bolus, due to the esophageal orifice not opening, result in inflow into the respiratory tract (Fig. 12, right). In organic disorders such as oral tumors, a mixture of the two types is most common and it is often the case that disorder of the oral stage becomes the cause of misdeglutition. Classification according to timing miss for the inflow of the bolus into the pharyn-

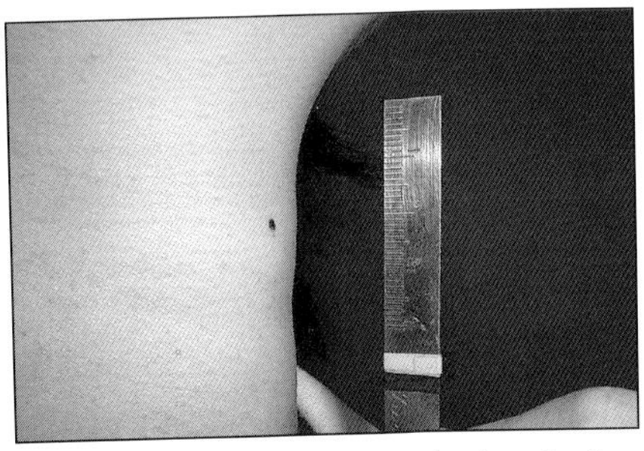

Fig. 10 RSST. When the marked projecting point of the thyroid cartilage has lifted 3 or more times in a 30-second period, deglutition is normal. A lift of 1cm or more is regarded as normal.

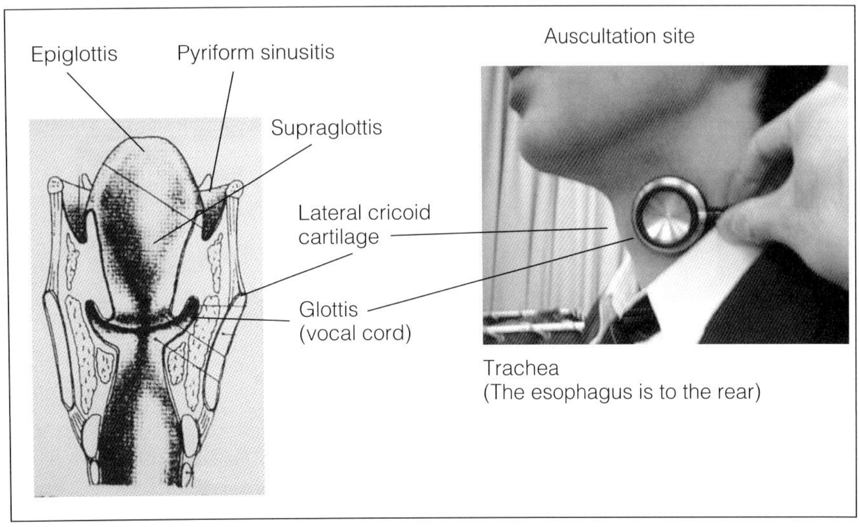

Fig. 11 Auscultation of neck.

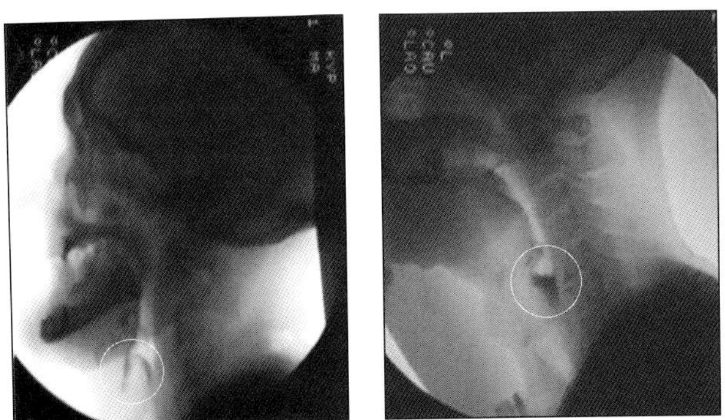

At the moment of "larynx-up" At the moment of "larynx-down"

Fig. 12 Videofluorography. Dysphagia classification according to swallowing reflex.

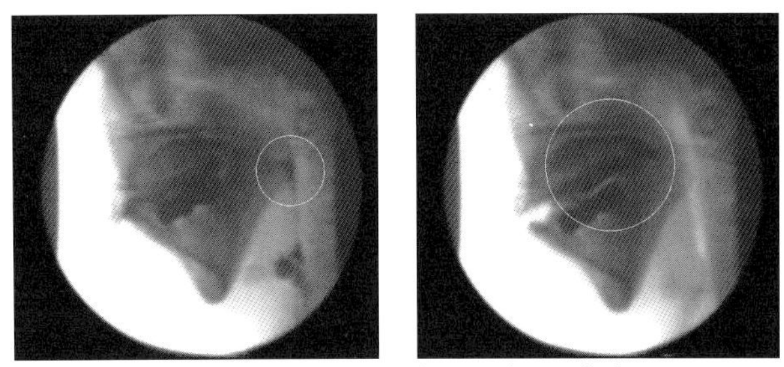

Early inflow Intraoral remainder (incomplete transfer of bolus)

Fig. 13 Videofluorography. Dysphagia classification according to timing of inflow into the pharyngeal cavity.

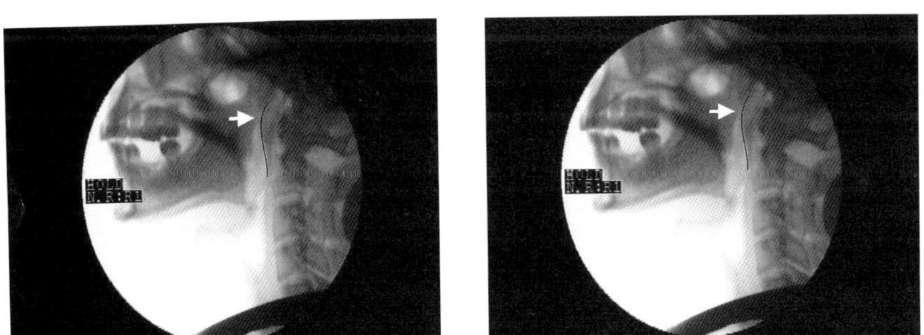

Fig. 14 Videofluorography. Assessment of soft palatal defect. *(left):* Movement of posterior pharyngeal wall and Passavant's ridge. *(right):* Regurgitation into nasal cavity.

Table 5 Guidelines for evaluation.

Grade 1	0 – 1 g
Grade 2	1 – 2 g (except for 1 g)
Grade 3	2 – 3 g (except for 2 g)
Grade 4	3 – 4 g (except for 3 g)
Grade 5	4 – 5 g (except for 4 g) or misdeglutition

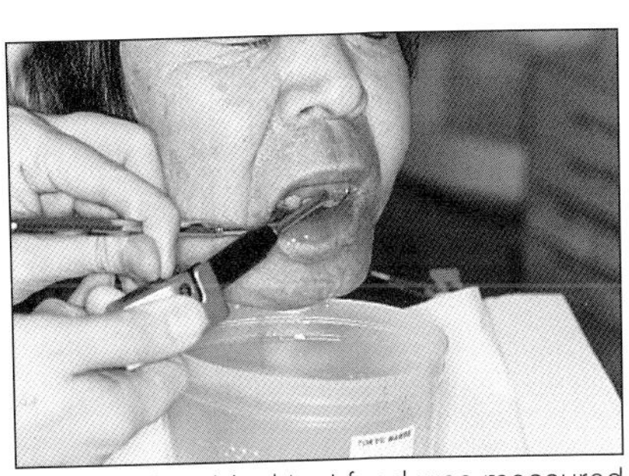

Amount of residual test food was measured by UV absorption of solution included in this food.

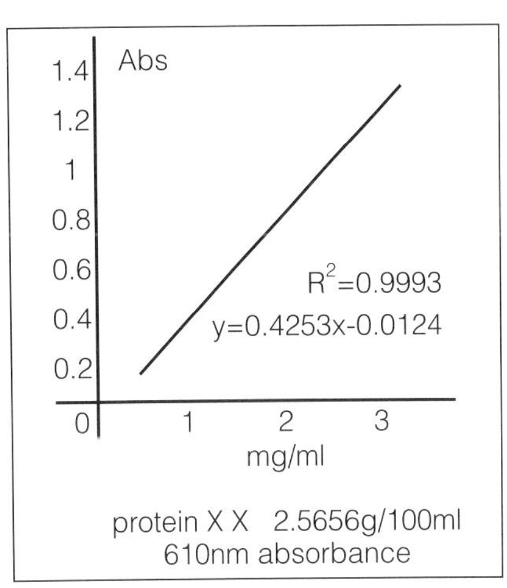

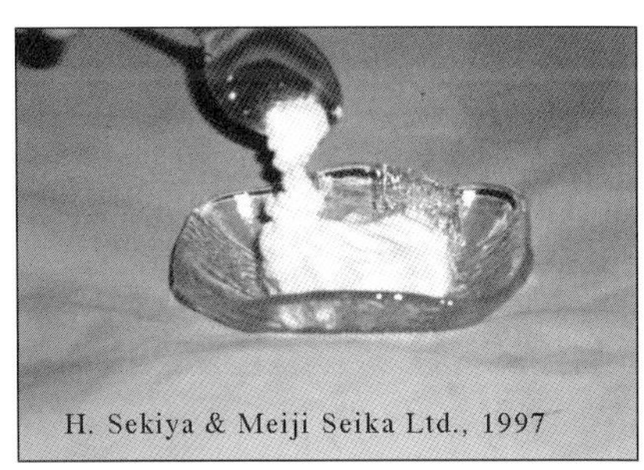

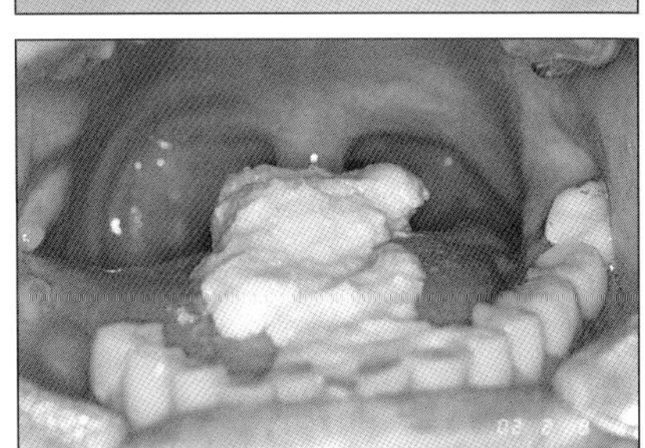

Fig. 15 Residual protein grade.

Table 6 Performance Status Scale.

Eating in public
100 No restriction of place, food, or companion (eats out at any opportunity)
75 No restriction of place, but restricts, diet when in public (eats anywhere, but may limit intake to less "messy" foods, e.g.. liquids)
50 Eats only in presence of selected persons in selected places
25 Eats only at home in presence of selected persons
0 Always eats alone
Understandability of speech
100 Always understandable
75 Understandable most of the time; occasional repetition necessary.
50 Usually understandable; face-to-face contact necessary
25 Difficult to understand
0 Never understandable; may use written communication
Normalcy of diet
100 Full diet (no restrictions)
90 Peanuts
80 All meat
70 Carrots, celery
60 Dry bread and crackers
50 Soft, chewable foods {e.g., macaroni, canned/soft fruits, cooked vegetables, fish, hamburger, small pieces of meat}
40 Soft foods requiring no chewing (e.g., mashed potatoes, apple sauce, pudding)
30 Pureed foods (in blender)
20 Warm liquids
10 Cold liquids
0 Non-oral feeding (tube fed)

Table 7 Oral Performance Status (OPS).

Deglutition (D)
D 0: possible to eat out
D 1: possible to eat special food
D 2: limit to eat fluid food
Conversation (C)
C 0: possible to talk over the telephone
C 1: possible to talk with his/her first meeting
C 2: limit to talk with his/her family or doctor
Aesthetic (A)
A 0: possible to meet his/her first meeting
A 1: possible to meet his/her acquaintance
A 2: limit to meet his/her family or doctor

OPS Grade	OPS	Status depended on OPS
0	D 0 C 0 A 0	same as preoperative status
1	D 1 C 0,1 A 0,1	status to recover into the public
2	D 1 C 2 any A	limit to recover into the public
3	D 2 any C any A	difficult to recover into the public

This grade was contrived based on deglutition

geal cavity (Fig. 13), includes early inflow because of the incomplete closure between the tongue root and palate, and the bolus remaining in the intraoral area because of incomplete transfer of the bolus. Inharmonious timing with respiration due to such problems causes misdeglutition.[7]

Also, this method can accurately provide control of movements of the posterior pharyngeal wall in soft palatal defect. Furthermore, the presence or absence of Passavant's ridge and the height of the maximum ridge can be observed. These provide references for the positioning of speech valves or palatal lifts. In addition, the extent of bolus regurgitation can be determined after positioning (Fig. 14).

• **Fiberscope:** The closure of the oropharyngeal cavity, epipharynx, epiglottis, and glottis is observed by direct viewing.

• **Protein remaining grade:** In this method the actual amount remaining intraorally is observed and the residual weight is measured by determination of absorbance following the eating of protein puree (Fig. 15 and Table 5).[1]

Relationships between articulatory and deglutitive functions

Although the restoration of articulation can be provided to some extent by contact between the palate and the tongue, the restoration of deglutition depends on the mobility of the residual and reconstructed tongue and pressure on the palate. Therefore, the restoration of deglutition is more difficult than the restoration of articulation.[1]

Subjective evaluations of conversational and eating functions

It is also necessary to take account of patients' subjective evaluations, using food questionnaires and the evaluation method by performance status[8] scale shown in Table 6. However, this classification has a defect because it is difficult to determine the functional status at first glance. Oral Performance Status Grade in respect of oral ADL including deglution and conversation are shown briefly as an appendix for reference (Table 7). This is our trial version.

References
1) Seto K., Sekiya H. : Functional Rehabilitation for Deglutition Disorders after Resection of Tumors. Fifth Meeting of the International Congress on Maxillofacial Rehabilitation Proceedings 127.
2) Hufnagle, J., Pullon, P., et al.: Speech consideration in oral surgery. Part II. Speech characteristics of patients following surgery for oral malignancies. Oral Surg. 46:354-361 1978.
3) Olson, M. L. and Shedd, D.P.: Disability and rehabilitation in head and neck cancer patients after treatment. Head & Neck Surg. 1:52-58 1978.
4) Manly RS., Shiere FR. : The effect of dental efficiency on mastication and food performance. Oral Surg Oral Med Oral Pathol 3 : 674-685 1950.
5) Hayakawa I, Watanabe I.,et. al.: A simple method for evaluating masticatory performance using a color changeable chewing gum. Int J. Prosthodont. 11: 173-176 1998.
6) Takahashi K., Groher ME., Michi K.: Methodology for detecting swallowing sounds Dysphasia9 : 54-62 1994.
7) Sekiya H., Sonoyama T., et. al. : Assessment of Rehabilitation Management Using Interim Palatal Augmentation Prosthesis (I-PAP) for Dysphasia Following Resection of Oral Malignant Tumors. Fifth Meeting of the International Congress on Maxillofacial Rehabilitation Proceedings 130.
8) List, M. A., Ritter-Stterr, C., et al.: A performance status scale for head and neck cancer patients. Cancer 66: 564-569 1990.

SECTION 2

Maxillary Defects

CHAPTER 4

Defect patterns and classifications of maxillary defects

Maxillary defects, mainly evident after removal of tumors, may also be caused by injuries or syphilis. Defects in the maxilla or soft palate make the shield between the nasal and oral cavities incapable and cause swallowing disorder, masticatory interference, and speech defects to develop. In addition, maxillary anterior defects result in alteration of face shape and cause serious aesthetic disturbances. Because surgery is performed using standard procedures, it is considered that such defects attributed to surgery can generally be classified into a few similar patterns. The authors et al. suggested HS classification for maxillary defects in 1979, and here describe a new, somewhat simplified, classification. It is desirable that the classification of defects should not only describe pathoses but also estimate the severity of disorders arising from defects, remedial difficulties related to prosthetic restoration, and the extent to which each disorder can be restored. The classification has already been shown from the results of previous reviews to be able to express up to a point the relationships between defects and the extent of functional recovery with jaw prostheses (maxillodental prostheses).

In HS classification, although the defective patterns of the hard palate and alveolus were previously divided to 8 categories, these have now been reduced to 7 categories by abolishing one division for which frequency of occurrence was low; defective patterns of the lateral pharyngeal wall have been included with the defective patterns of the soft palate. Disturbances of mouth opening have been divided into 3 categories, and the numbers of missing teeth have been divided into 4 categories.

HS classification of maxillary defects

The following 4 items are assessed to express the pathosis of maxillary defects:

1. Defects of the hard palate and alveolus (H);
2. Defects of the soft palate (S);
3. Mouth-opening range (D);
4. Number of remaining teeth (T).

The modifications we determined for the previous HS classification to create the new classification are the elimination of "maxillary anterior and posterior defects", formerly in H_5, the inclusion in the new H_5 of items corresponding to those in the previous H_6, some changes in the contents of S_2, S_3 and, S_4, and elimination of measurement of the extent of mouth-opening area [D]; this is now described as the extent of mouth-opening disturbance.

1. Defects of the hard-palatal alveolar area (H)

H_0: No defect
H_1: Defect limited to alveolus
H_2: Defect limited to hard palate
H_3: Defect extending from alveolus to a portion of the hard palate within the hemilateral side
H_4: Maxillary hemilateral defect
H_5: Greater-than-hemilateral alveolar and palatal defects
H_6: Complete defect

2. Defects of the soft palate (S)

S_0: No defect
S_1: Defect of anterior soft-palatal margin
S_2: Defect limited to posterior soft-palatal margin, and less-than-hemilateral defect extending to posterior margin
S_3: Greater-than-hemilateral defect extending to posterior margin
S_4: Defect extending to posterior margin with defect of lateral pharyngeal wall

3. Mouth-opening range (D)

D_0: No disturbance of mouth opening
D_1: Moderate disturbance of mouth opening
D_2: Severe disturbance of mouth opening
D_x: Impossible to determine

4. Number of remaining teeth (T)

T_0: Seven or more teeth remaining for retention
T_1: Four, five, or six teeth remaining for retention
T_2: One, two, or three teeth remaining for retention
T_3: No teeth

* When a defect has been reconstructed, a postscript should be added as RH (+) or RS (+) at the end of the classification.

RH (+): The hard palate has been reconstructed.
RS (+): The soft palate has been reconstructed.

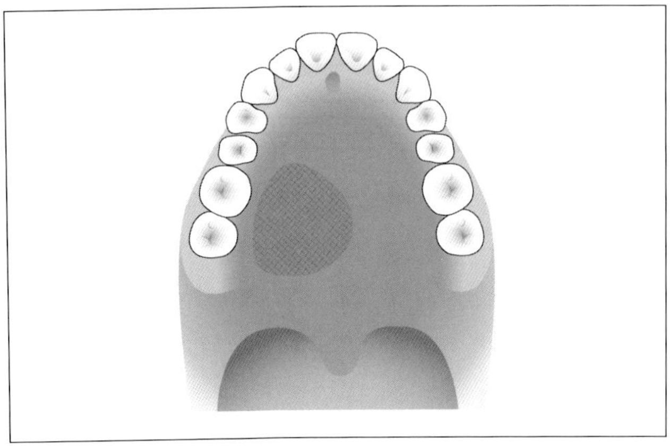

Fig. 1 This defect is limited to the hard palate and there is no defect of the soft palate. Fourteen teeth remain and there is no disturbance of mouth opening. This is described as $H_2S_0D_0T_0$. according to the defect classification.

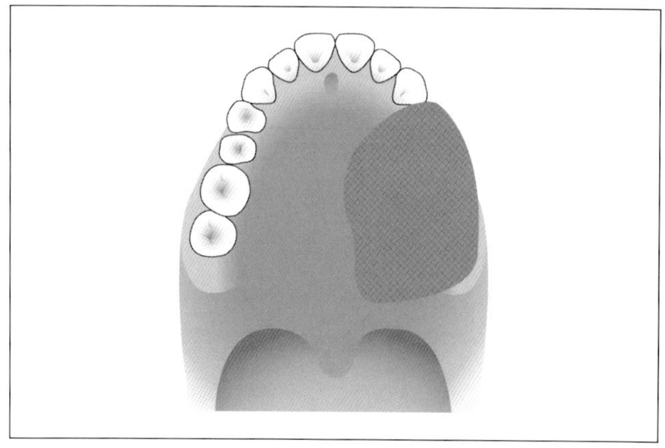

Fig. 2 There are within-hemilateral alveolar and hard palatal defects. Though the defect extends to the soft palate, the posterior soft-palate margin is preserved. Disturbance of mouth opening is slight; 10 teeth remain. This is described as $H_3S_1D_1T_0$ according to HS classification.

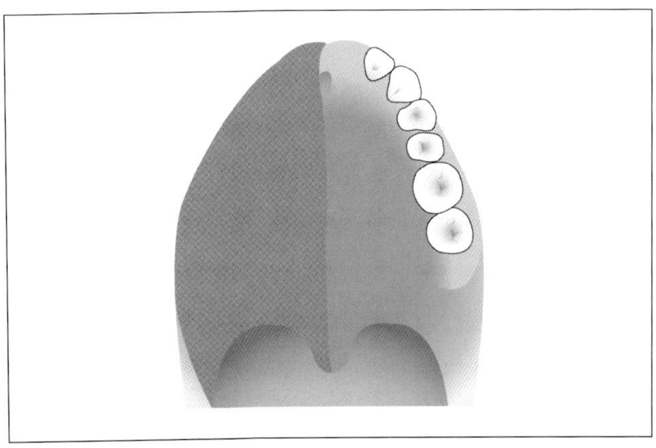

Fig. 3 This is a maxillary hemilateral complete defect, with a less-than-hemilateral defect extending to the posterior margin of the soft palate. Disturbance of mouth opening is moderate and 6 teeth remain. This is described as $H_4S_2D_1T_1$ according to HS classification.

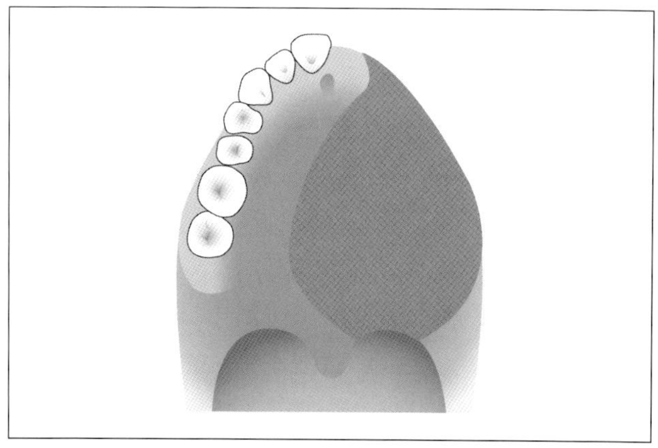

Fig. 4 This is a maxillary greater-than-hemilateral defect and there is a greater-than-hemilateral defect extending to the posterior margin in part of the soft palate. Disturbance of mouth opening is serious and 7 teeth remain. This is described as $H_5S_3D_2T_0$ according to HS classification.

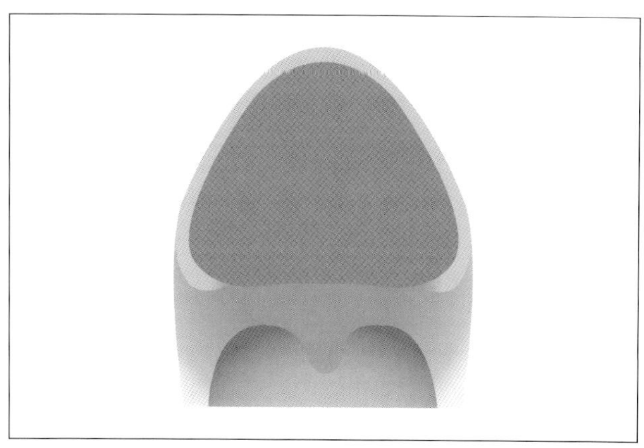

Fig. 5 Although this is a complete defect, the soft palate is preserved. The mouth-opening range is impossible to determine because of lack of maxillary anterior teeth, and no teeth remain. This is described as $H_6S_0D_xT_3$ according to HS classification.

The examples described are shown in Figs. 1 to 5.

Fig. 1 $H_2S_0D_0T_0$
Fig. 2 $H_3S_1D_1T_0$
Fig. 3 $H_4S_2D_1T_1$
Fig. 4 $H_5S_3D_2T_0$
Fig. 5 $H_6S_0D_xT_3$

Classification of maxillary defects

It is convenient to represent maxillary defect patterns as the proportion of the defect range relative to the total area of the alveolar-hard palatal region. An alveolar-hard palate defect is expressed as a ratio relative to the total alveolar-hard palate area, which is shown as 6, and a soft palate defect is expressed as a ratio relative to the total soft palate area, which is shown as 4. Each denominator is expressed as 6 or 4 respectively. This is referred to as "6-4 classification".

In the alveolar-hard palatal region, as shown in Fig. 6, if there is no defect it is shown as 0/6 (Fig. 7), and a defect of approximately one-sixth of the total area of the alveolar-hard palate is expressed as a 1/6 defect (Fig. 8). Even if the defect is located in the center of the hard palate (Fig. 9), the defect pattern is determined only from the size of the defective area without reference to the site of the defect. A defect of one-third of the total area is expressed as a 2/6 defect (Fig. 10). Likewise, the defect pattern is determined as shown above even if the site is located in the anterior position (Fig. 11).

A maxillary hemilateral defect, the most common pattern, is expressed as a 3/6 defect (Figs. 12 and 13). A defect of two-thirds of the total area is expressed as a 4/6 defect (Figs. 14 and 15). A defect extending over the entire alveolar-hard palatal area is expressed as a 6/6 defect (Fig. 16).

This simple classification may facilitate the communications between surgeon and MF prosthesis.

Defect patterns and classification of soft palate

Defect pattern classification is proportionate, comparing the defective range with the total area of the soft palate. Basically, this will be shown with the alveolar-hard palate defect. Alveolar-hard palate defects are indicated by numbers up to 6, with 6 as the denomina-

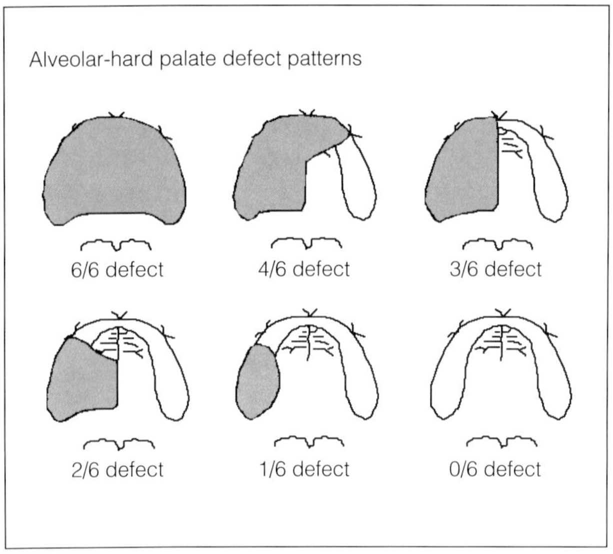

Fig. 6a Maxillary defect patterns (6 classification of 6-4 classification).

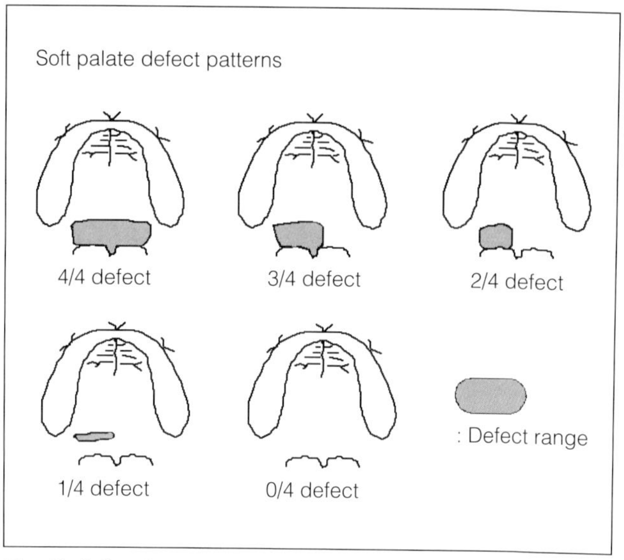

Fig. 6b Soft palate defect patterns (4 classification of 6-4 classification.

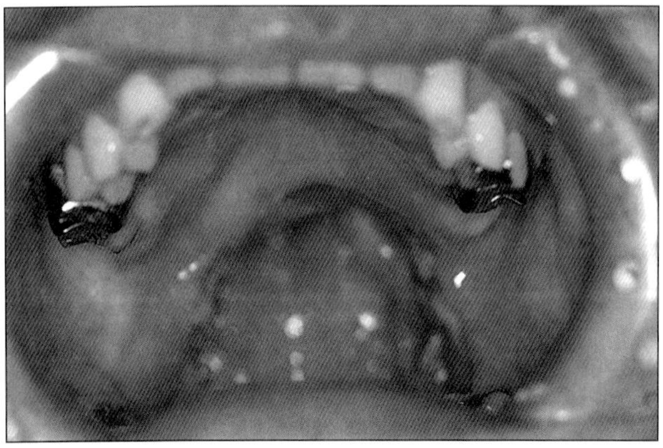

Fig. 7 0/6 - 2/4 defect. No defect in the alveolar-hard palate. A defect in the soft palate.

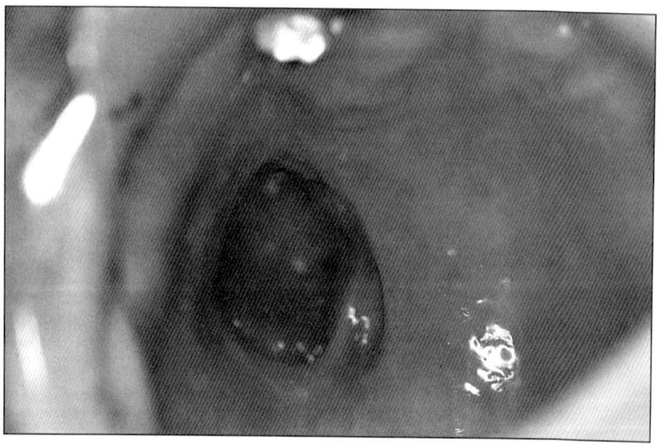

Fig. 8 1/6 - 0/4 defect. The defect range is approximately 1/6 of the entire hard palate. No defect in the soft palate.

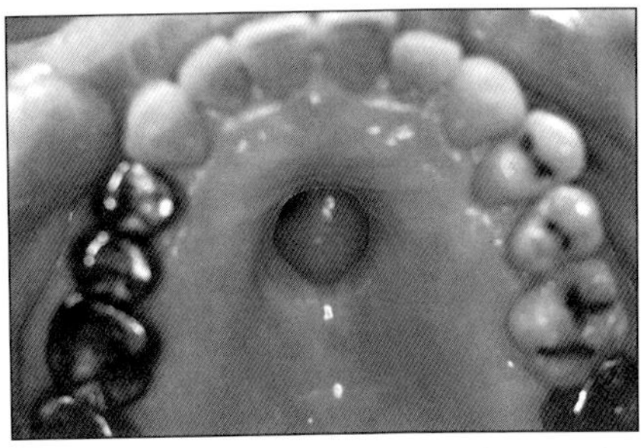

Fig. 9 1/6 - 0/4 defect. A defect in the center of the hard palate. The defect range is 1/6 or less of the entire hard palate. No defect in the soft palate.

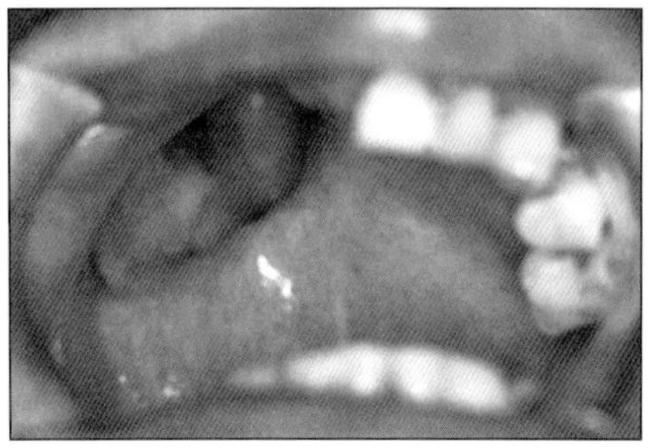

Fig. 10 2/6 - 0/4 defect. The defect range is about 1/3 of the hard palate. No defect in the soft palate.

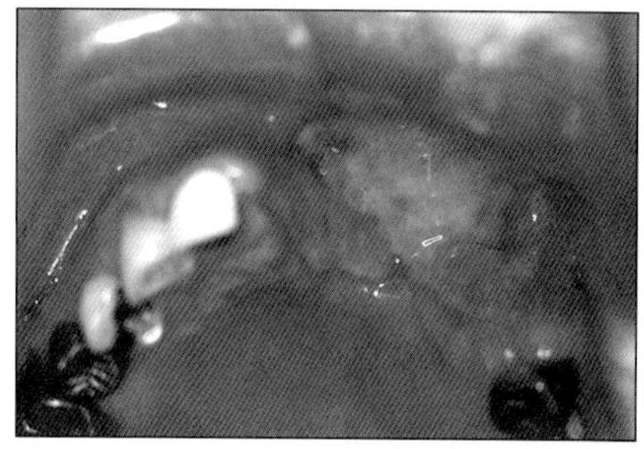

Fig. 11 2/6 - 0/4 defect. Even though the defect is in the anterior region, the defect is determined as a 2/6 defect when the defect range is about 1/3 of the whole.

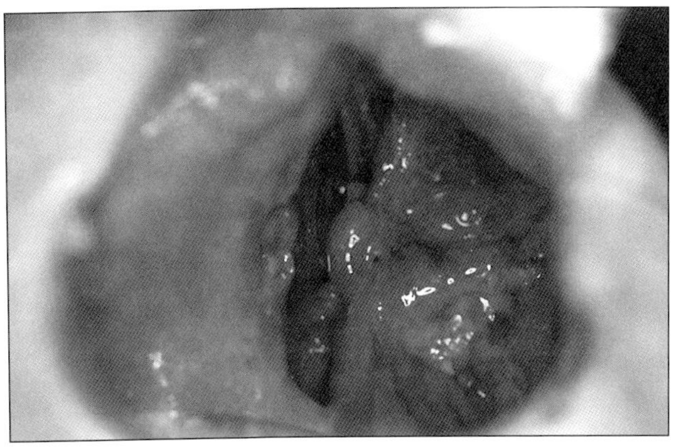

Fig. 12 3/6 - 1/4 defect. A maxillary hemilateral defect is expressed as a 3/6 defect. The soft palate has a defect only of the anterior margin; this defect is expressed as a 1/4 defect.

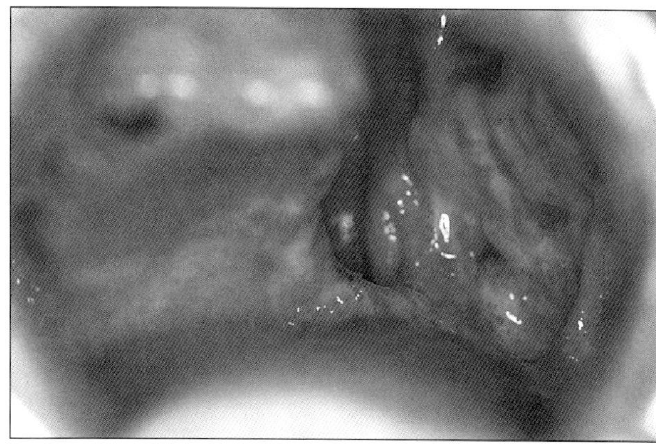

Fig. 13 3/6 - 0/4 defect. Whether on the right or left side, this is expressed as a 3/6 defect when the defect is hemilateral. No soft palate defect in this case.

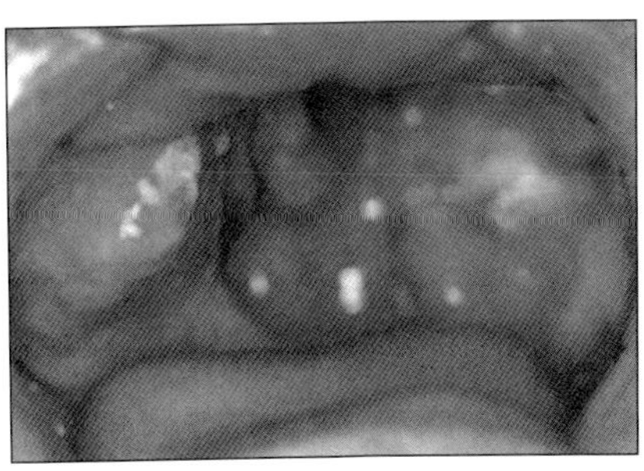

Fig. 14 4/6 - 0/4 defect. Expressed as a 4/6 and 0/4 defect when the defect covers two-thirds of total hard palate area.

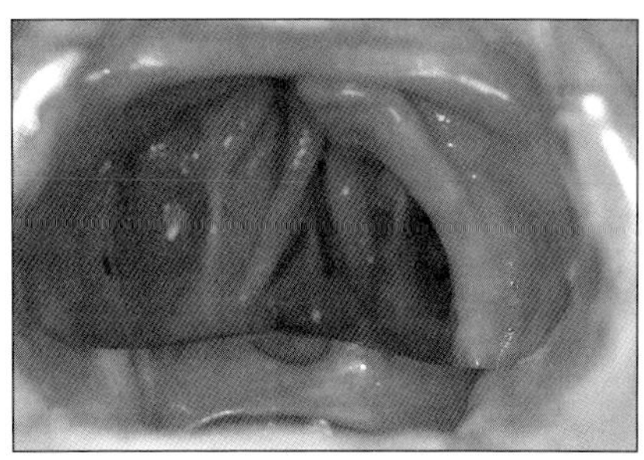

Fig. 15 4/6 - 1/4 defect. The hard palate defect is 4/6. The soft palate defect is 1/4.

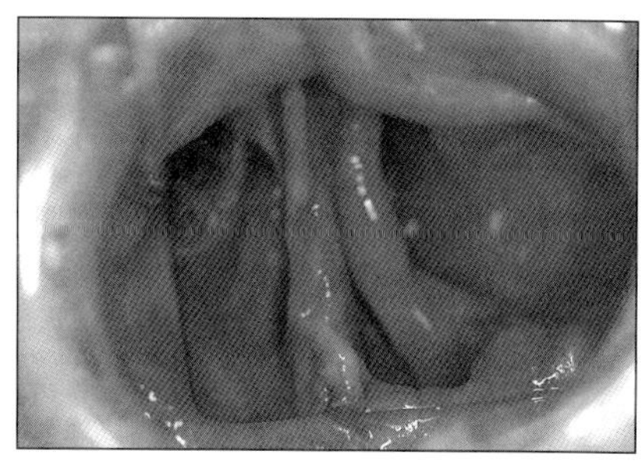

Fig. 16 6/6 - 0/4 defect. A complete maxillary hard palate with alveolar process defect is expressed as a 6/6 and 0/4 defect.

tor, and soft palate defects are indicated by numbers up to 4, with 4 as the denominator. This is referred to as "6-4 classification" as described previously (Fig. 6a, b).

A case in which there is no defect of the soft palate is expressed as a "0/4 defect" (Fig. 17), and a defect of the anterior margin in the soft palate (frequently extending from an alveolar-hard palate defect) is expressed as a 1/4 defect (Fig. 18). Considering the uvula as a standard, a defect extending to the posterior free margin of the soft palate but not including the uvula is expressed as a 2/4 defect (Figs. 19 and 20). Flap reconstruction to the pharyngeal lateral wall may be performed in the case of 2/4 defect. Fig. 19 is an example of resection alone in its left side, and Fig. 20 is an example of flap reconstruction to the right lateral wall. A soft palate defect extending to the posterior free margin including the uvula is expressed as a 3/4 defect (Fig. 21), and a defect of the entire soft palate is expressed as a 4/4 defect (Figs. 22 and 23).

In Fig. 23, flap reconstruction to the pharyngeal lateral wall has been done.

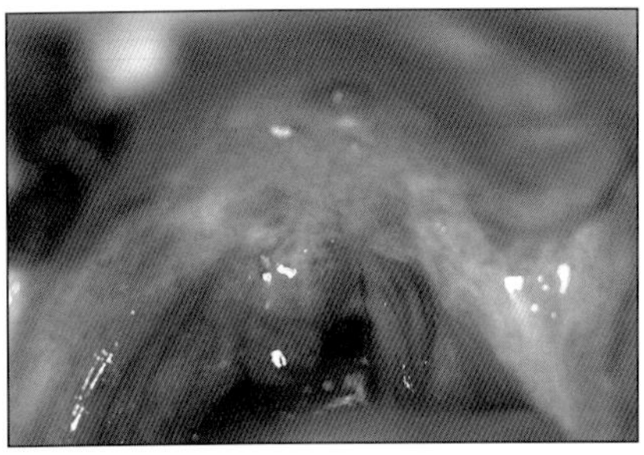
Fig. 17 1/6 - 0/4 defect.

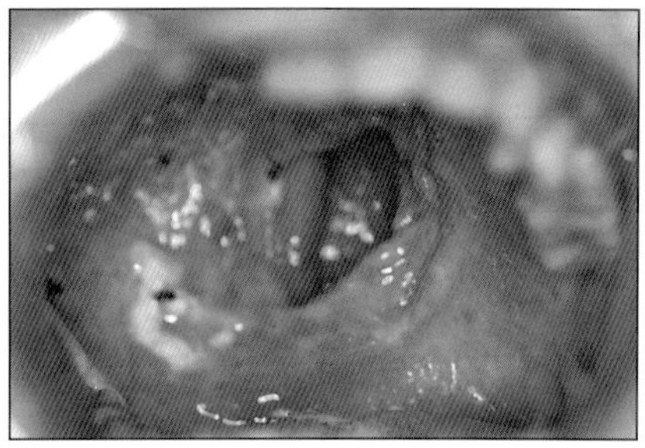
Fig. 18 4/6 - 1/4 defect.

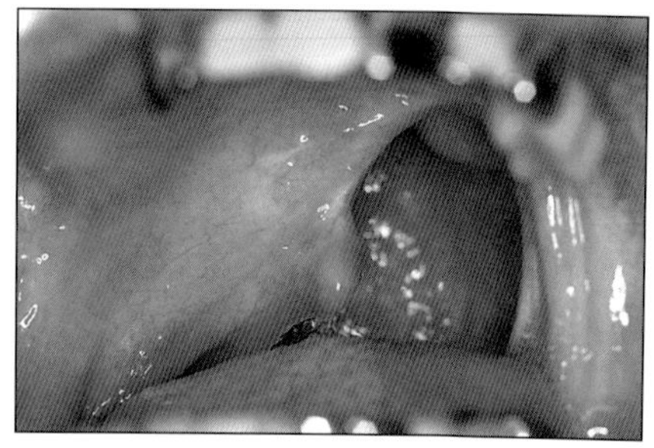
Fig. 19 2/6 - 2/4 defect.

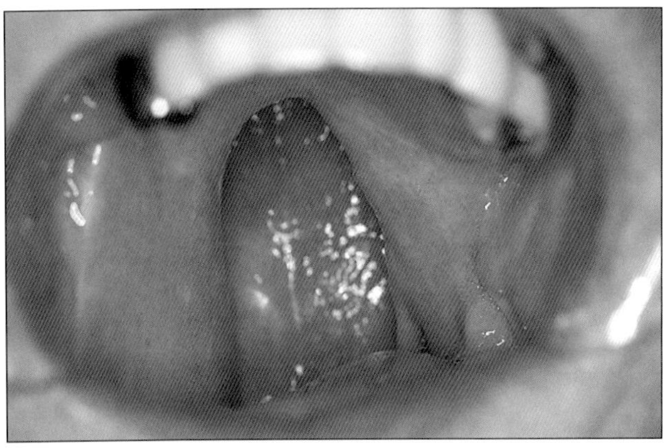
Fig. 20 1/6 - 2/4 defect. Flap reconstruction to lateral wall.

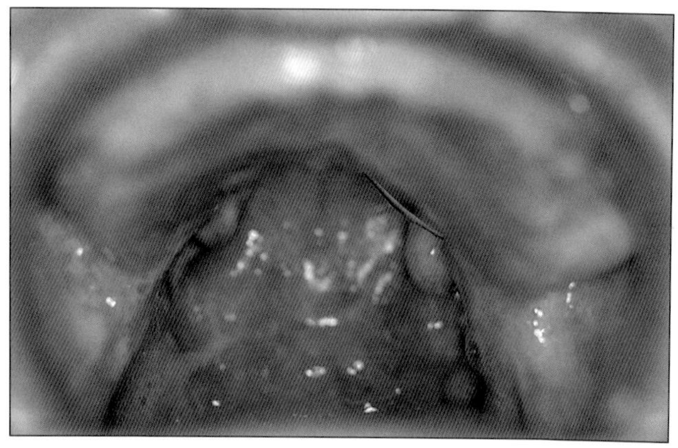
Fig. 21 1/6 - 3/4 defect.

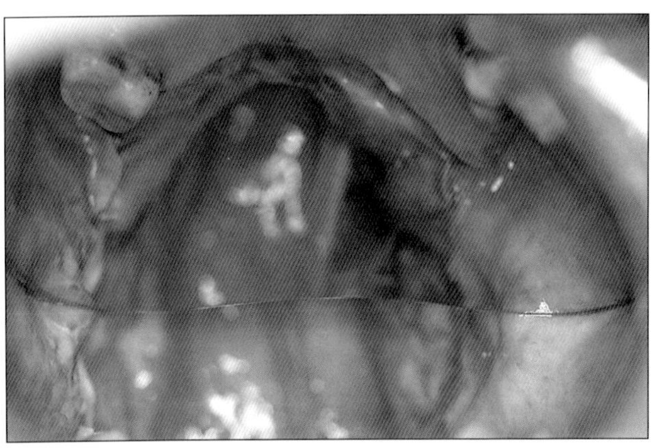
Fig. 22 0/6 - 4/4 defect.

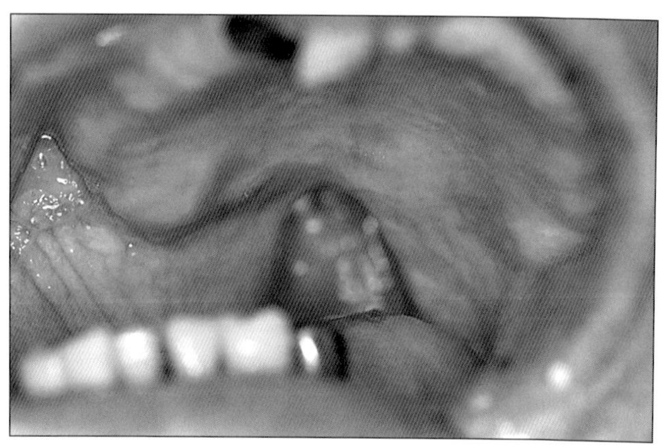
Fig. 23 0/6 - 4/4 defect. Flap reconstruction to lateral wall.

CHAPTER 5

Structures and names of parts of maxillodental prosthesis

Due to the variety of maxillary defects caused by tumors, injuries, and malformations, the forms of prostheses for functional and esthetic restoration cover a fairly broad spectrum. This chapter describes maxillodental prostheses for sequential defects after the treatment of maxillary tumors.

The maxillodental prosthesis structure consists of an obturator, a denture base, and retainers.

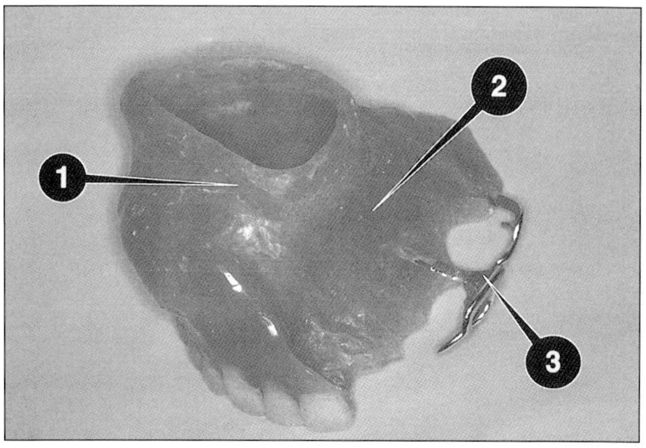

Fig. 1 Common structures and names of maxillodental prosthesis parts.

Table 1 General structures and names of parts of maxillodental prostheses.

① Obturator	Part that is inserted to close defective regions and reconstruct the oral cavity proper. There are various forms.
② Denture base	The part that is the denture-base section in common dentures; it makes contact with residual hard palate and alvelus.
③ Retainer	Clasp, Konus crown, magnet, ball or bar attachment, etc.

Advantages and disadvantages of resin plates and metal plates

The general features of resin and metal plates as materials for maxillodental prostheses are shown in Table 2. Resin plates are likely to become contaminated. On the other hand, metal plates are unlikely to degenerate and their frames are durable and remain clean (Figs. 2 and 3). However, the disadvantage of metal plates is that repairs are difficult when maxillodental prostheses become ill-fitting due to intraoral changes.

Table 2 General features of resin and metal plates as material for maxillodental prostheses.

	Advantages	Disadvantages
Resin plate	1) Materials are inexpensive and available anywhere. 2) Easy handling 3) Repair and rebase are easy because of good adhesion of heat curing resin and self (room-temperature) curing resin	1) Because it deteriorates easily and absorbs water, it is likely to become contaminated. 2) Lower wear resistance 3) Thinning leads to fracturing because of lower mechanical strength.
Metal plate	1) Higher mechanical strength 2) Unlikely to deteriorate.	1) Fabrication takes a long time. 2) If a fracture or crack occurs, refabrication is required because repair is impossible. 3) Weight is heavy.

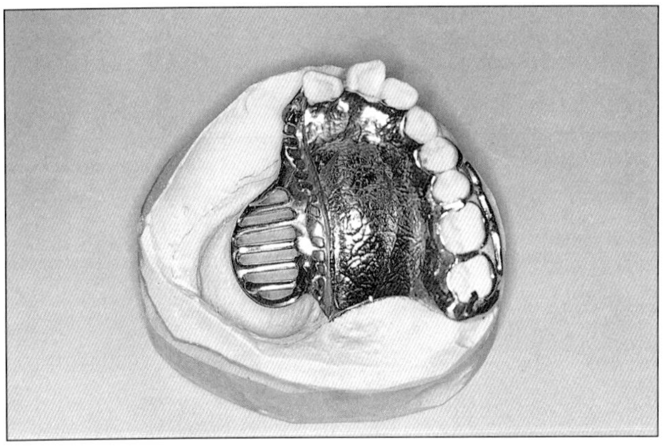

Fig. 2 Fabrication of metal frame (plate).

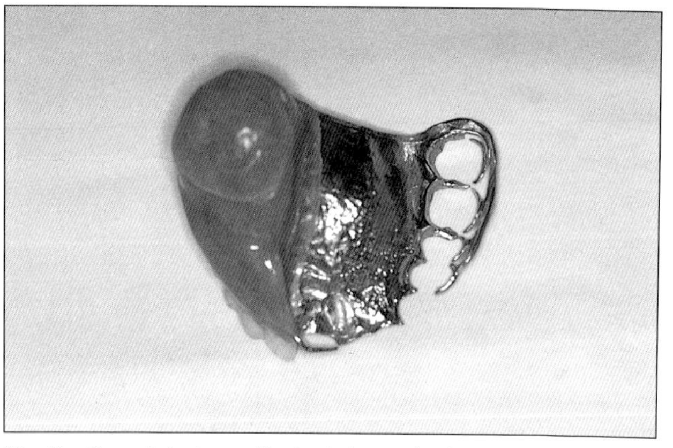

Fig. 3 Completed maxillodental metal plate prosthesis with open type obturator with removable lid.

CHAPTER 6

Measures for treatment of disturbance of mouth opening

Though prosthetic treatment of maxillary defects was previously said to be very difficult in those cases where the mouth opening range was below 20mm, out of 520 cases of maxillary defects treated from 1981 to 2001, 82 cases (16%) had mouth opening ranges of 11-20mm, and in 25 cases (5%) it was below 10mm; combined, these cases were equivalent to 20% of the total (Table 1). However, in almost all of these cases it was possible to fabricate a maxillodental prosthesis.

The goals when fabricating jaw prostheses are better settled on the basis of convenience, simplification, and possible light weight. The design of maxillodental prostheses should be simplified in ways such as the use of one-arm clasps as retainers, the buccal impressions of non-defective sites should be limited as far as is needed, and the resultant average height of the top part of the obturator was as little as 13.7mm, making it unnecessary to take a high-position impression of the maxillary defect.

The above are the distinctive features of impression taking for these cases.

Factors affecting the ease of access to the maxillary defect are the same as those regulating the extent of working space for taking impressions and for the insertion and removal of jaw prosthesis; these factors include extension of the lip-buccal region, at scar bundles maxillary defect and the presence of upper and lower residual teeth and of the defect ridge itself. Experience has shown that even though the mouth opening is small, it is possible to fabricate a jaw prosthesis when Access Route Width Ball No. 2, shown in the photograph in Fig. 1, can be inserted into the oral cavity. In short, if any space allowing access to the maxillary defect exists, maxillodental prostheses can be created by using this space.

Table 1 Mouth opening range.

Range	Cases	%
– 10mm	25	5
11 – 20	82	16
21 – 30	143	28
31 – 40	89	17
41 –	164	32
Not measurable	17	3

Mouth opening ranges in maxillary defect cases experienced from 1981 to 2001 (520 cases)

Access to working space

These measuring instruments indicate Access Route Width (ARW) and are used to measure the space for reaching the maxillary defect from the lip without interference by the upper and lower residual teeth and the residual alveolar ridge.

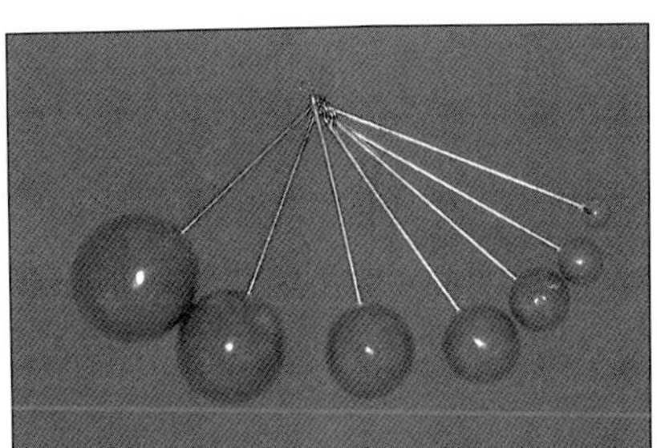

Fig. 1 This instrument consists of 7 different balls: at the left side is a ball 4cm in diameter and at the right side is a ball 1cm in diameter. Ball sizes decrease by 0.5cm por ball from left to right. The ARW number shows the maximum ball diameter that can be inserted from the lip to the maxillary defect.

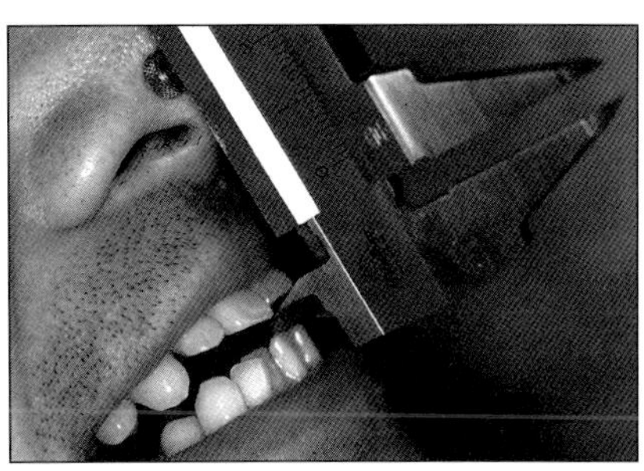

Fig. 2 Measurement of mouth opening range. Measuring mouth opening range with calipers. The mouth opening range is about 5mm at #21, 31.

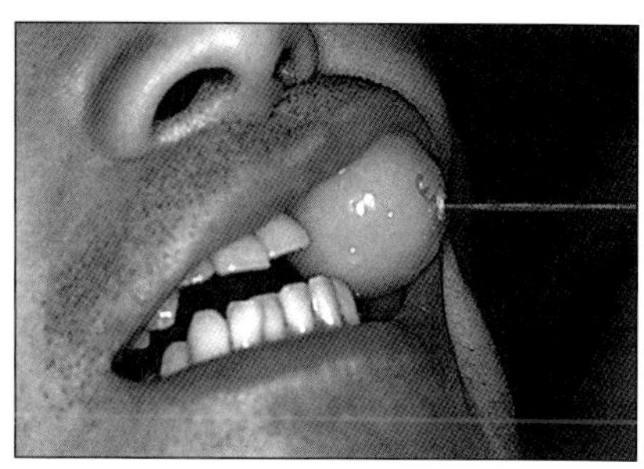

Fig. 3 Measurement of ARW. The ARW measurement was No. 3.

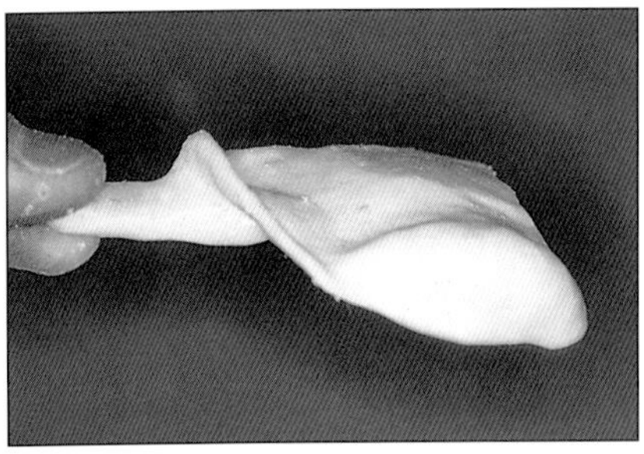

Fig. 4 Custom tray. This is the insertable custom tray used in this case; its height is very low.

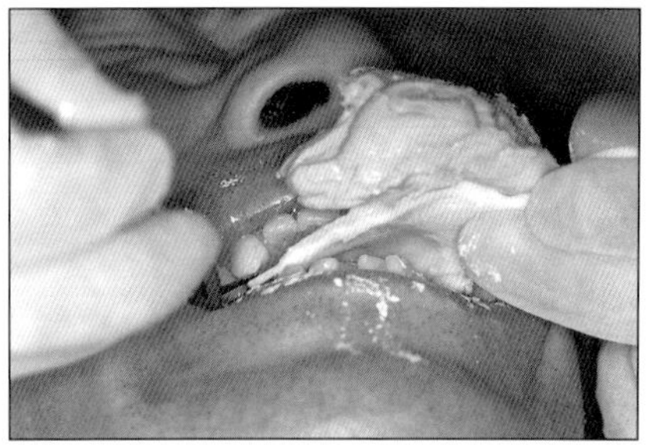

Fig. 5 Taking of impression. The final impression is taken using this custom tray.

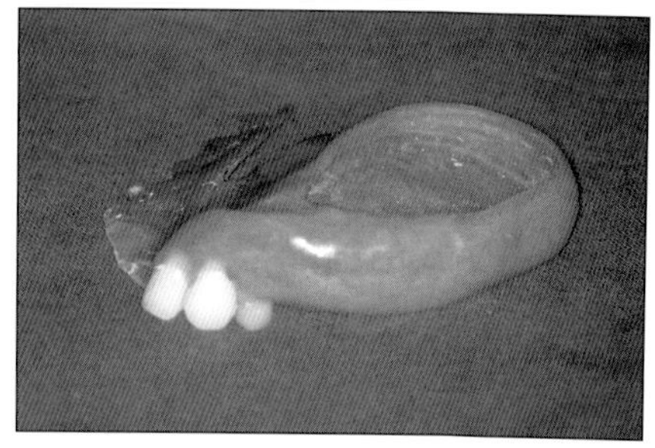

Fig. 6 Maxillodental defect prosthesis. Maxillodental prosthesis with open type obturator for a patient who is partially edentulous. The height is quite low, to match the ARW. Part of the denture plate has been omitted to avoid interference by residual anterior teeth during insertion.

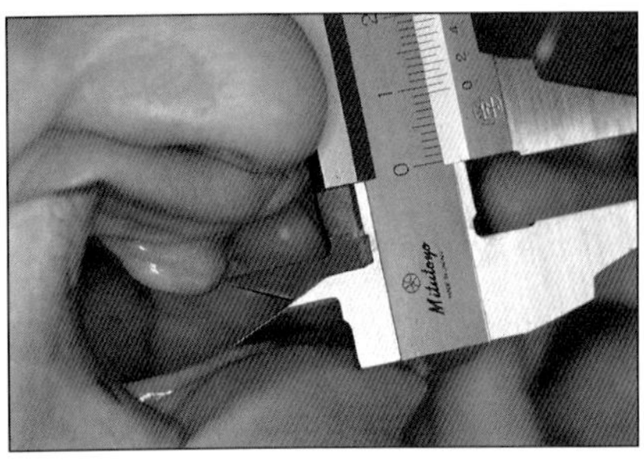

Fig. 7 Measurement of mouth opening range. Measuring the mouth opening range with calipers. The mouth opening range is about 9mm at #21, 31.

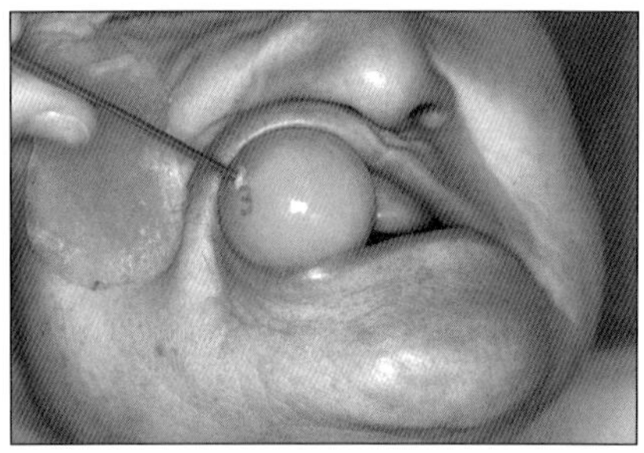

Fig. 8 The ARW measurement was No. 3.

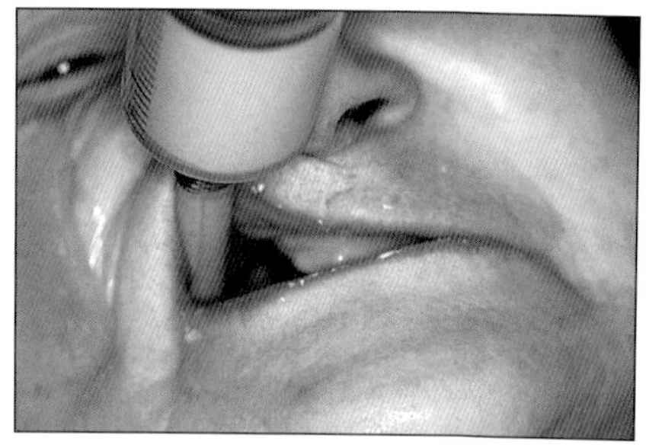

Fig. 9 Taking impression. In addition to the use of a custom tray, impression material coating may sometimes be applied directly to the oral cavity using a spatula, or an injector may be used.

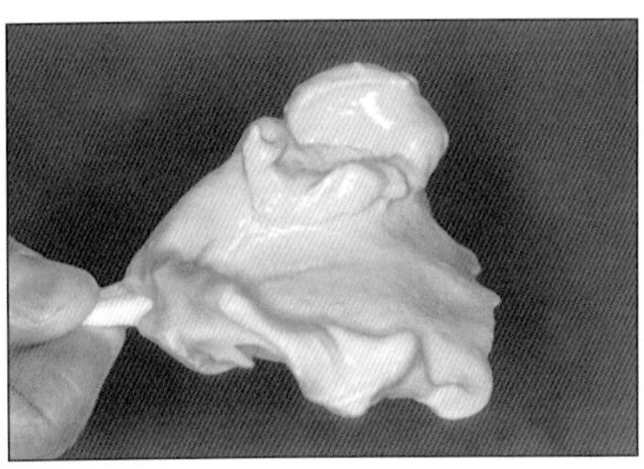

Fig. 10 Taking of final impression. Taking of impression is possible when ARW is No.3 even when the mouth opening range is 9mm.

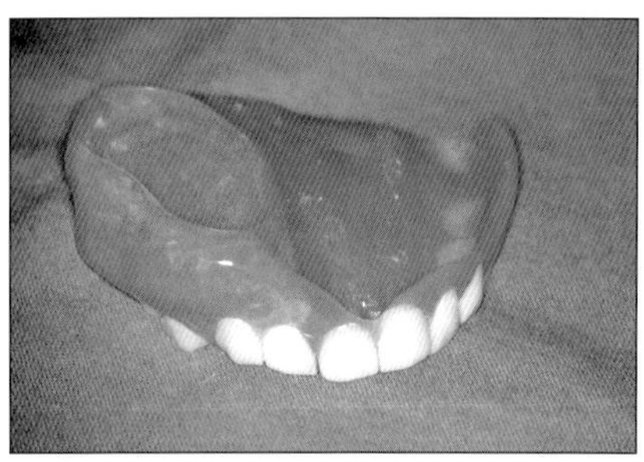

Fig. 11 Maxillodental prosthesis. Maxillodental prosthesis with open type obturator for a patient who is totally edentulous. The flange is quite low. Artificial anterior teeth were arranged on the frontal surface of the residual alveolar ridge to secure the path for ingestion.

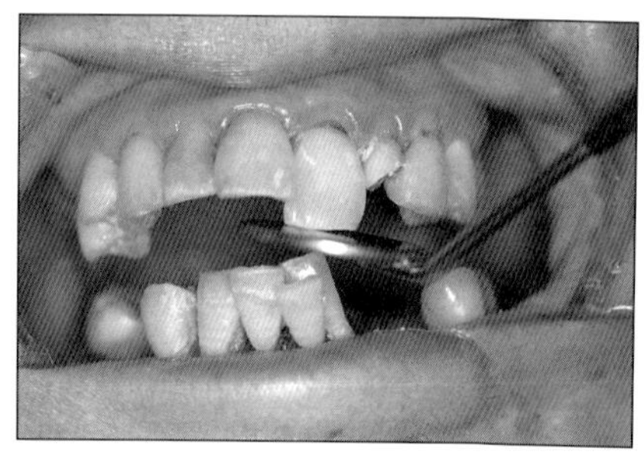

Fig. 12 Example of serious disturbance of mouth opening. The disturbance of mouth opening is only the thickness of a dental mirror.

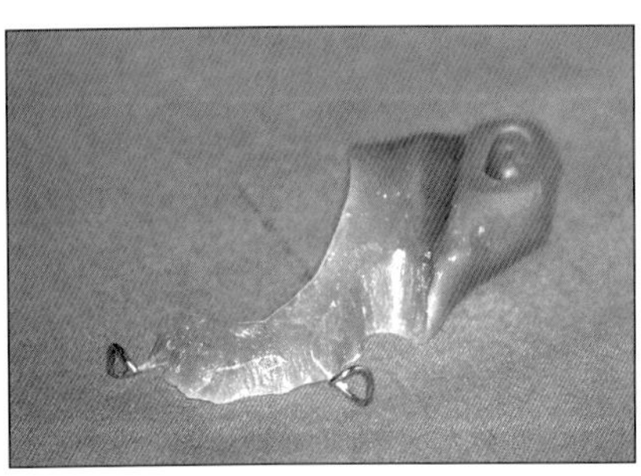

Fig. 13 Maxillodental prosthesis. Since the insertion path is affected by residual teeth, the maxillodental prosthesis was created in this atypical form. Articulation, speech, and feeding were improved sufficiently.

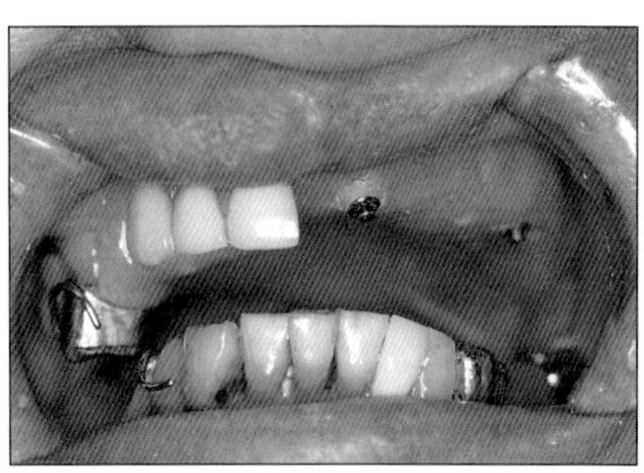

Fig. 14 Sectional maxillodental prosthesis. When the mouth opening range is small, the part of anterior teeth on the maxillodental prosthesis can be of the removable type, to secure a path for ingestion by removing the anterior section for eating.

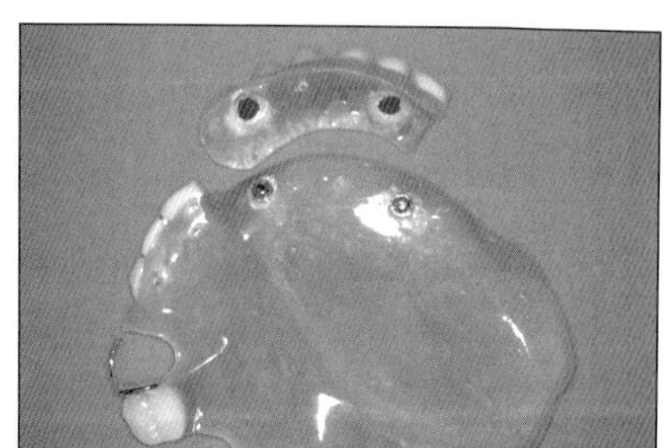

Fig. 15 A sectional maxillodental prosthesis. The anterior section remains in place at times other than while the patient is eating. Two root attachments were used to make detachment possible. (GPC stud attachments from Hader, Germany).

CHAPTER 7

Impression taking

The author's usual techniques for fabrication of maxillodental prostheses, maxillodental prostheses with open type obturator and maxillodental prostheses with open type obturator with lids are described here.

1. Fabrication of maxillodental prosthesis with open type obturator: (Fig. 1)

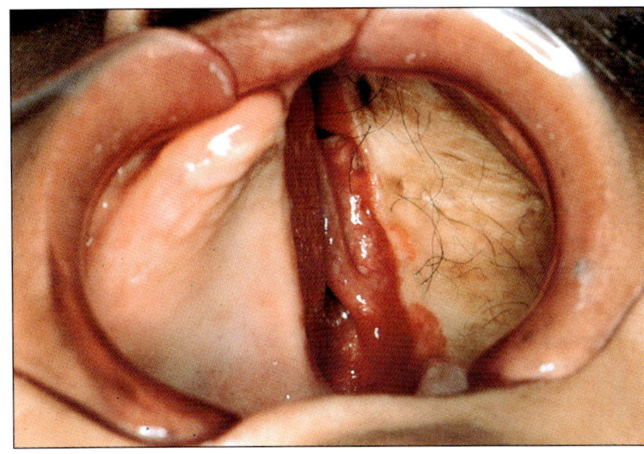

Fig. 1 This case is a 60-year-old woman with edentulous hemi-maxillary defect (HS classification: H_4T_4) status.

Snap impression

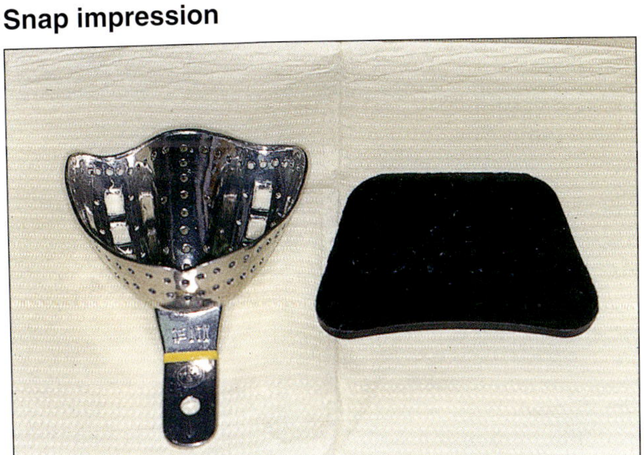

Fig. 2 Standard (ready-made) tray and black compound for snap impression.

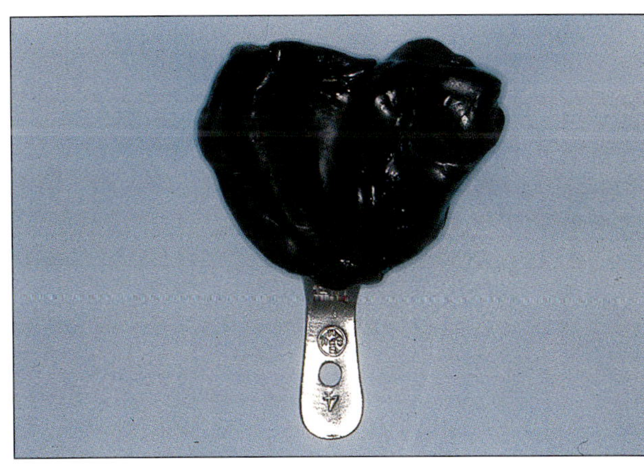

Fig. 3 The defect space and residual hard palate are roughly shaped with softened black compound.

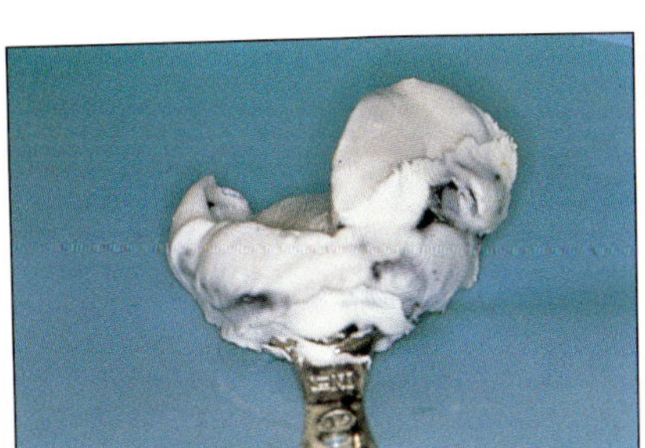

Fig. 4 Preliminary impression is taken intraorally using alginate impression material.

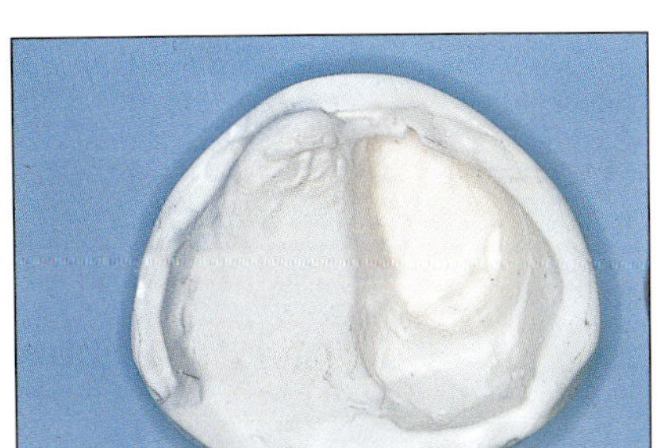

Fig. 5 A study cast, on which an individual resin-tray will be made, is fabricated.

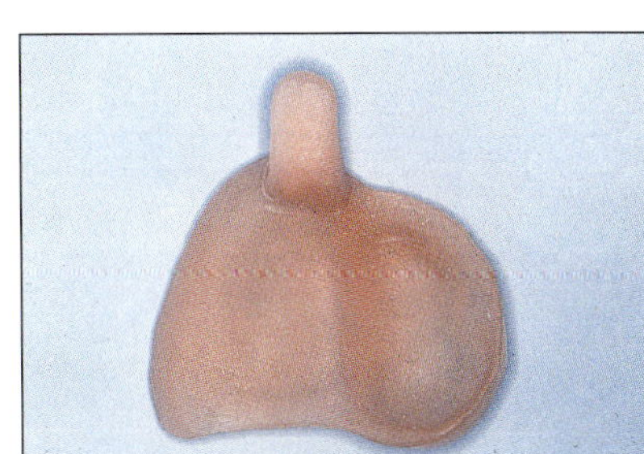

Fig. 6 Individual resin-tray.

Impression for trial denture

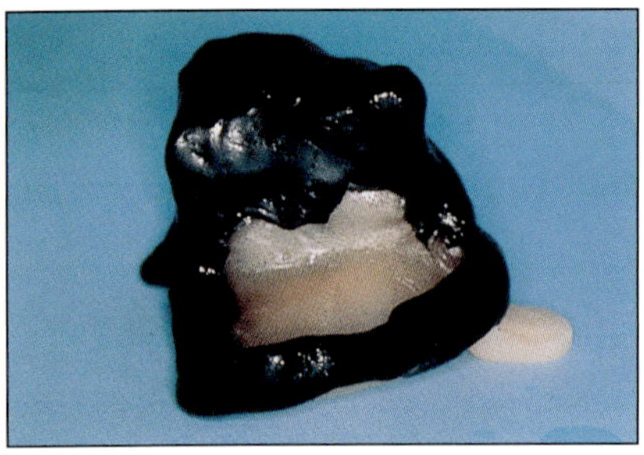

Fig. 7 Using the individual resin-tray and black compound, the defect space and residual hard palate are roughly shaped, more precisely than the snap impression.

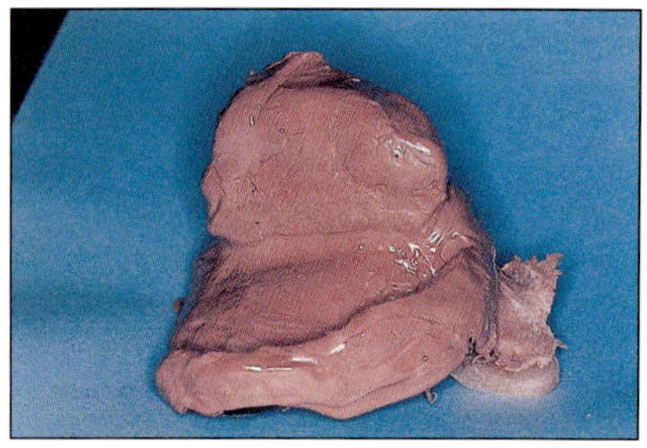

Fig. 8 Following the application of Poly-sulfid rubber impression material to the entire tray, intraoral impression is taken.

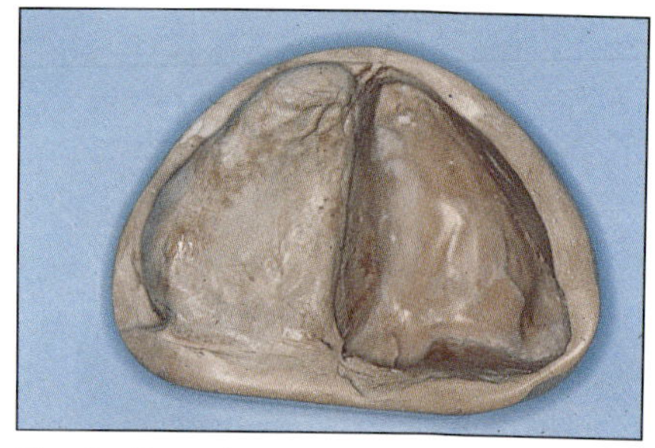

Fig. 9 Dental stone is poured onto the surface of the impression taken to fabricate a working cast.

Registration of interocclusal relation

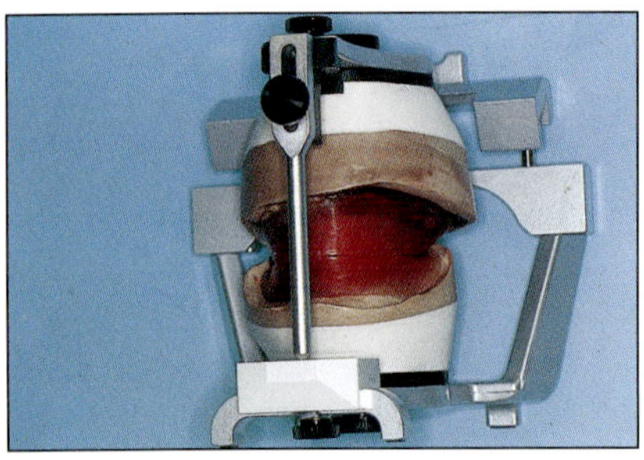

Fig. 10 First, occlusion plates are made on the working cast, then registration of interocclusal relation are taken by the usual method. They are then mounted on an articulator.

Arrangement of artificial teeth

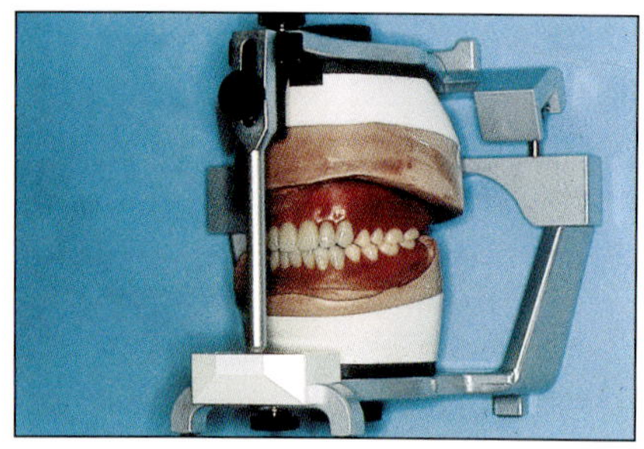

Fig. 11 After registration of the interocclusal relation, artificial teeth are arranged on the articulator.

Final impression using wax maxillodental-prosthesis

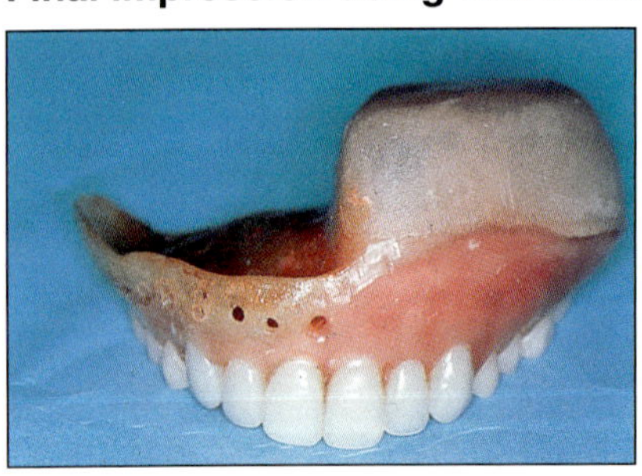

Fig. 12 Arrangement of artificial teeth on the wax maxillodental-prosthesis is corrected in the oral cavity, then the final impression is taken using the wax maxillodental-prosthesis.

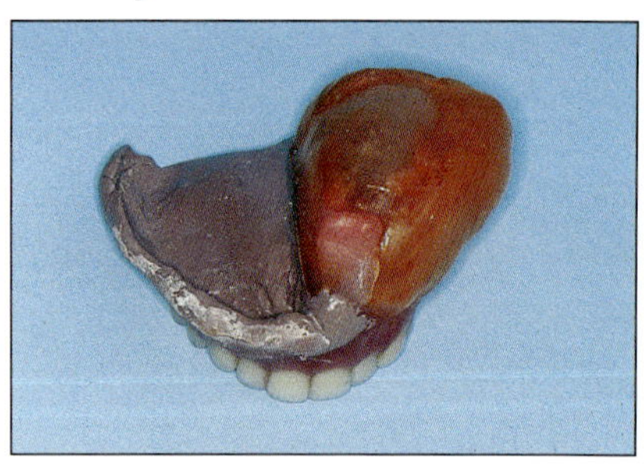

Fig. 13 First, several holes for retention and spillway of impression material are made in the anterior flange of the wax maxillodental-prosthesis. After applying a small amount of high melting-point paraffin wax around the obturator and adjusting the form of the obturator in order to stabilize the wax maxillodental-prosthesis to some extent, the impression of the denture base is taken under occlusal stress, using Poly-sulfid rubber impression material.

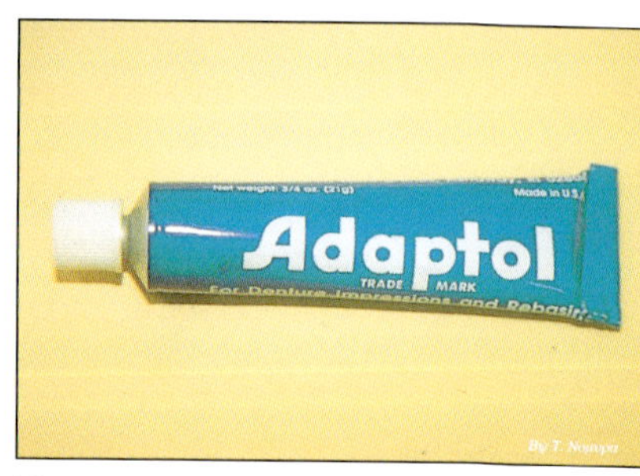

Fig. 14 Movement of the buccal cicatrical tissue bands during function should be marked as precisely as possible on the buccal wall of the obturator using Adaptol® (Jelenko Co., NY) wax impression material.

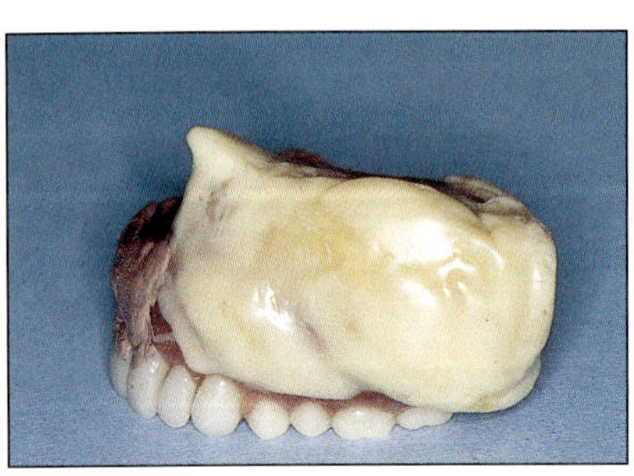

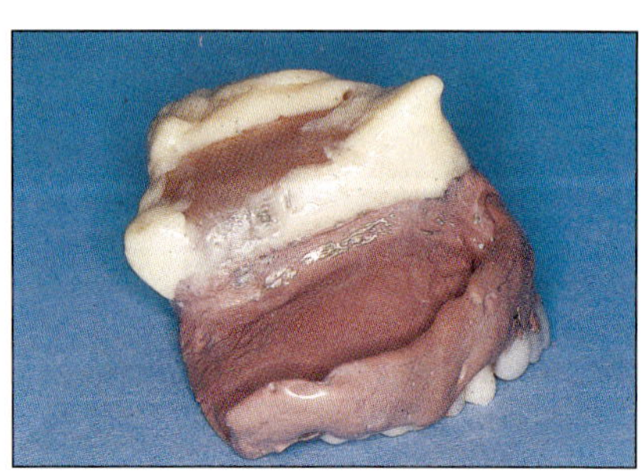

Fig. 15 *(left)* With gradual movement during function, impressions of the center, anterior region, and posterior region of the obturator are taken in sequence.
Fig. 16 *(right)* The protrusions on the anterior and posterior regions of the obturator are fitted by Adaptol® and retentive stability is confirmed, followed by completion of the final impression.

Curing and completion of maxillodental prosthesis

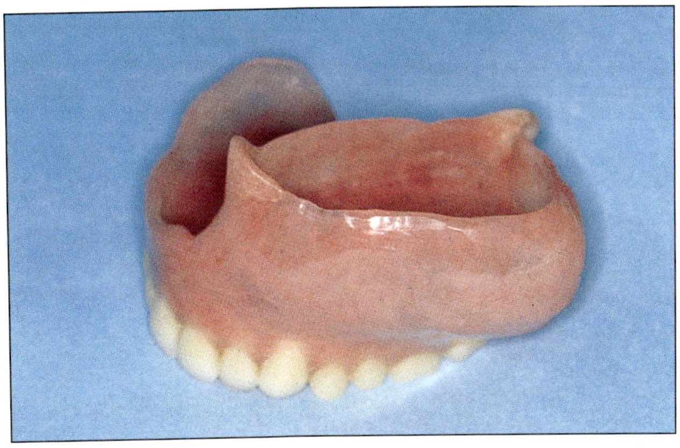

Fig. 17 With the final impression completed, the wax maxillodental prosthesis is invested into a flask, in which resin curing is performed in the conventional manner, then the resin of the inner walls of the obturator and the inner surfaces of artificial teeth is ground off until the weight of the prosthesis becomes less than 20g.

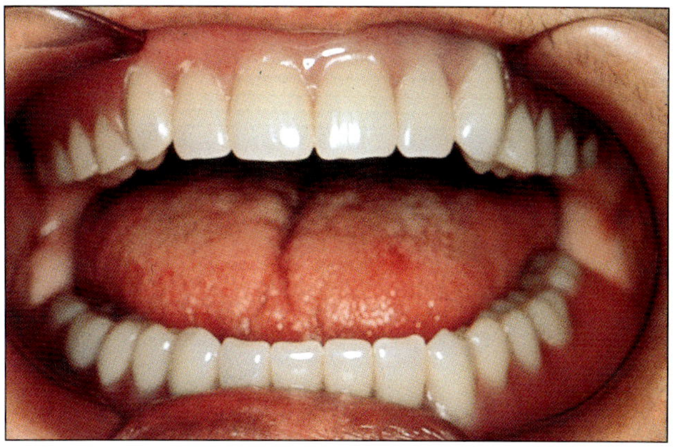

Fig. 18 With exactly the same form as in the final impression, the completed maxillodental prosthesis is lighter in weight (weight: 18.5g), has good retentive stability and will not fall off even when the mouth is opened widely.

2. Fabrication of maxillodental prosthesis with open type obturator with removable lid: (Fig. 19, 20)

Since maxillodental prostheses with open type obturator with lid are fabricated after resin-curing of maxillodental prostheses with open type obturator, descriptions overlapping those already shown above have been omitted.

3. Preparation for fabrication of removable lid and mounting device: (Fig. 21 – 26)

A flared section 5mm wide is fabricated around the upper inside of the obturator to receive the lid, which is fabricated to conform to this opening after fabrication of the maxillodental prosthesis with open type obturator. The lid should be adjusted to fit the flared section perfectly.

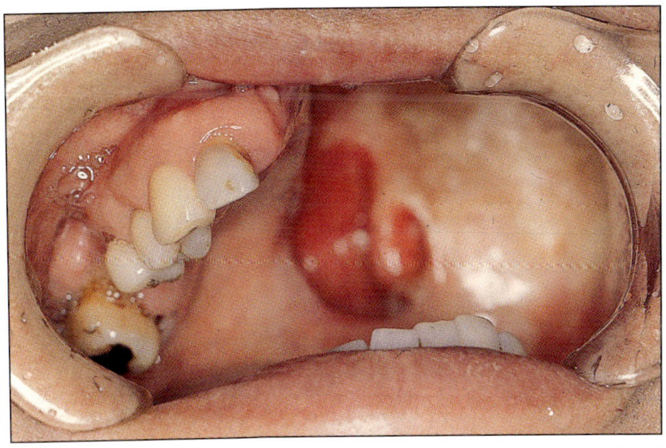

Fig. 19 This case is a 60-year-old woman with dentulous hard palatal hemilateral defect (HS classification: H_4T_1) status.

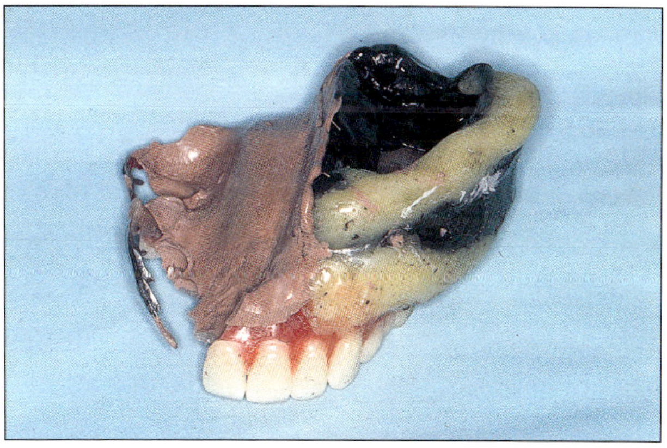

Fig. 20 The final impression of the denture base has been taken with Polysulfid rubber impression material and that of the obturator has been taken with black compound and a wax impression material, after arrangement and trial of the wax maxillodental-prosthesis.

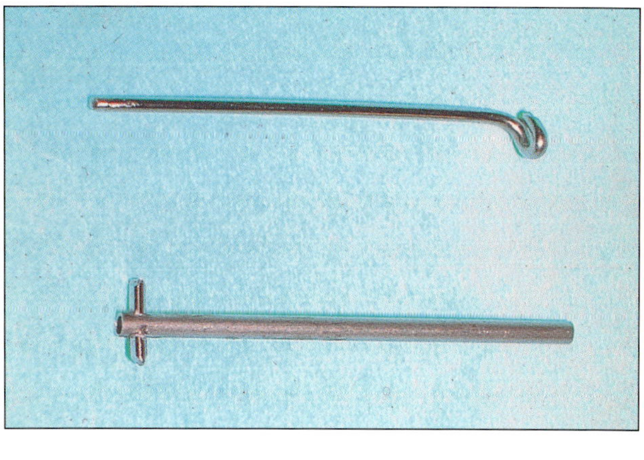

Fig. 21 Three wires of 0.8 to 1.0mm in diameter to be mounted on the lid, and three hollow metal tubes with internal diameters of 1.0 to 1.2mm to be mounted on the base of the obturator are prepared to fabricate a detachable lid. Upper: One end of each wire is bent into a loop about 5mm in diameter, to be fixed on the inside of the lid using self-curing resin. Lower: A hole about 0.8 mm in diameter is drilled into one end of each hollow metal tube. A wire of the same diameter is inserted, then cut to about 7mm in length to be fixed on the inside of the obturator by self-curing resin.

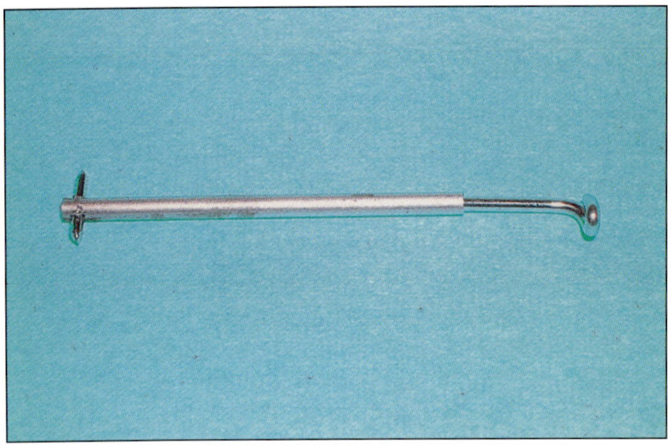

Fig. 22 The wires and the hollow metal tubes are checked to confirm that the wires fit into the tubes. Fabrication of detachable lid: The positions for the hollow metal tubes to be fixed on the base of obturator are marked, then the length of each section is determined.

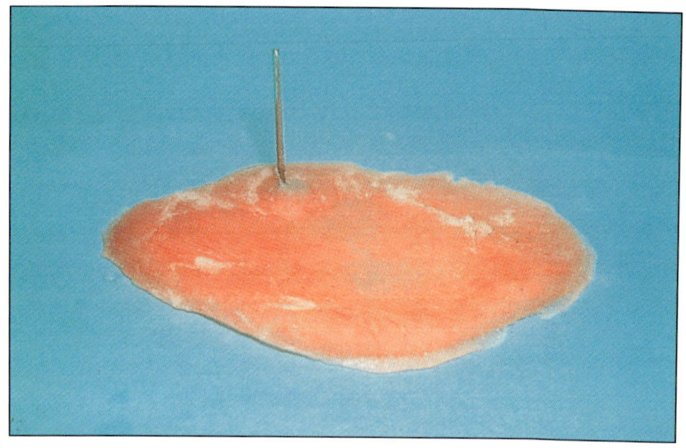

Fig. 23 First, the wires are fixed on the inside of the lid.

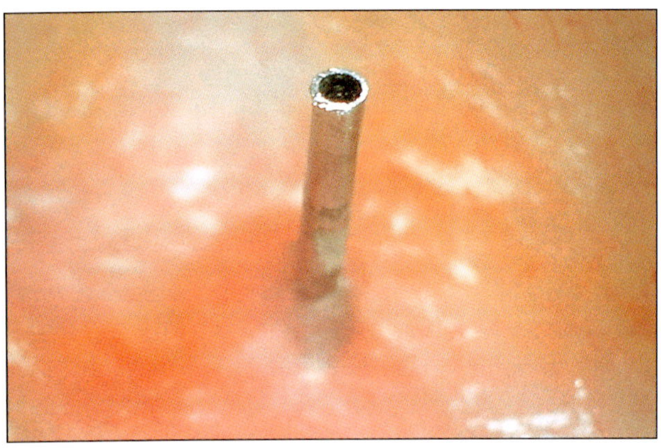

Fig. 24 Each hollow metal tube is slid onto a wire and self-curing resin is applied to the areas where the wires are fixed, each hollow metal tube is fixed to the base of the obturator.

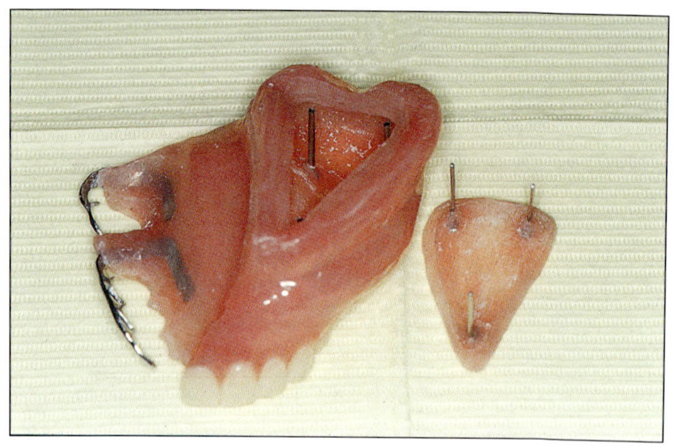

Fig. 25 Completed maxillodental prosthesis with open type obturator with removable lid.

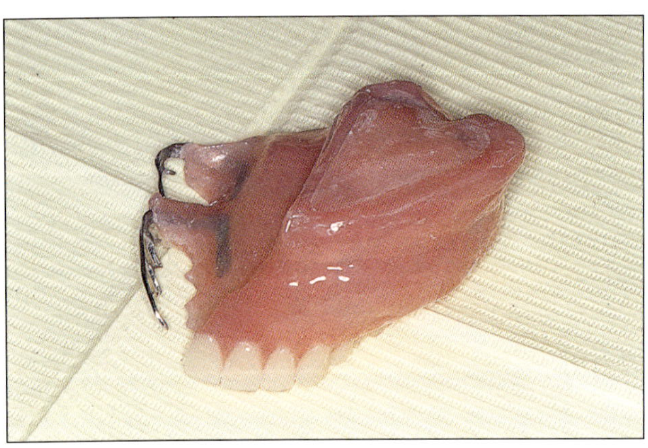

Fig. 26 A removable lid has been incorporated on the upper part of a maxillodental prosthesis with open type obturator.

CHAPTER 8

Forms of maxillodental prostheses and features of obturators

The forms of maxillodental prostheses are divided broadly into 4 categories: the maxillodental prosthesis with solid obturator (Fig. 1), maxillodental prosthesis with hollow obturator (Fig. 2), maxillodental prosthesis with open type obturator (Fig. 3), and maxillodental prosthesis with open type obturator with removable lid (Figs. 4 and 5). The distinctive features of each type are shown in Table 1. The maxillodental prosthesis with hollow obturator is good due to its light weight and cleanliness, and is commonly fabricated as the most standard form. However, the weight of this type may gradually increase for such reasons as the external resin of the obturator increasing in thickness after repairing and rebasing, or the invasion of dirty water and contaminants into the obturator after several years of use, as shown in Figs. 6 and 7. To remove this, cleaning or cutting the resin of the obturator is required, and these procedures are complicated. Because of its many advantages, including easy cleaning to remove water and food residue and the weight reduction provided by cutting the thickened resin off the interior surface after repairing and rebasing, the maxillodental prosthesis with open type obturator or with open type obturator with removable lid is excellent for long-term use.

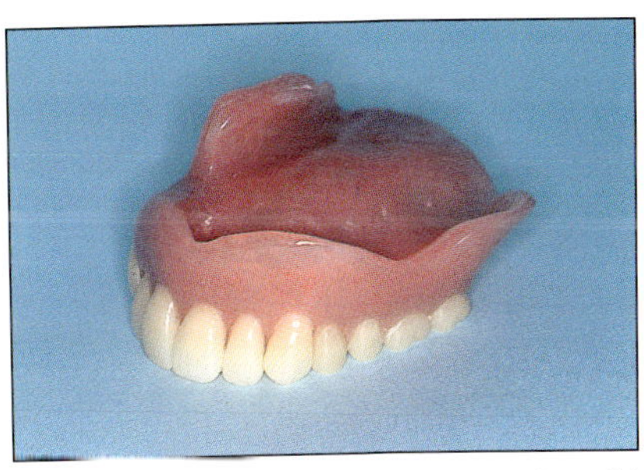

Fig. 1 Maxillodental prosthesis with solid obturator.

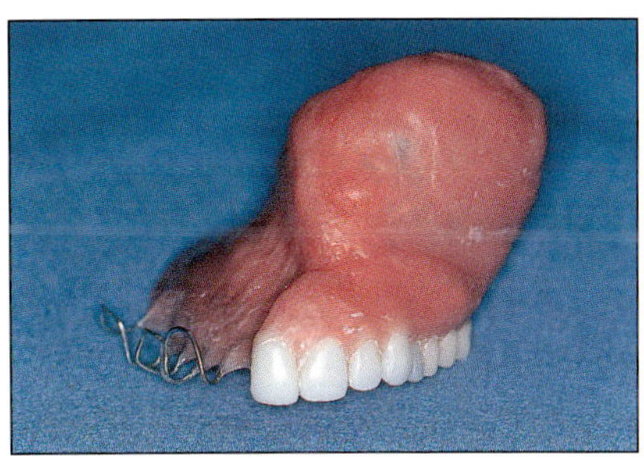

Fig. 2 Maxillodental prosthesis with hollow obturator.

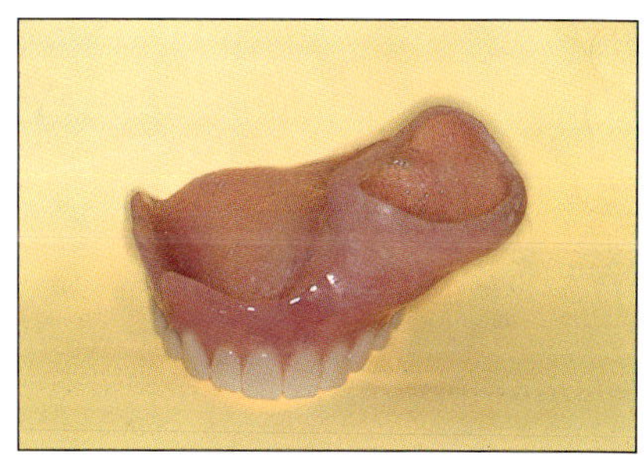

Fig. 3 Maxillodental prosthesis with open type obturator.

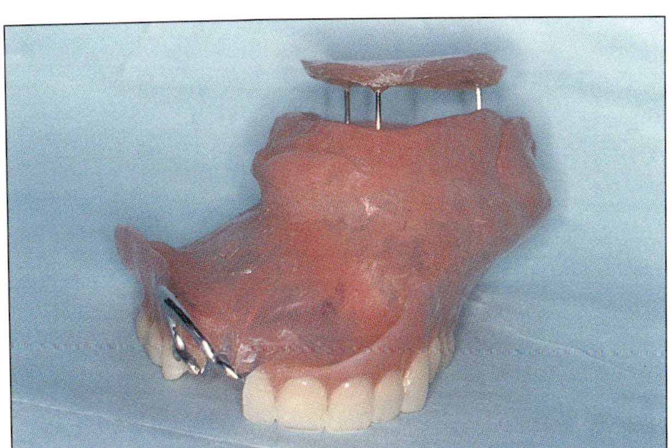

Fig. 4 Maxillodental prosthesis with open type obturator with removable lid (during incorporation).

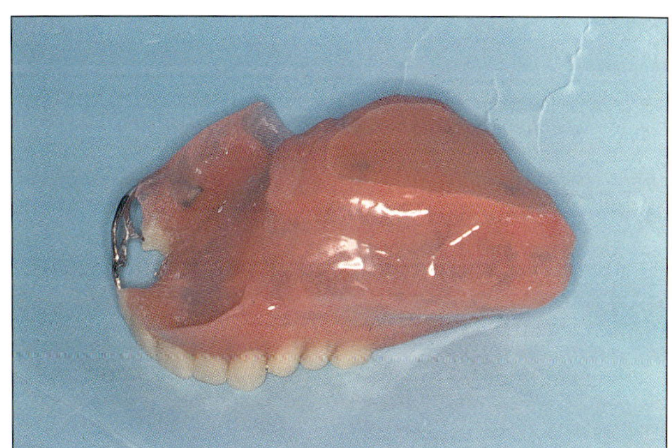

Fig. 5 Maxillodental prosthesis with open type obturator with removable lid (incorporation completed).

Table 1 Features for each form of obturator.

Form of obturator	Features of form	Advantages	Disadvantages
1) Solid obturator	The entire obturator is fabricated of resin. Used mainly for small defects.	Easy fabrication	Weight is greater (than that of hollow obturator).
2) Hollow obturator	The inside is hollowed out to lighten the weight of the obturator. Conventional method.	Lighter in weight than solid obturator.	① Water and contaminants may invade the inside. The fabrication process to prevent the intrusion of water and contaminants is complicated and increases obturator weight. ② Time-consuming since the invasion of contamination requires cleaning which involves cutting the hollow region open. ③ The external resin becomes thicker with repair and rebase, and weight gradually increases.
3) Open type obturator, buccal flange obturator	The upper section of the obturator is open.	① The open type obturator is of lower height than the hollow obturator, making it easier to insert and remove. ② Lighter in weight than the hollow type because there is no lid. ③ Because resin can be ground from the inside after doing repairs and rebase, weight-saving can be done at any time. ④ Cleaning is simple.	Water and food debris may accumulate in the obturator.
4) Open type obturator with removable lid	The top of the open type obturator has a detachable lid.	① Water and food debris are not likely to accumulate inside the obturator. ② Periodic cleaning keeps the interior clean. ③ Because resin can be ground from the inside after repair and rebase, weight-saving can be done at any time.	Increase of weight due to addition of lid

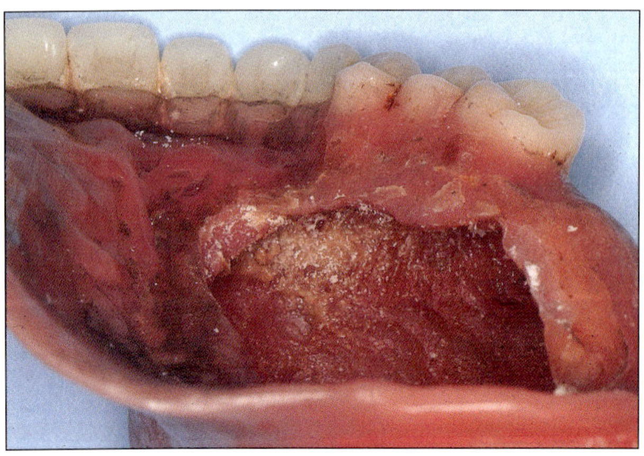

Fig. 6 Opening of interior of hollow obturator with invasion of contamination.

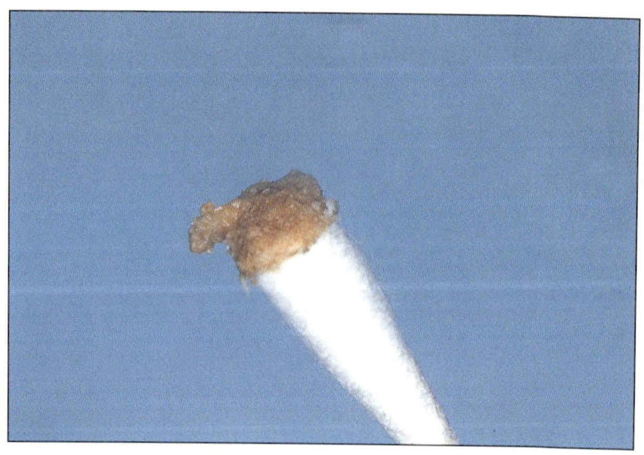

Fig. 7 Contamination from interior of hollow obturator adhering to swab.

CHAPTER 9

Retention of maxillodental prostheses

Intraoral conditions after the removal of maxillary tumors show various patterns ranging from simple palatal defects to complex conditions resulting from combined reconstruction surgeries. While some reconstruction surgeries provide intraoral retentive sources for maxillodental prostheses that are effective for retention, bulky flaps fail to provide retentive sources for maxillodental prostheses, instead hanging down within the oral cavity and interfering with retention, producing forces that cause prostheses to drop off (Fig. 1: red arrow). To oppose the forces in various falling directions, it is absolutely essential to make skillful use of the anatomical conditions of residual tissue and the periphery of the defect cavity (Fig. 1: green arrow).

Factors to be considered concerning retention of maxillodental prostheses include intraoral retentive sources based on the postoperative anatomical form, retentive actions based on the forms of maxillodental prostheses to make effective use of these sources, retainers for residual teeth, the weight of maxillodental prostheses, and the placement of implants in the oral cavity to provide artificial retentive sources.

Intraoral retentive sources and forms and retainers with which maxillodental prostheses are endowed:

Intraoral retentive sources for patients with maxillary defects, and corresponding forms of maxillodental prostheses and retentive actions, are shown in Table 1. Residual teeth are the most powerful retentive sources. For edentulous patients, however, it is necessary to make use of the residual hard palate, residual nasal septum, within the defect (a) and undercuts suited onto the nasopharyngeal site of the residual soft palate (b), and the buccal cicatrical tissue, as retentive sources, as shown in Fig. 2. Retentive forms of maxillodental prostheses corresponding to these are shown in Fig. 3. In particular, providing processes as retentive sources at the front and rear of the obturator (a, b) is effective for preventing the detachment of maxillodental prostheses. Therefore, the providing of these forms for edentulous patients is a key point in the fabrication of maxillodental prostheses with good retention stability.

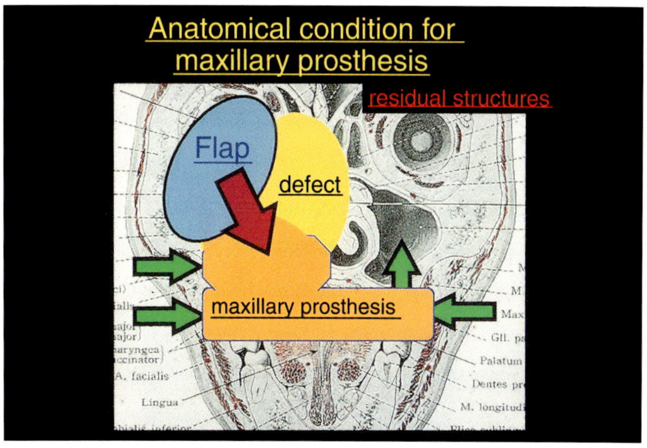

Fig. 1 Conditions for maxillodental prosthesis within the defect.

Weight and retention of maxillodental prostheses in edentulous maxillary defective patients

In addition to the above-mentioned forms of maxillodental prostheses, weight is a major factor in the insertion of maxillodental prostheses with good retention stability, essential for the restoration of deglutitive, masticatory, and speech functions for edentulous patients with maxillary defects. The increase in weight of a maxillodental prosthesis is chiefly due to an increase in the weight of the obturator, which means that in the weight distribution of maxillodental prostheses the weight bias is toward the obturator. For edentulous patients with maxillary defects, retention through the defective-side circumferential tissue decreases as the weight of the obturator increases, and this leads to detachment. Consequently, it is considered that separation of the denture base from tight contact with the residual hard palate and the diminishment of adsorptive power by negative pressure will result in the complete detachment of a maxillodental prosthesis.

We studied the relationship between the weight and retention of dentures for defective maxilla, and sequential changes in retention, from 2 weeks to a maximum of one year and 5 months after insertion.

Table 1 Intraoral retentive sources and forms of maxillodental prostheses, and corresponding retentive actions.

Intraoral retentive sources	Forms and retainers provided for maxillodental prostheses	Retentive actions
① Residual teeth	Retainers for use with teeth: clasps, Konus crowns, magnets, ball or bar attachments, etc.	Mechanical retention
② Residual hard palate	Denture base of maxillodental prosthesis is tightly adhered to hard palate.	Absorption by negative pressure
③ Residual nasal septum	Inner wall of obturator is made higher in the detachable range (about 10mm).	Maintaining of negative pressure, or prevention of sideways rolling
④ Defect space	Processes project to the undercuts of the anterior and posterior within the defect (a; anterior nasal apature and b; onto the nasopharyngeal site of residual soft palate)	Mechanical retention in detachment of maxillodental prosthesis
⑤ Buccal cicatrical tissue	Buccal wall of obturator is contoured.	Retention by cicatrical tissue and flap tissue pressure

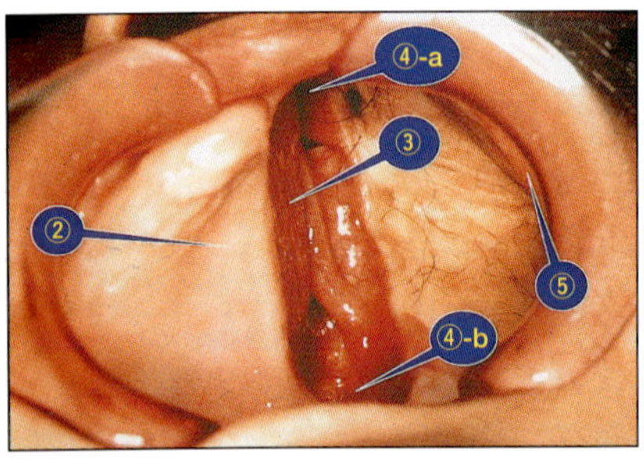

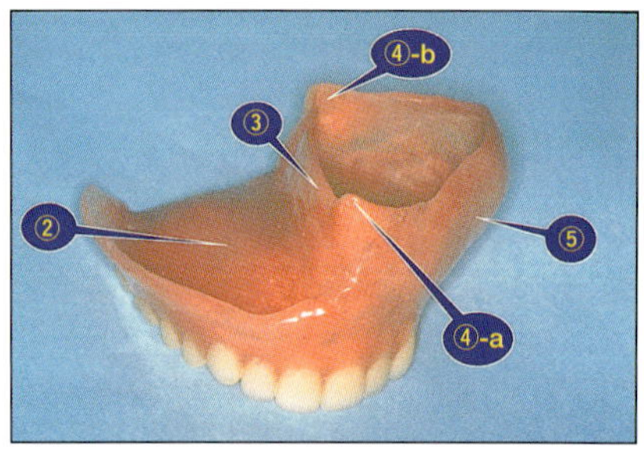

Fig. 2 *(left)* Intraoral retentive sources in patient with edentulous maxillary defect.
Fig. 3 *(right)* Retentive forms on maxillodental prosthesis corresponding to intraoral retentive sources.

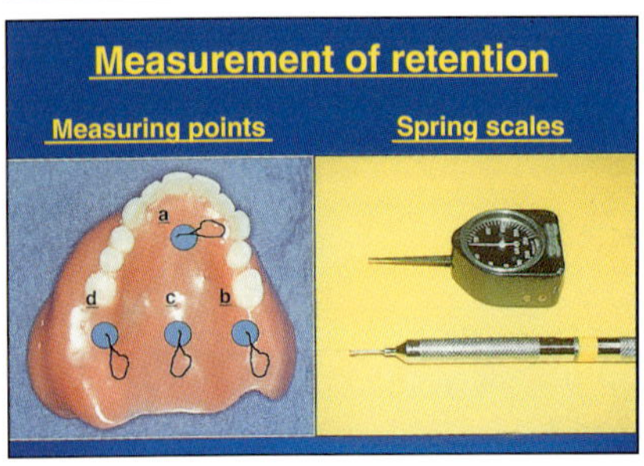

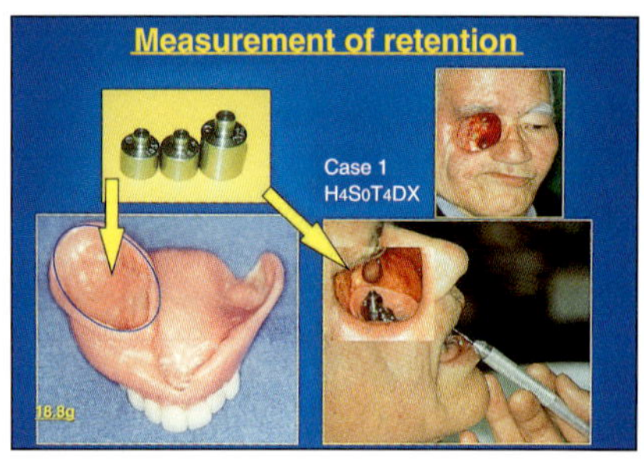

Fig. 4 *(left)* Points for measurement of retention of maxillodental prosthesis, and spring scales.
Fig. 5 *(right)* Measurement of retention of maxillodental prosthesis; 10g weights are placed into the obturator one after another to increase its weight (left); the maxillodental prosthesis is pulled as vertically as possible from below (right).

Relationship between weight and retention of maxillodental prostheses:

The subjects were 5 patients with edentulous maxillary hemilateral defects; the mean weight of the maxillodental prostheses inserted was 18.7g (15.6g to 21.0g). Measurement of retention was conducted at 4 points, a to d, on each maxillodental prosthesis as shown on the left in Fig. 4, using the 2 spring scales shown on the right in Fig. 4, pulling as directly below as possible to determine the force at the instant of falling off. Measurements were done three times at each point to calculate the mean value, regarded as the retention value for each measuring point. In addition, the mean retention value for the 4 points was regarded as the retention value for the maxillodental prosthesis. Regarding the effect of the weight of maxillodental prostheses on retention, 10g weights were placed sequentially inside an open type obturator from the top, as shown in Fig. 5, to increase its weight. The retention of each maxillodental prosthesis was calculated using the above-mentioned procedures to determine the force at detachment, called "retention weight". Fig. 6 shows the results. The vertical axis shows retention and the horizontal axis shows the weights of maxillodental prostheses. When the weight of the maxillodental prostheses was 19g, retention of the maxillodental prosthesis in each case was between 1.8N and 4.8N. Retention decreased on average by 2N with a 10g increase (total weight: 30g), and the mean value of retention decreased to half or less than half of primary retention with a 20g increase (total weight: 40g). Therefore, it seems desirable to keep the weight of maxillodental prostheses under 20g.

Sequential changes of retention in edentulous maxillary defective patients:

The subjects were 10 patients with edentulous maxillary hemilateral defects. The vertical axis shows retention and the horizontal axis shows the follow-up period (Fig. 7). Even cases with retention greater than 40N at insertion of maxillodental prostheses showed a considerable decrease in retention 2 months later, and the retentive average for these cases dropped almost to one-half of retention at the time of insertion. In contrast, cases with (initially) poor retention, less than 3N, showed (relatively) undiminished retention with a tendency for all of these cases to converge at about 1N to 2N in 6 months. Therefore, all edentulous maxillary defective patients seem to require rebase about once a year.

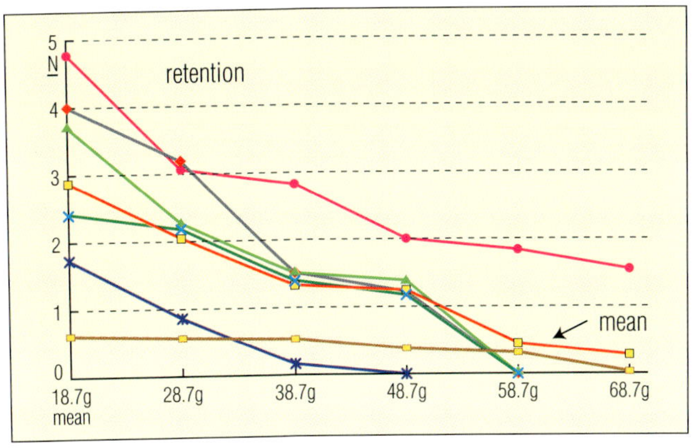

Fig. 6 Relationship between weight and retention of maxillodental prostheses in patients with edentulous maxillary defects.

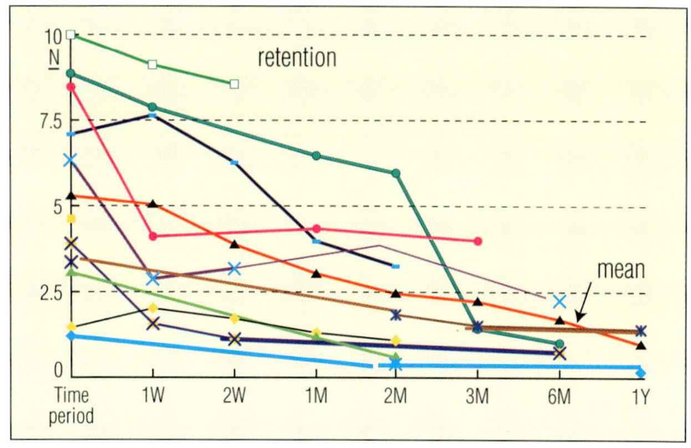

Fig. 7 Sequential changes in retention of maxillodental prostheses in edentulous maxillary defective patients.

Clinical Case

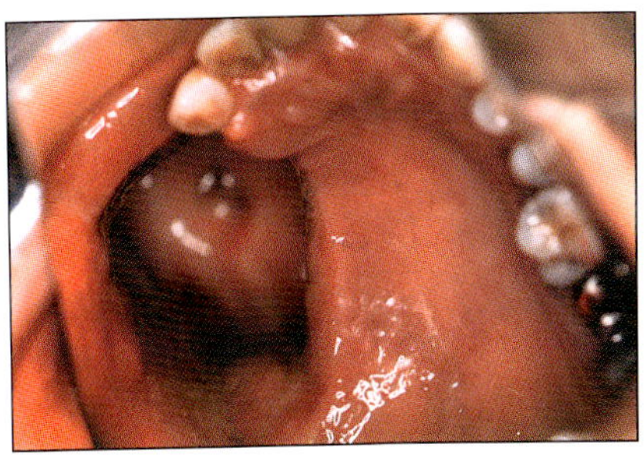

Fig. 8 Intraoral view. Twenty-one days after right partial maxillectomy.
Residual teeth were #13–28. Mouth opening range was 40mm. HS classification was $H_3S_0D_0T_0$ (#11, 41). 6-4 classification was 2/6, 0/4 defect.

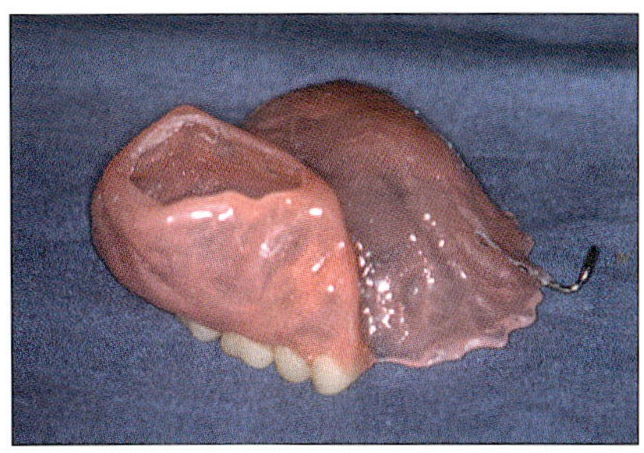

Fig. 9 Maxillodental prosthesis with open type obturator for a patient who is partially edentulous. The wire clasp is useful as a retainer.

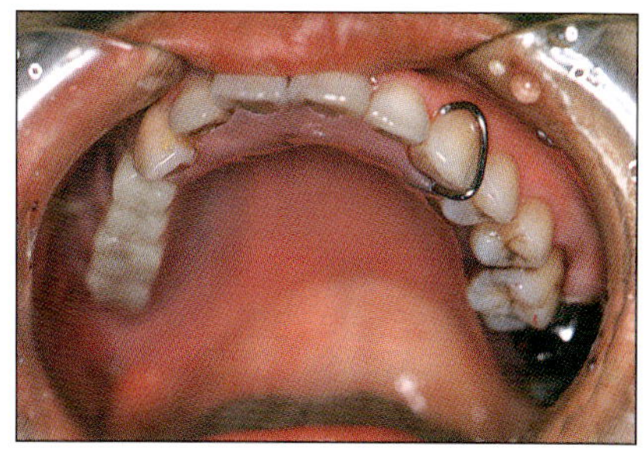

Fig. 10 Maxillodental prosthesis with open type obturator for a patient who is partially edentulous with a one-arm wire clasp attached to #23.

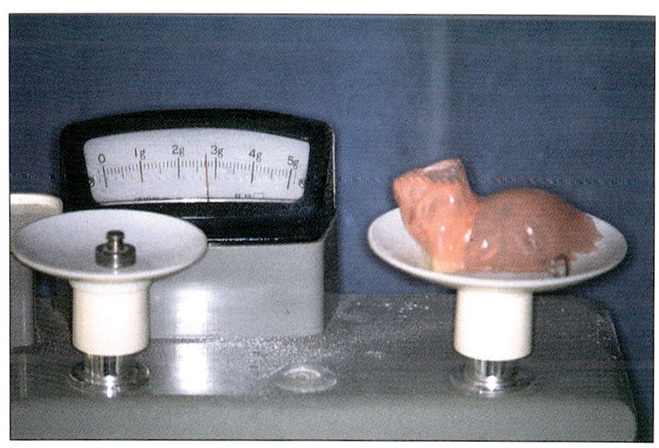

Fig. 11 Maxillodental prosthesis with one wire clasp as retainer. The non-impression surface of the jaw prosthesis is ground down to reduce weight (weight: 7.8g).

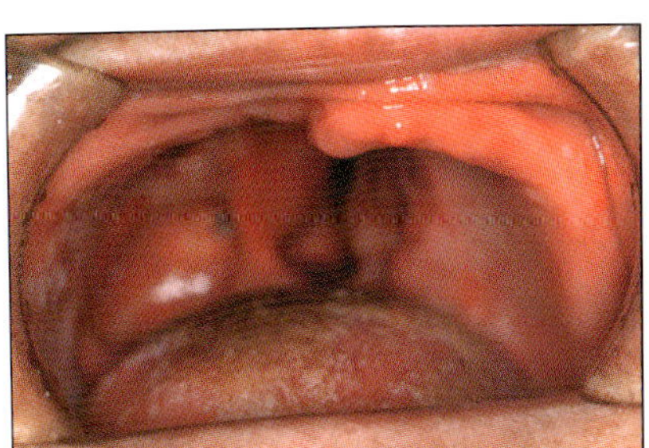

Fig. 12 Right partial maxillectomy, Mouth opening range was 45mm. No residual teeth. HS classification was $H_3S_1D_0T_4$ (#21, 31). 6-4 classification was 3/6, 1/4 defect.

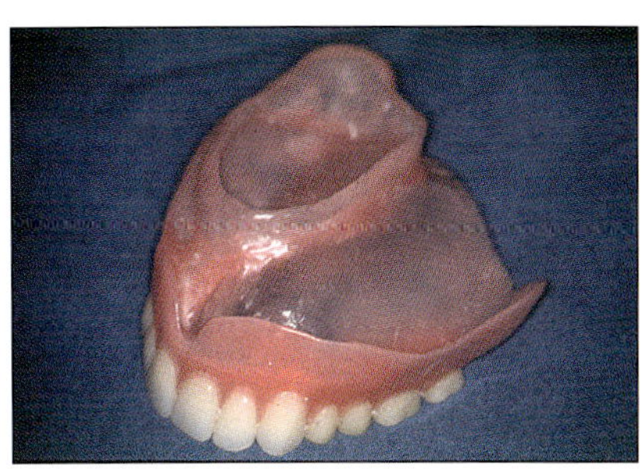

Fig. 13 Maxillodental prosthesis with open type obturator for a patient who is totally edentulous.

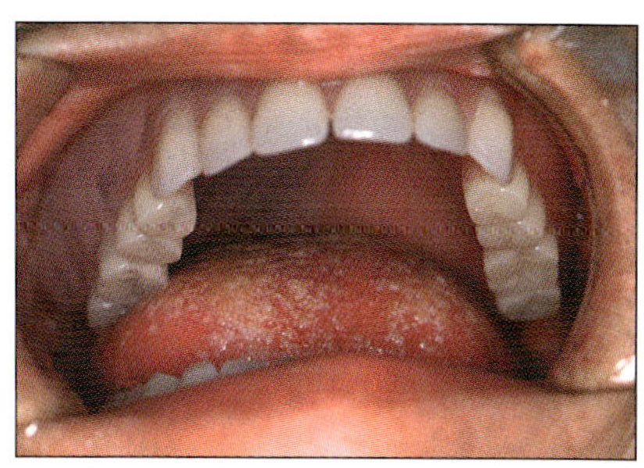

Fig. 14 Maxillodental prosthesis with open type obturator for a patient who is totally edentulous. (weight: 9.7g).

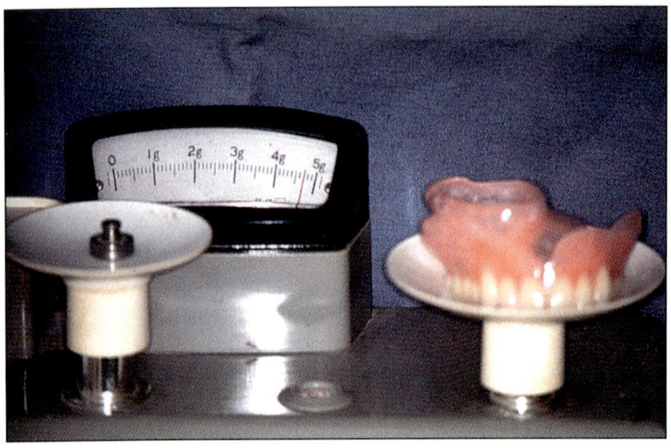

Fig. 15 Maxillodental prosthesis similar to that shown in the previous illustration.

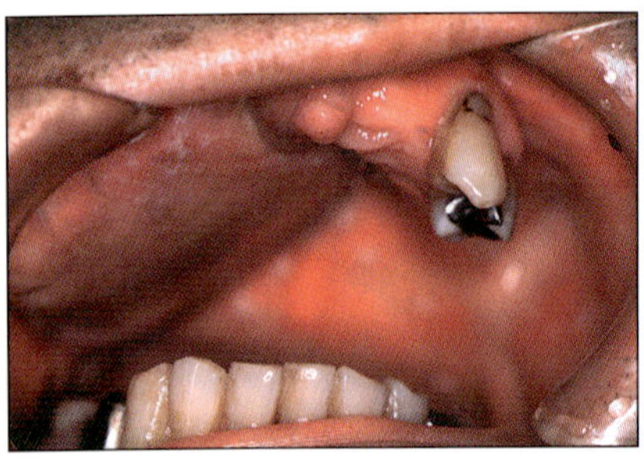

Fig. 16 A free rectus abdominis MC flap is filled to the defect after total resection of the right maxilla. HS classification was $H_6S_0D_2T_3P$ (#23, 33). 6-4 classification was 4/6, 0/4 defect. The only remaining teeth were #23, 24. Mouth opening range was 26mm.

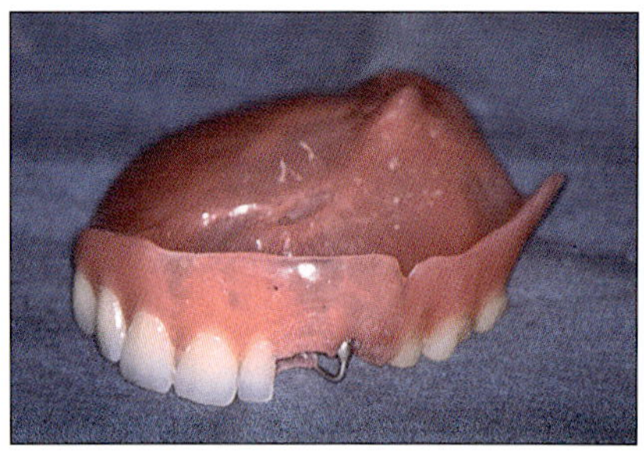

Fig. 17 A ball clasp was used since the existing skin flap made the maxillodental prosthesis unstable when the patient's mouth was open. Maxillodental prosthesis with open type obturator for a patient who is partially edentulous.

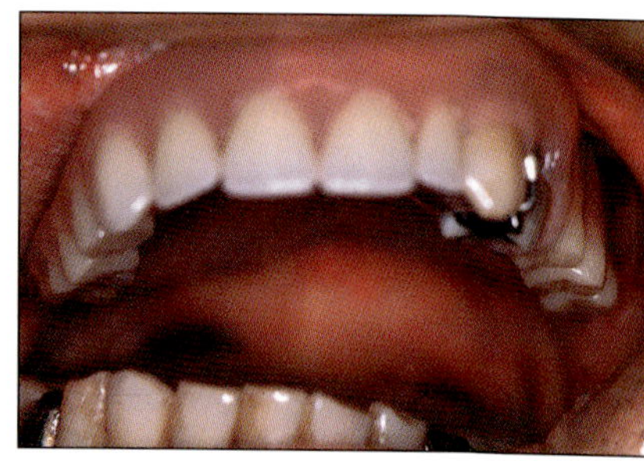

Fig. 18 This maxillodental prosthesis is stabilized by a ball clasp between #23, 24.

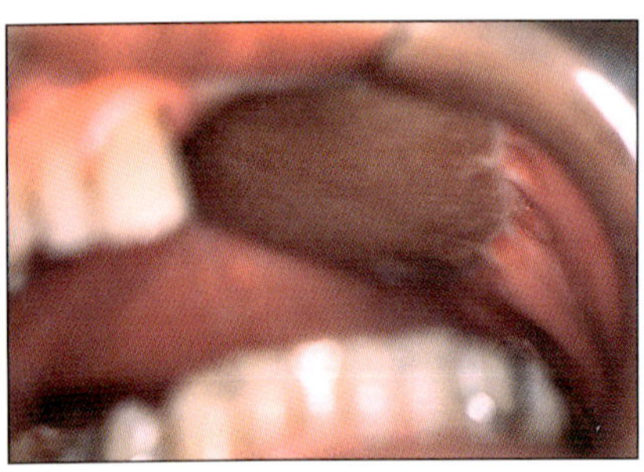

Fig. 19 Lt. maxillectomy defect is closed with a free rectus abdominis MC flap. Residual teeth were #11–14. Mouth opening range was 17mm. HS classification was $H_4S_0D_3T_2PF$ (#11, 41). 6-4 classification was 3/6, 0/4 defect.

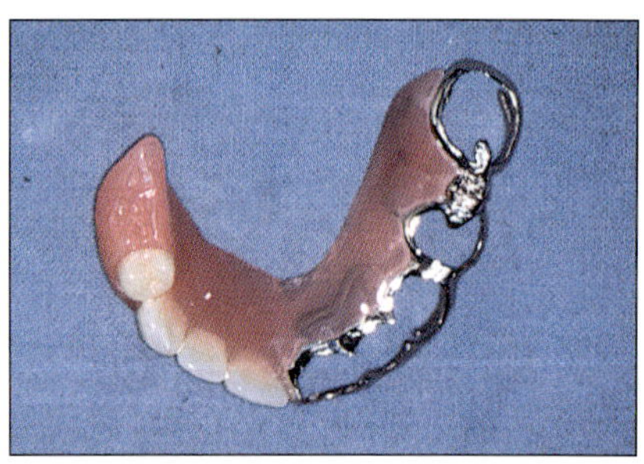

Fig. 20 A cast continuous clasp surrounding all residual teeth was used for the maxillodental prosthesis with open type obturator for a patient who is partially edentulous.

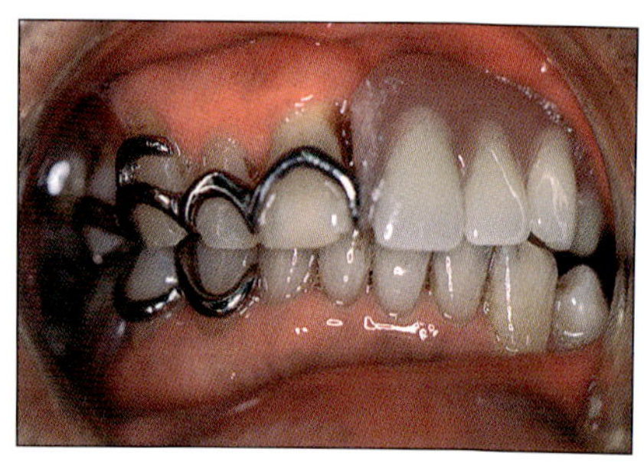

Fig. 21 This maxillodental prosthesis is retained by a cast continuous clasp.

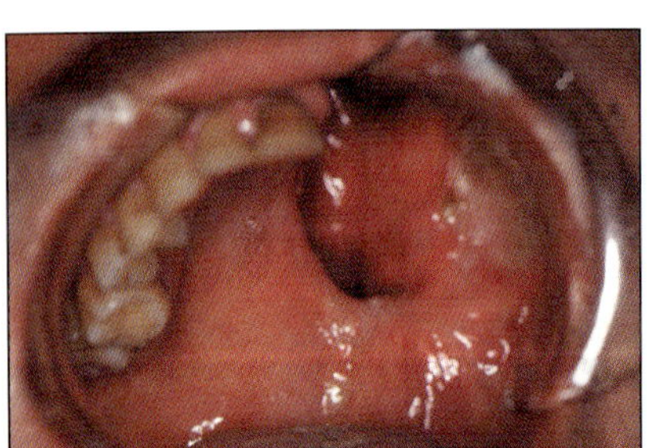

Fig. 22 Lt. hemi-maxillectomized. HS classification was $H_3S_0D_0T_0$ (#11, 41). 6-4 classification was 3/6, 0/4 defect. Residual teeth were #41–47 and mouth opening range was 42mm.

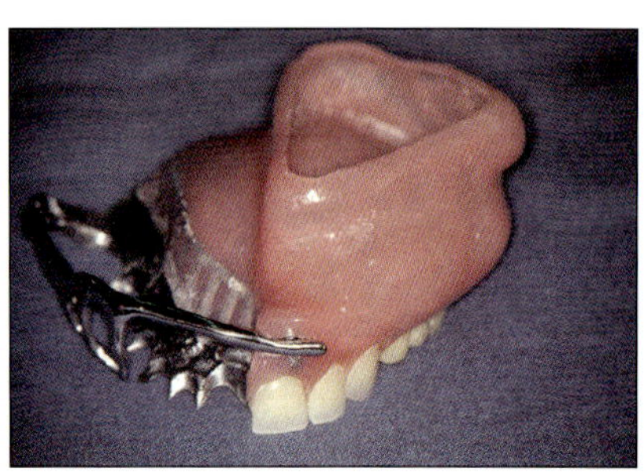

Fig. 23 A swing lock attachment was used for this maxillodental prosthesis with open type obturator for a patient who is partially edentulous.

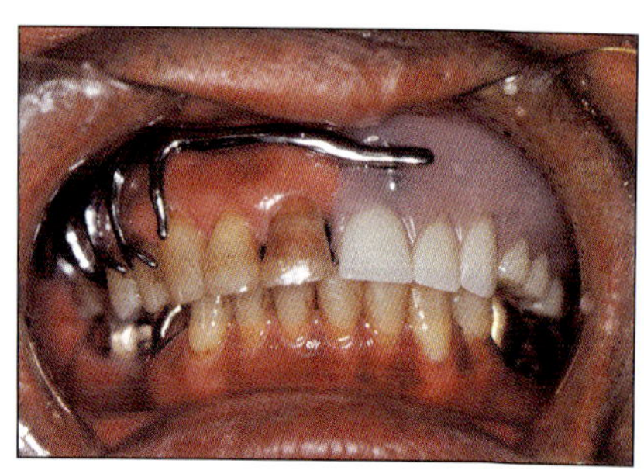

Fig. 24 Using a swing lock attachment, the maxillodental prosthesis is sufficiently retained by the unaffected residual teeth.

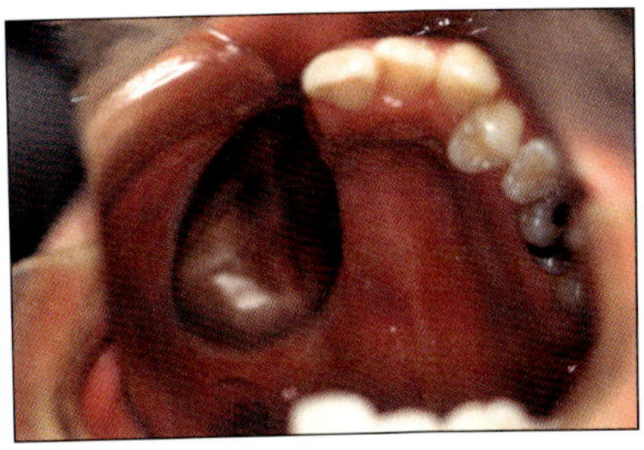

Fig. 25 Rt partial maxillectomized. HS classification was $H_3S_0D_3T_0$ (#21, 31) (mirror image). 6-4 classification was 3/6, 0/4 defect. Mouth opening range was 17mm. Residual teeth were #21–27.

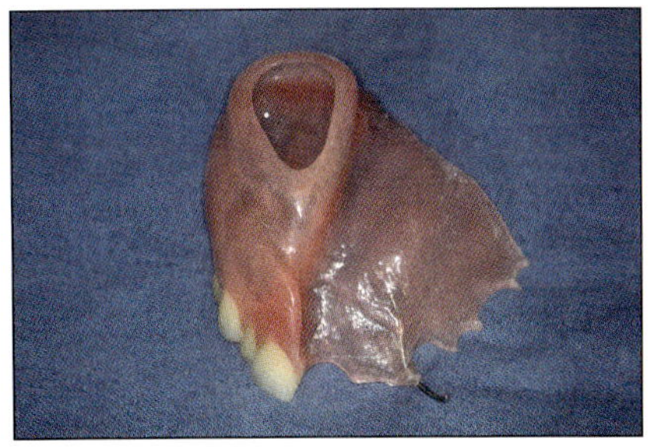

Fig. 26 Maxillodental prosthesis with open type obturator for a patient who is partially edentulous. A wire clasp was intentionally left at the base.

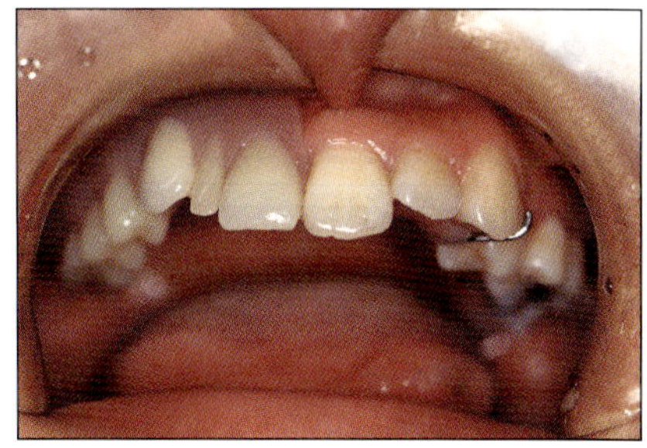

Fig. 27 This clasp left on the base is an auxiliary part to aid in insertion and removal of the maxillodental prosthesis, and does not function as a clasp.

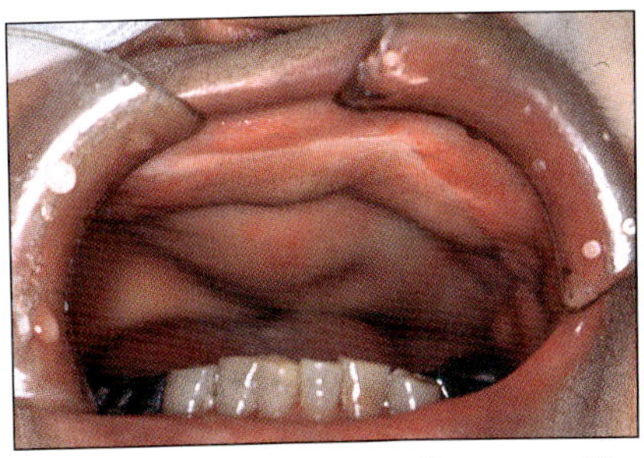

Fig. 28 Bilateral total maxillectomy. The palate was closed by a free rectus abdominis MC flap. HS classification was $H_6S_0D_0T_4F$ (#21, 31). 6-4 classification was 6/6, 0/4 defect. No residual teeth. Mouth opening range was 40mm.

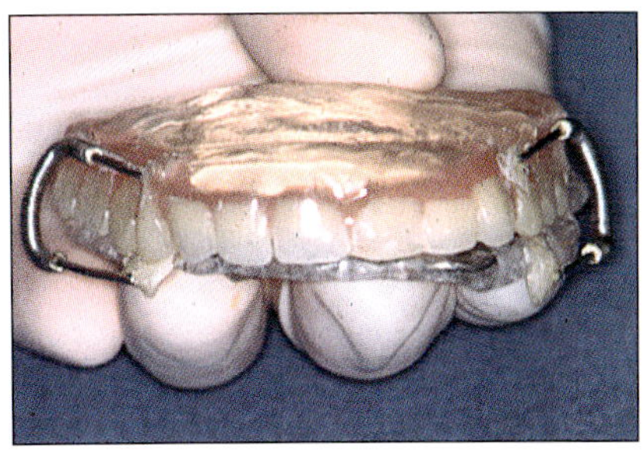

Fig. 29 Due to reconstruction of the palate with the skin flap, there are no sites which bear the maxillodental prosthesis. The structure called a "spring denture" uses counter-occlusal teeth for anchorage.

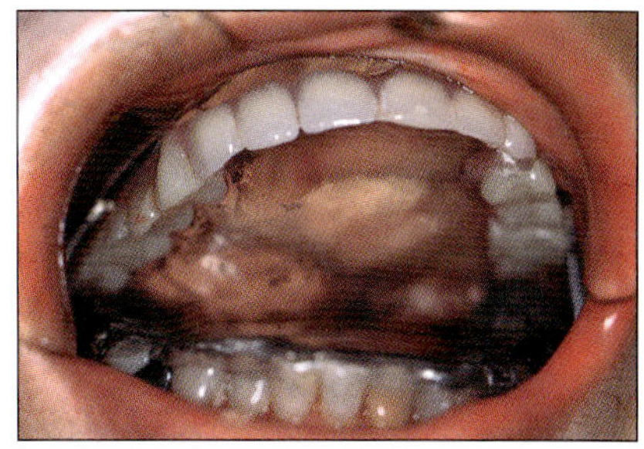

Fig. 30 Occlusion is established between the upper artificial and lower teeth.

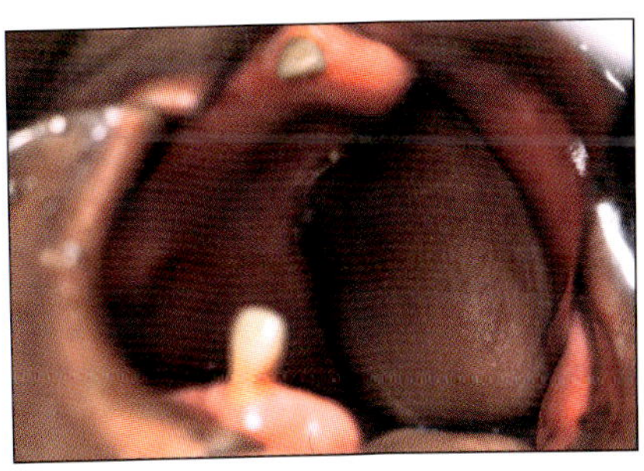

Fig. 31 Lt. total maxillectomy. The palatal region was closed by a free rectus abdominis MC flap (mirror image). HS classification was $H_3S_0D_2T_4F$ (#12, 42). 6-4 classification was 3/6,0/4 defect. The only residual tooth was #12. Mouth opening range was 28mm.

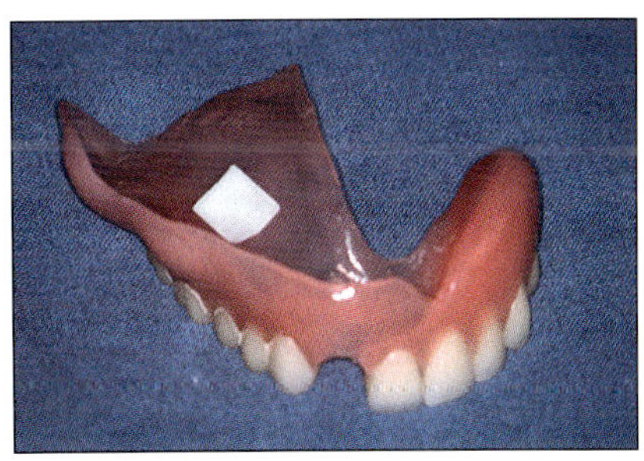

Fig. 32 Use of a sheet of adhesive tape to the remaining maxillary masticatory mucous membrane is planned.

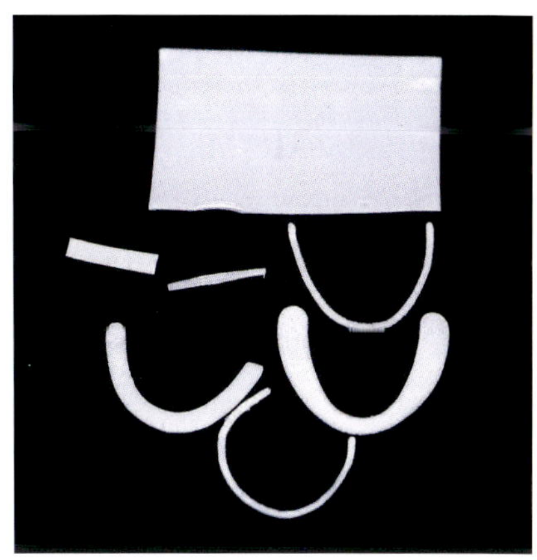

Fig. 33 Product name: Touch Correct 2 from Kyowa Co., Ltd. Distributed by Shionogi & Co., Ltd.

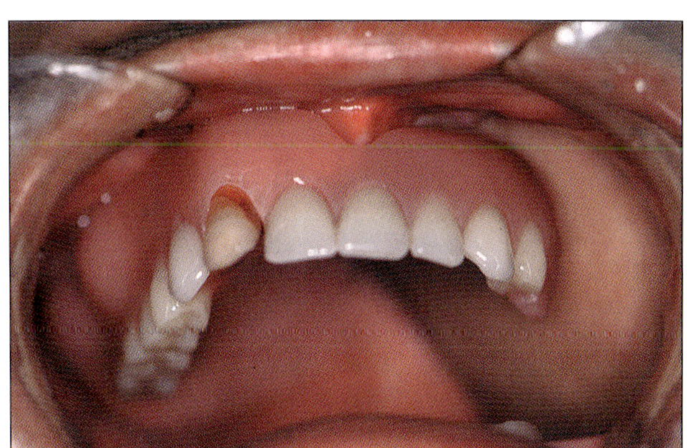

Fig. 34 Occlusion and mastication are made possible by designing the maxillary prosthesis to avoid the highly compressible reconstructed region.

CHAPTER 10

From placement of implants to insertion of upper structures

1. A case with implants placed into residual maxilla for a maxillodental prosthesis after tumor resection

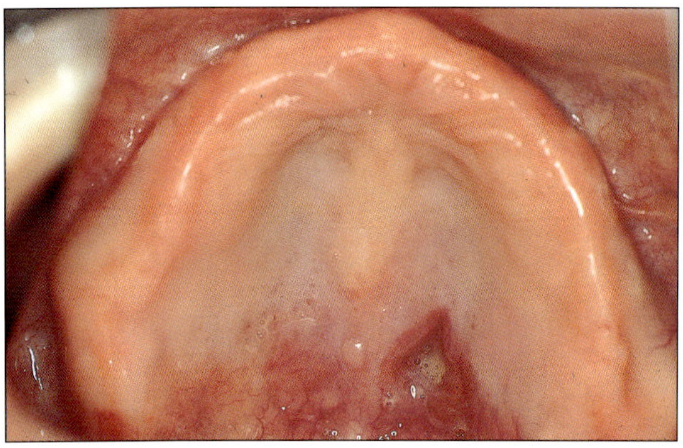

Fig. 1 The patient was a 60 year-old woman who had an ulcer in the palate and was diagnosed by histopathological examination as having adenoid cystic carcinoma. 30Gy radiotherapy and chemotherapy were performed preoperatively.

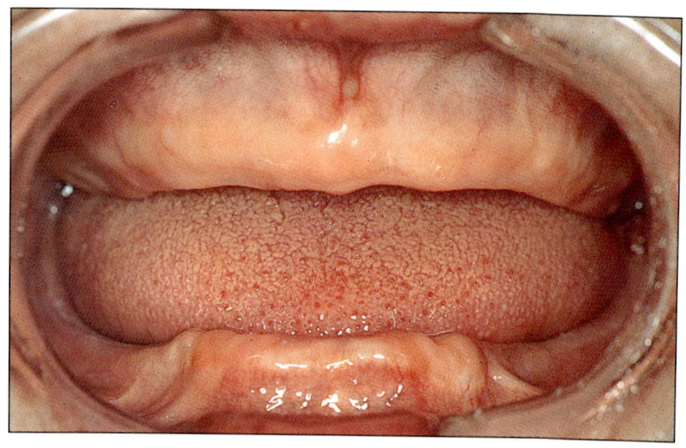

Fig. 2 Both the maxilla and mandible were edentulous, with resorption of the alveolar bones.

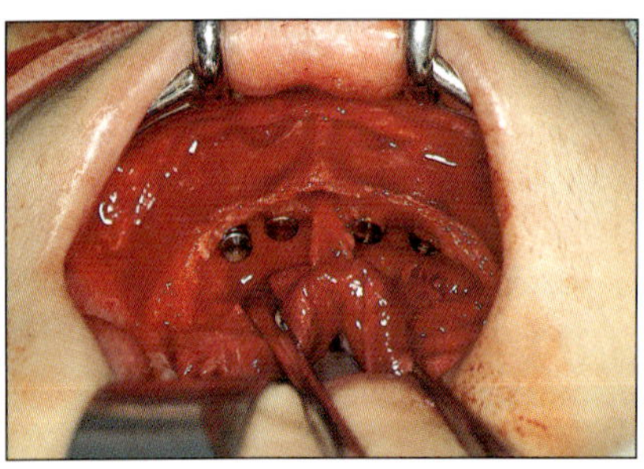

Fig. 3 For the retention of a maxillodental prosthesis after tumor resection, the placement of implants into the residual maxilla was planned, and this was done at the time of resection of the tumor. Four osseointegrated-implants were placed in the site at an appropriate distance from the location of the tumor.

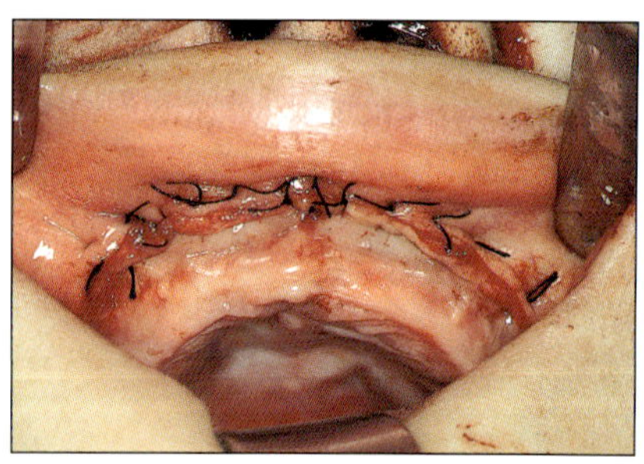

Fig. 4 The maxillary mucosa was sutured.

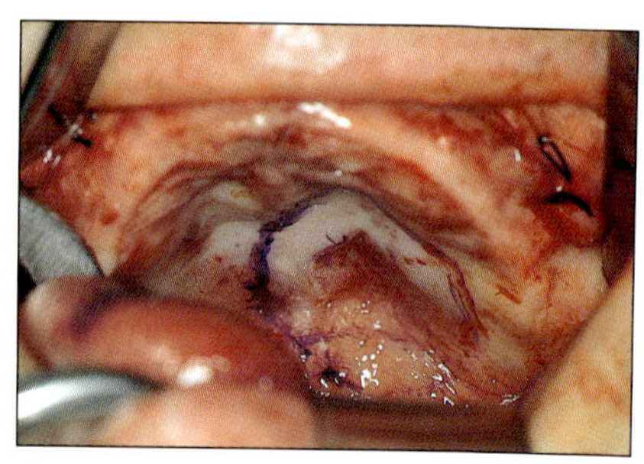

Fig. 5 The resection area of the palatal tumor was established.

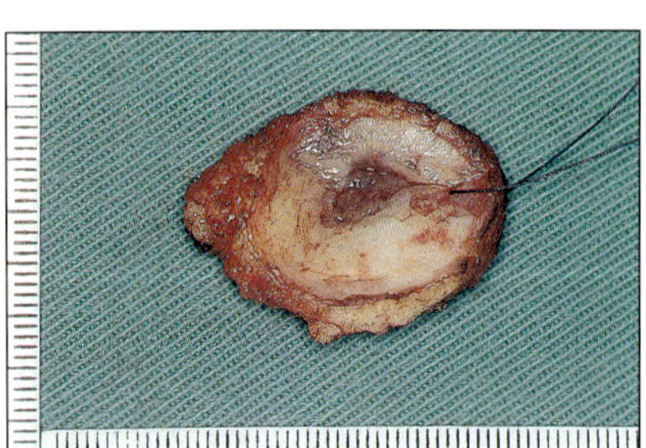

Fig. 6 Specimen after resection of palatal tumor.

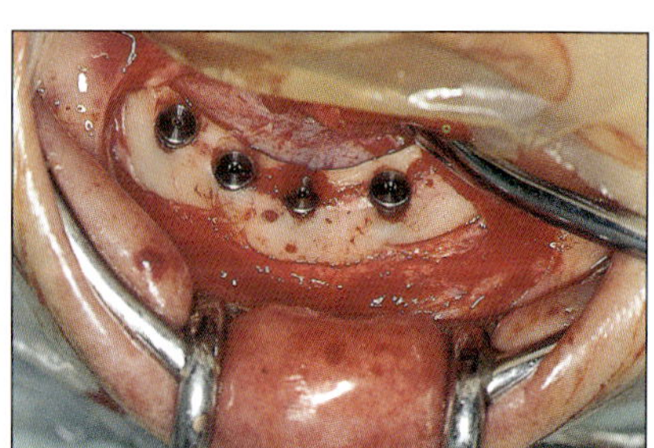

Fig. 7 The mandible was also edentulous, and 4 implants were placed in it for stabilization of the lower denture.

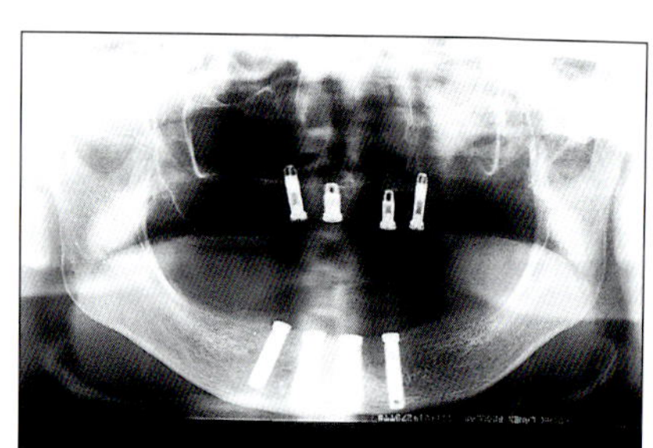

Fig. 8 Four implants are placed in the maxilla and mandible in the panoramic radiograph.

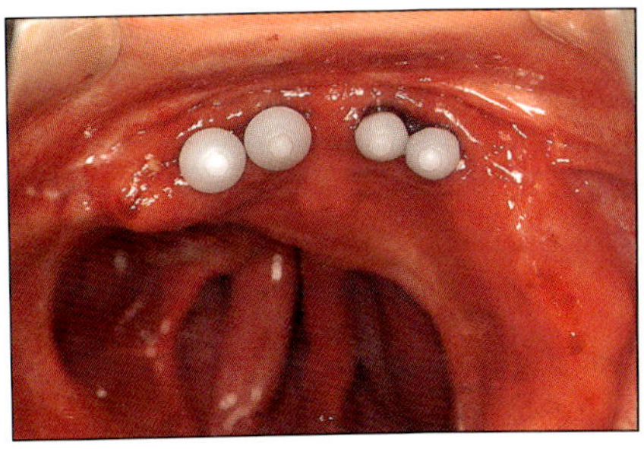

Fig. 9 A secondary operation to connect the abutments was done 6 months after the tumor resection. The mucosal surface of an old denture was ground to prevent direct contact between the healing caps and the denture, on which a soft lining material for shock absorption was applied to permit its use as a temporary denture.

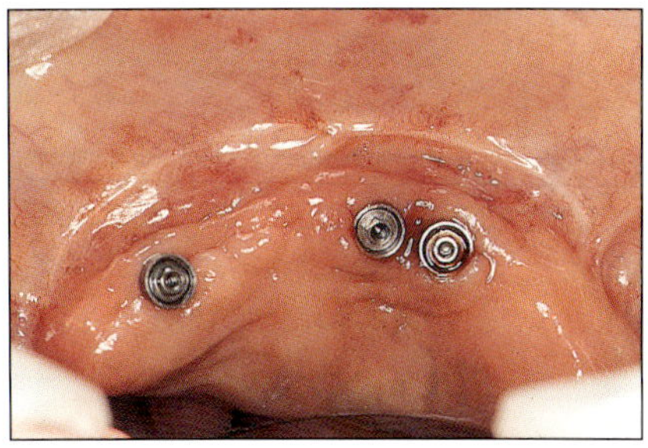

Fig. 10 Following the secondary operation, one implant was lost. The cause seemed attributable to the total of 70Gy of pre- and postoperative radiotherapy.

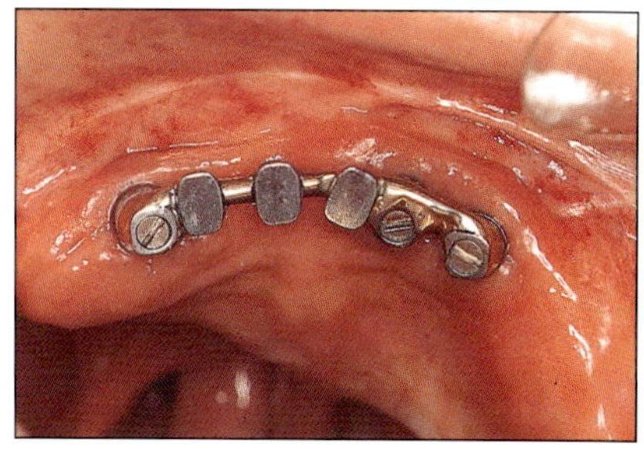

Fig. 11 On the maxilla, the 3 implants were connected by a bar, along which 3 magnet keepers were soldered.

Fig. 12 *(left)* The abutments for the 4 implants placed in the mandible were connected.
Fig. 13 *(right)* For the maxillodental prosthesis, magnets were placed in the mucosal surface of the denture base corresponding to the residual alveolar ridge. A buccal flange type obturator was used for the obturator portion of the maxillodental prosthesis.

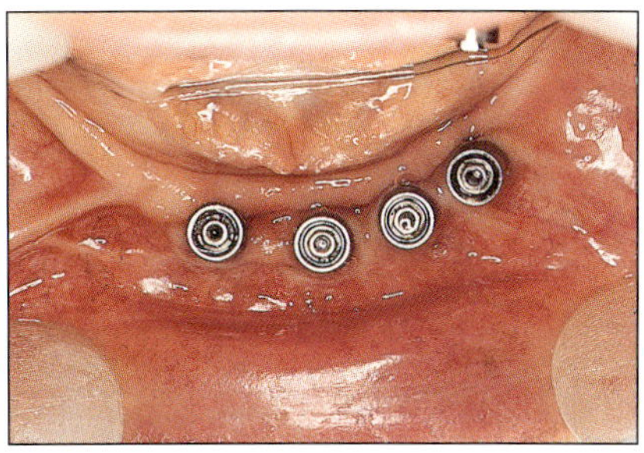

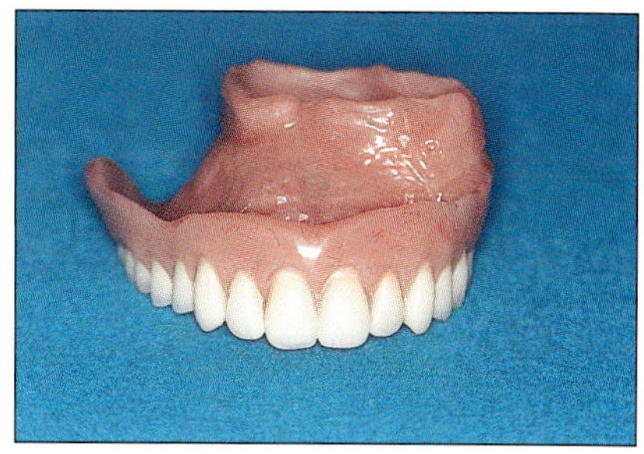

Fig. 14 *(left)* A fixed implant-prosthesis was attached to the mandible.
Fig. 15 *(right)* The retention of prosthesis supported with dental implants on both the maxilla and mandible was excellent, and masticatory function was significantly restored. The maxillodental prosthesis prevented leakage to the nasal cavity, and speech function was also excellent.

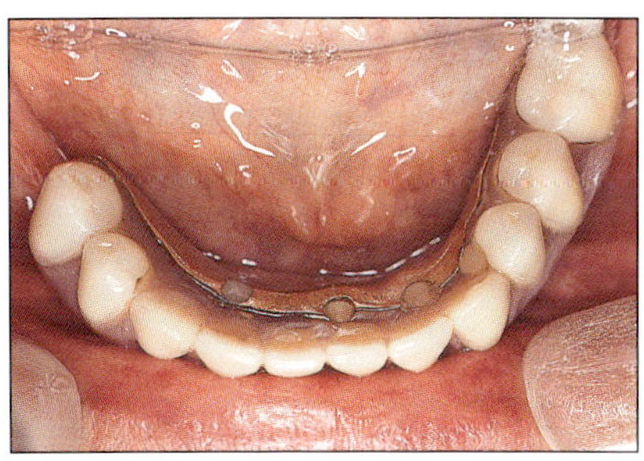

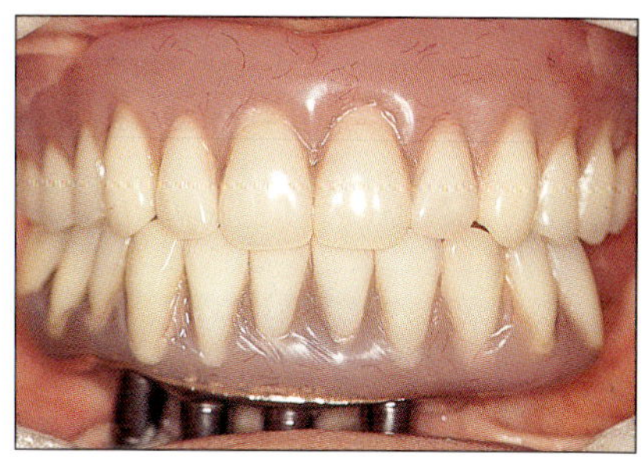

2. Case in which a maxillary prosthesis supported by a dental implant was positioned after bone grafting into the floor of the maxillary sinus on the non-resected site

Fig. 16 *(left)* Intraoral photograph of case of gingival carcinoma of the left maxilla in a 66-year-old woman.
Fig. 17 *(right)* The left side of the maxilla was partially resected.

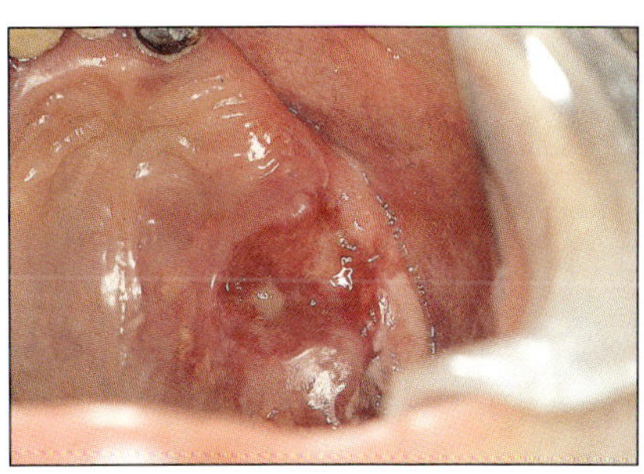

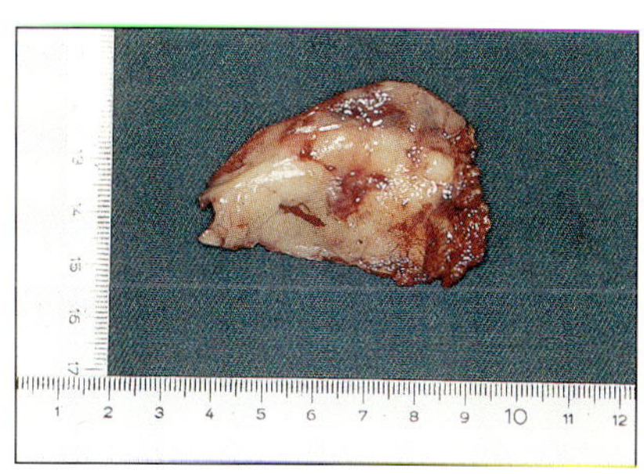

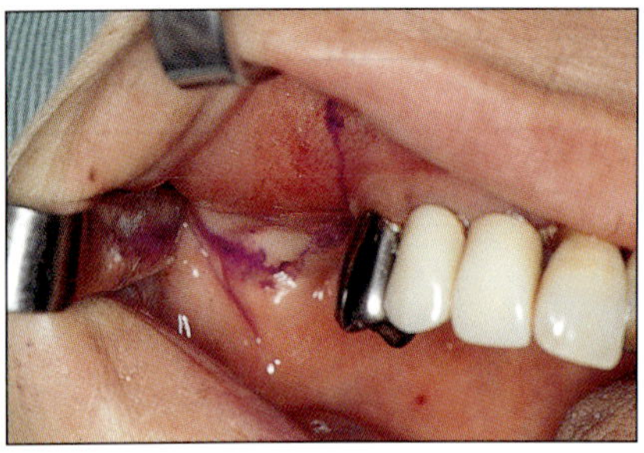

Fig. 18 Postoperatively, with maxillodental prosthesis retained by clasps on residual teeth, implant placement in the right posterior region was planned because the remaining teeth had begun to become mobile. A bone graft was applied into the right maxillary sinus floor due to alveolar-bone resorption of the residual maxilla.

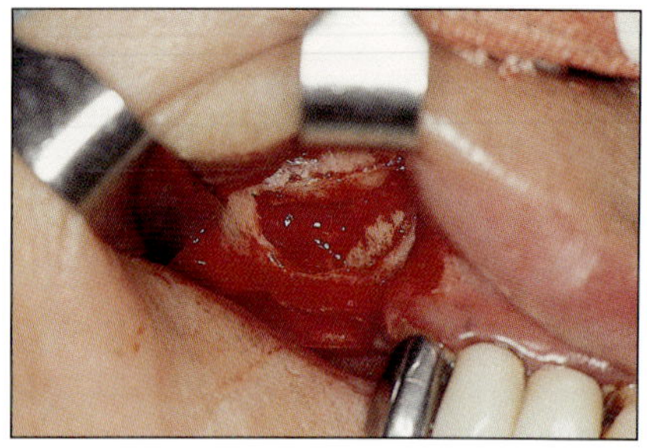

Fig. 19 Marsupiarization of anterior wall of maxillary-sinus. A quadrangular groove was formed into the anterior wall of maxillary-sinus at a depth that caused no damage to the sinus membrane. The sinus membrane was reflected by a raspatory, and the anterior wall was folded to the inside of sinus to ensure space for the bone grafting.

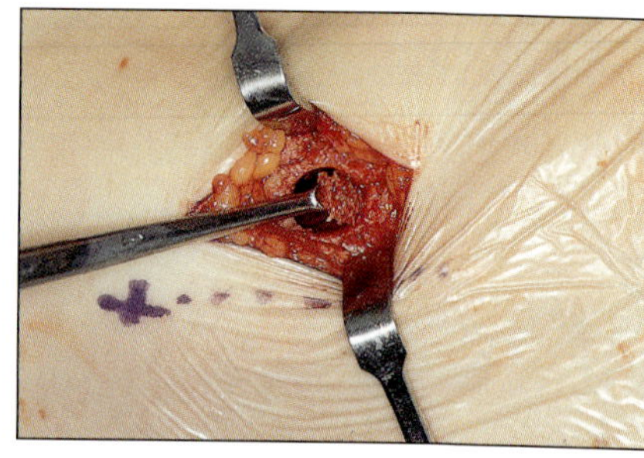

Fig. 20 6ml of bone collected from the iliac crest was grafted into the maxillary sinus floor. As a result, the maxillary sinus floor was elevated about 20mm.

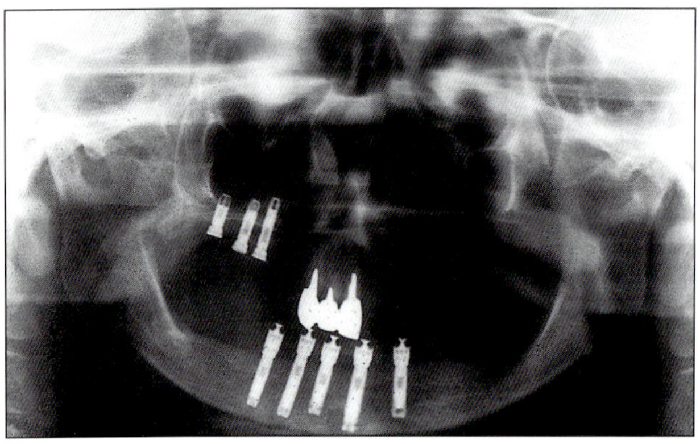

Fig. 21 Three implants were placed 4 months after the maxillary sinus was lifted with a bone graft. At this point, the grafted bone had been resorbed about 15mm. In addition, 5 implants were placed in the edentulous mandible.

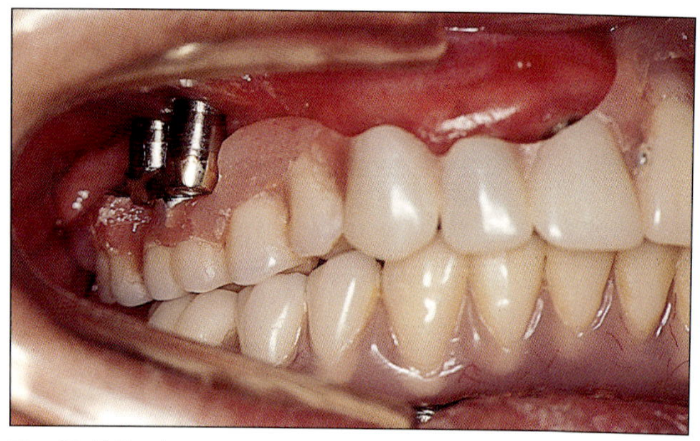

Fig. 22 Following crown reduction of the residual maxillary teeth, root caps were inserted into those which had started to become mobile. The implants were then connected by a bar and CM rider attachments were inserted into the inner surface of the prosthesis for retention of a removable implant-denture.

3. Application of zygomatic implant to maxillodental prosthesis

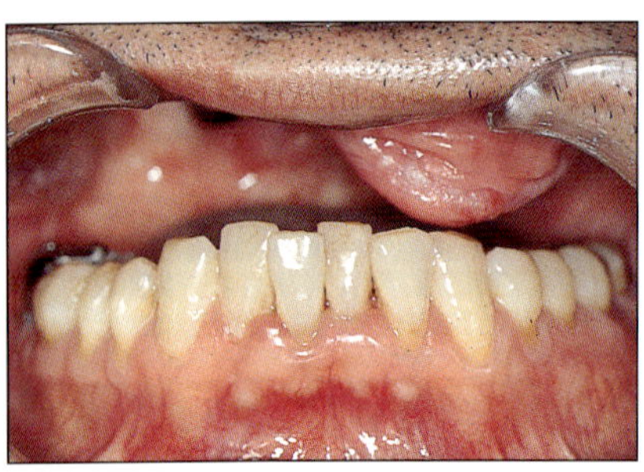

Fig. 23 Hemi-maxillectomy on the right side, which was edentulous, had been conducted due to gingival cancer. The maxillary left posterior alveolar ridge was found to have severe resorption. The right zygomatic bone was also partially resected.

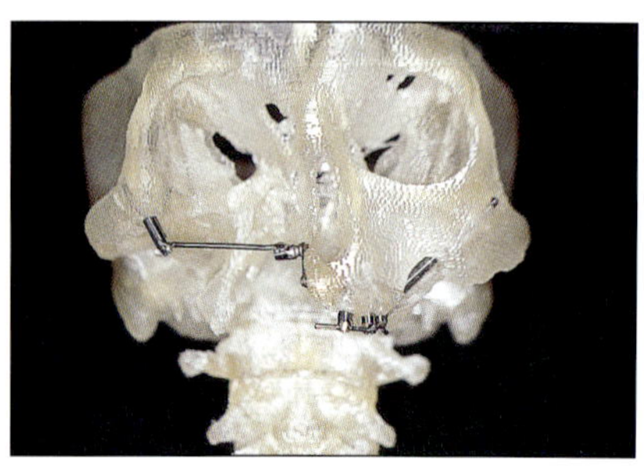

Fig. 24 Preoperative simulation of the positions and the lengths of implants was done using a photo-curable plastic skull model using the patient's CT data. In addition, the simulation was carried out in respect of retainers for a maxillodental prosthesis.

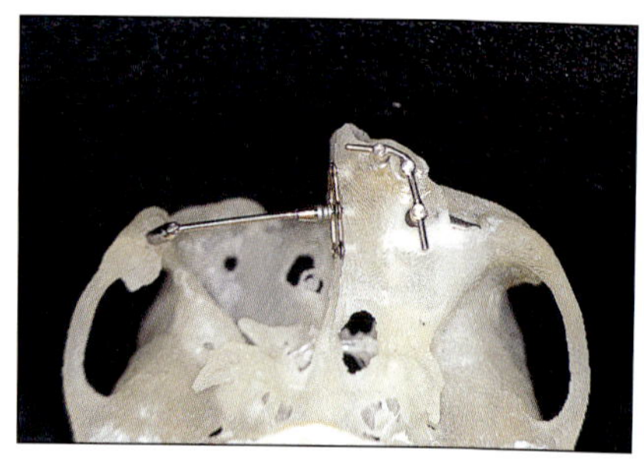

Fig. 25 The plan was to place two dental implants, each 13mm in length, in the anterior region on the unresected side (left) and a zygomatic implant, 45mm in length, between the premolar region and the zygomatic bone. These 3 implants were to be connected by a bar and used as retainers for a maxillodental prosthesis. The placement of a dental implant of 15mm in length in the right residual zygomatic bone and of an Epitec carrier plate (Leibinger Co. Ltd) between the palatal bone and the nasal septum were also considered. The Epitec carrier plate was connected to an implant to be placed into the right zygomatic bone and the bar to stabilize retention of the maxillodental prosthesis on the resected side.

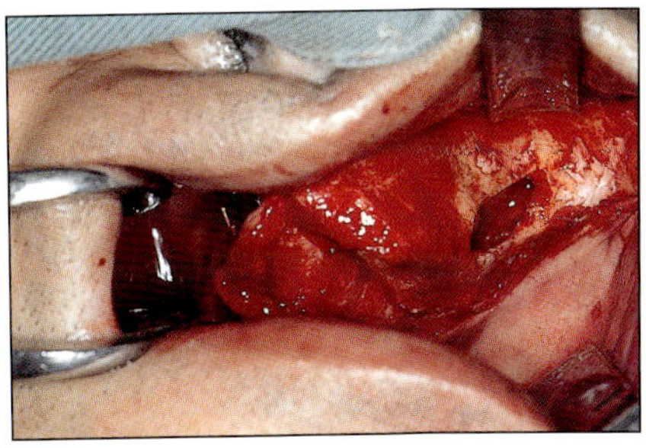

Fig. 26 The zygomatic implant was placed from the palatal side of the alveolar crest toward the body of the zygomatic bone in the vicinity of the second premolar. On this occasion, marsupialization of the posterior part of the maxillary sinus was done to confirm the direction for placement of the implant.

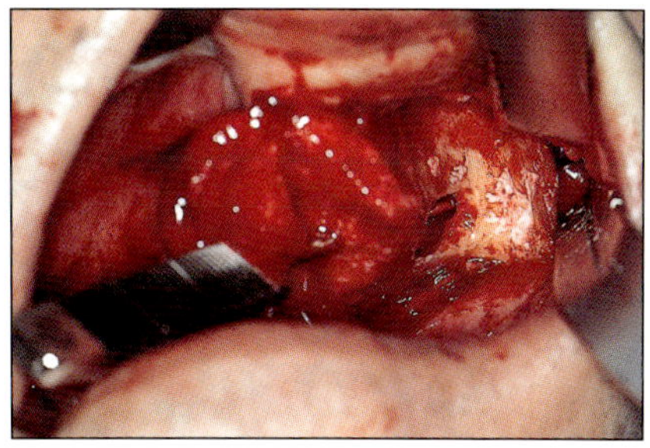

Fig. 27 Placement of the zygomatic implant was performed in the direction of the retractor applied to the angle making the transition from the body of the zygomatic bone to the zygomatic arch. In this case, a zygomatic implant 45mm in length was used.

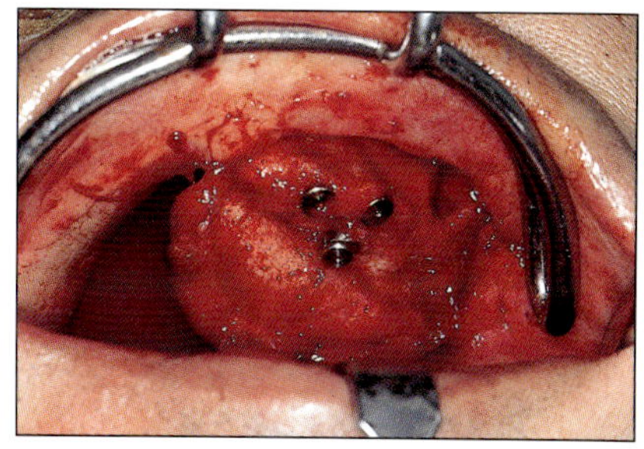

Fig. 28 Two implants, each 13mm in length were placed in the anterior region of the maxilla.

Fig. 29 *(left)* The right zygomatic bone had been partially removed in resecting the maxilla, so a 15mm implant was placed in the residual zygomatic bone.
Fig. 30 *(right)* An Epitec carrier plate was placed in position between the palatal bone and the nasal septum.

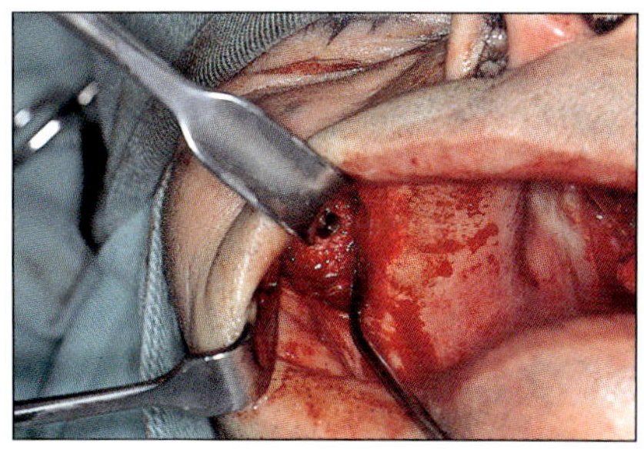

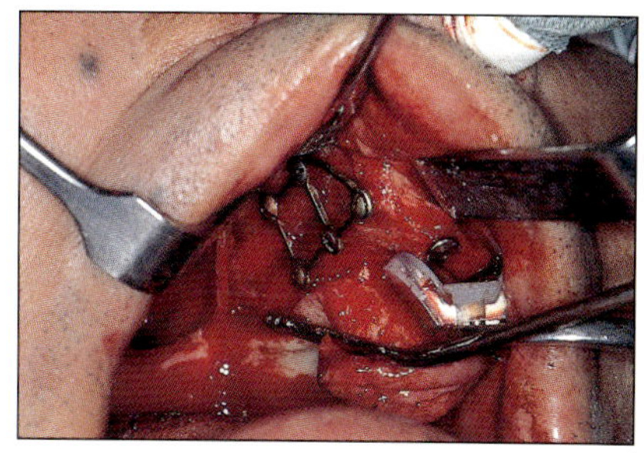

Fig. 31 *(left)* A second operation was conducted after 4 months to position an abutment.
Fig. 32 *(right)* Since a flap was grafted into the buccal region (at the time of tumor resection), the thickness of the flap was reduced to make it as thin as possible, to expose the abutment.

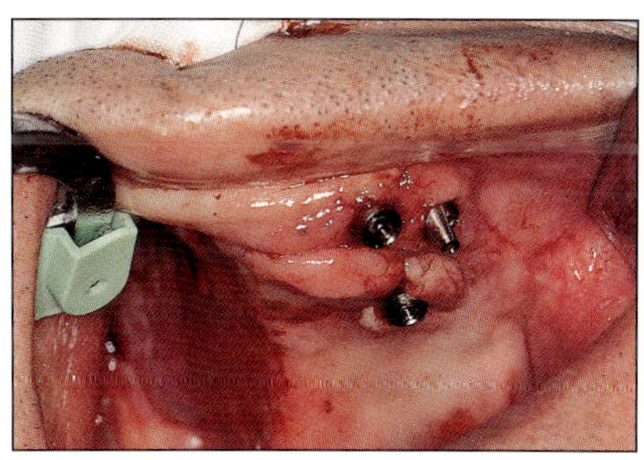

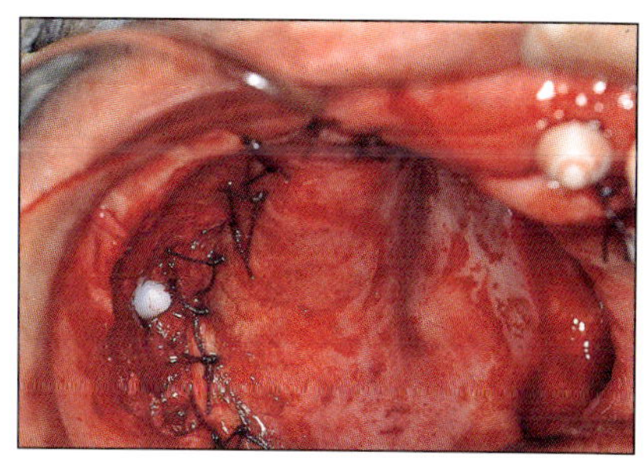

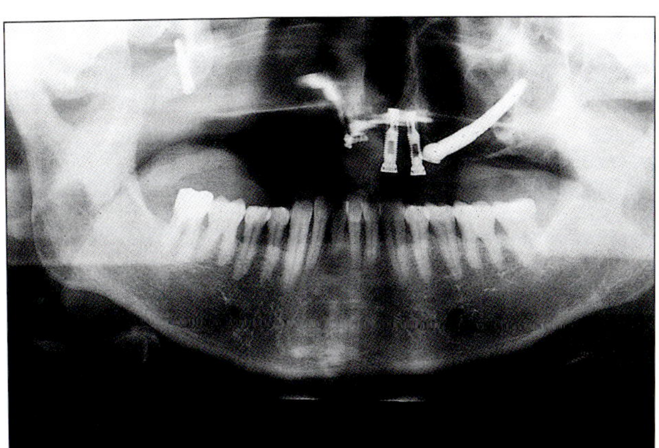

Fig. 33 Panoramic radiograph after placement of implants.

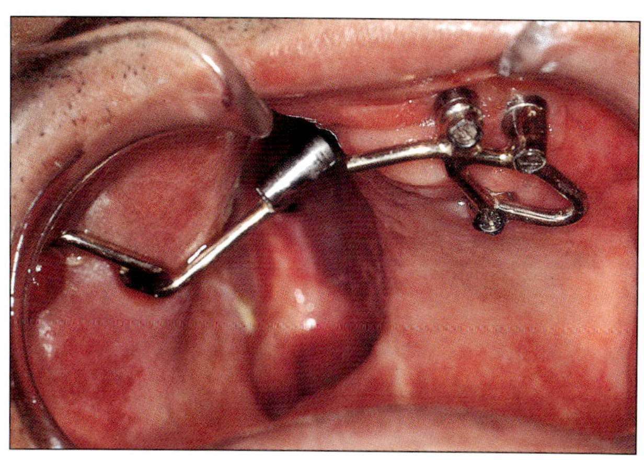

Fig. 34 The abutment of the dental implant positioned into the zygomatic bone and the Epitec carrier plate attached to the nasal septum on the resected side, were connected by means of bars, and the 3 abutments on the non-resected side were also attached by another bar.

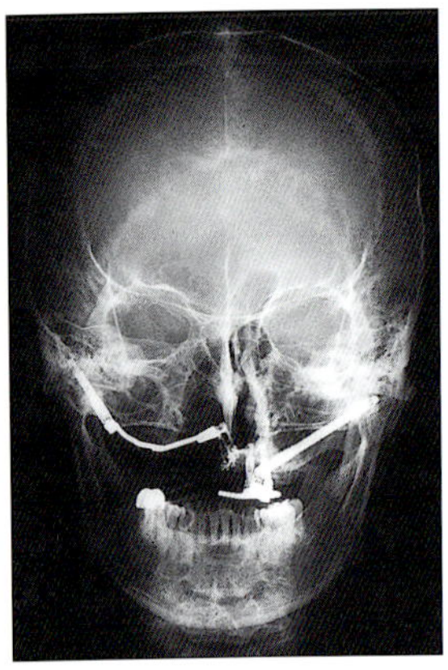

Fig. 35 Frontal radiograph after connection by bars.

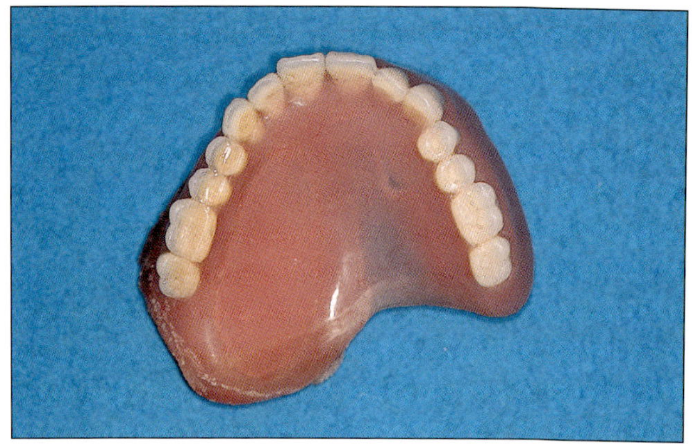

Fig. 36 Occlusal view of the maxillodental prosthesis.

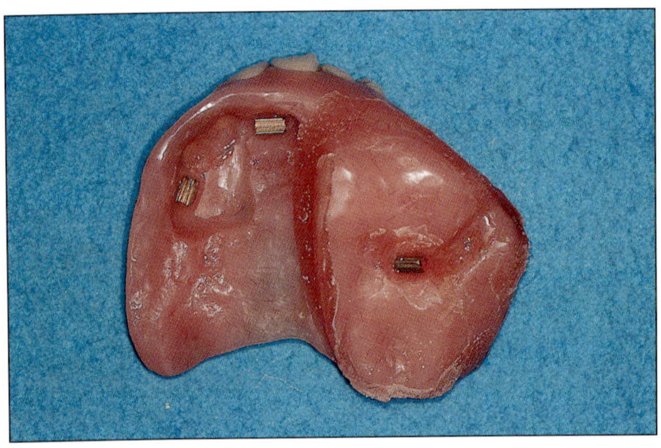

Fig. 37 On the mucosal aspect of the prosthesis, CM rider attachments connected by bars were placed in the alveolar region and in the obturator.

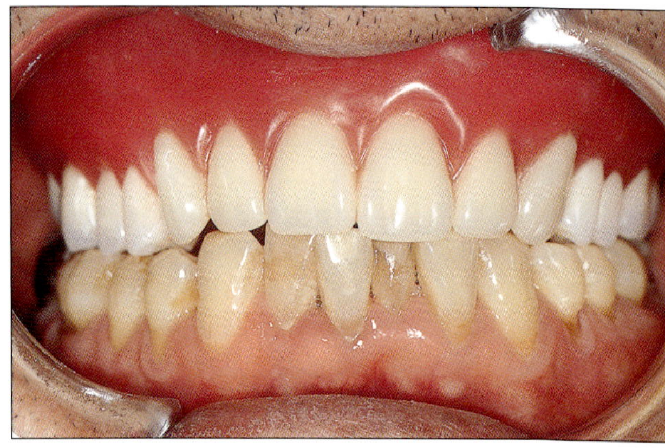

Fig. 38 Intraoral findings at the insertion of a maxillodental prosthesis. The prosthesis was prevented from sinking on the resected side during occlusion, was observed to allow almost no water-leakage to the nasal cavity, and allowed occlusal stress on the resected side.

4. Use of ITI Bonefit solid screw implants for retention of maxillodental prosthesis

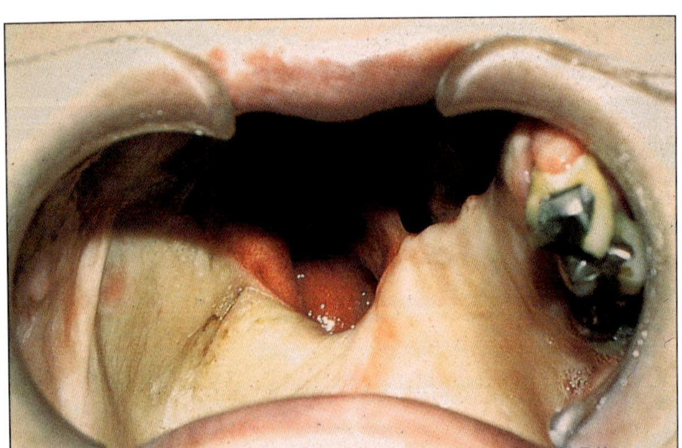

Fig. 39 This case is a 58-year-old woman with an extensive maxillary defect with residual teeth; the soft palatal posterior region was reconstructed with a forearm flap (HS classification: H_4T_2. R).

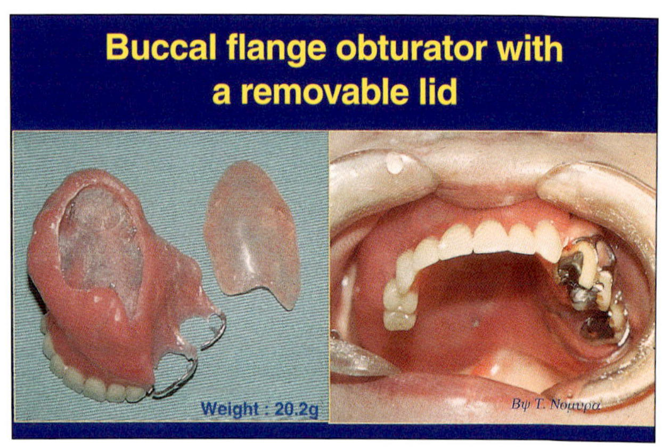

Fig. 40 Left: the maxillodental prosthesis fabricated immediately after surgery was a maxillodental prosthesis with open type obturator with removable lid and cast clasps using residual teeth as retentive sources. Right: The retentive, masticatory, and speech functions of the maxillodental prosthesis were good, but extraction of the residual teeth after 2 years because of their significant mobility resulted in the patient's maxilla becoming edentulous. Consequentially, the loss of the intraoral retentive sources for the maxillodental prosthesis caused its retentive stability to decrease, resulting in swallowing disorder, a speech defect, and interference with mastication.

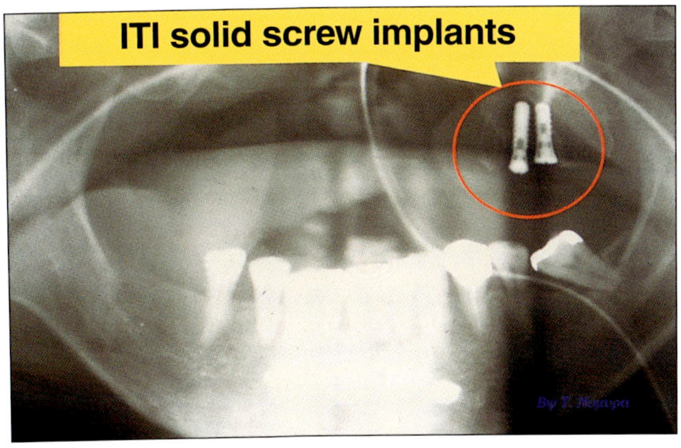

Fig. 41 Two ITI solid screw implants were inserted into the residual alveolar ridge as new sources for the maxillodental prosthesis to improve these conditions.

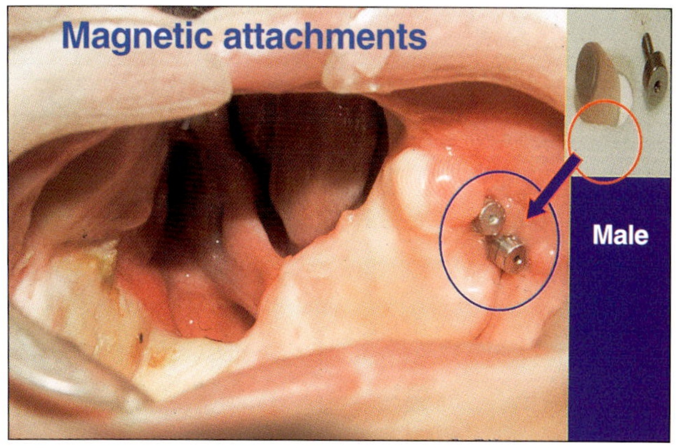

Fig. 42 After 4 months, receivers for magnetic attachments were placed on the tops of the implants.

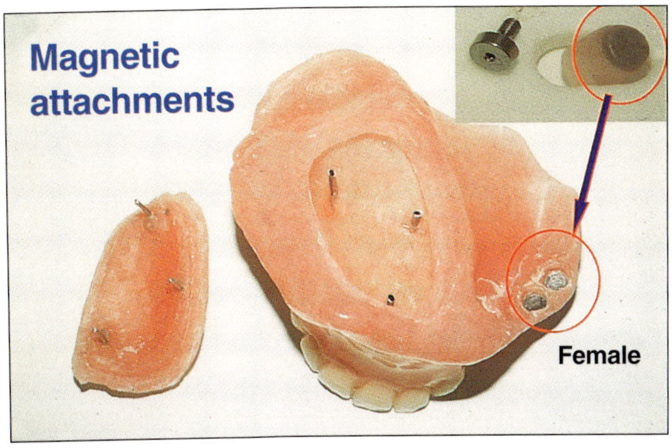

Fig. 43 Magnets were fixed on the inside of the maxillodental prosthesis.

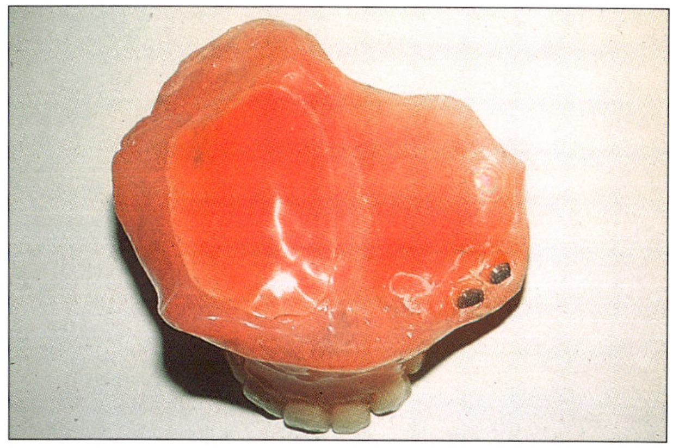

Fig. 44 A maxillodental prosthesis with open type obturator with lid was completed.

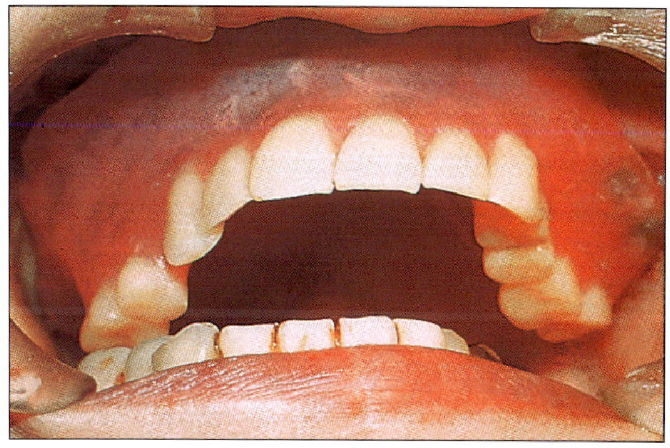

Fig. 45 Retention of the maxillodental prosthesis, and oral functions, have again become good.

CHAPTER 11

Immediate postoperative start of prosthetics and rapid fabrication of maxillodental prostheses

On immediate postoperative starting of maxillodental prosthesis production

As the role of maxillary prosthetic techniques in functional rehabilitation for the stomatognathic area, particularly for maxillary defects, has become clear, demand for prosthetic reconstructions has gradually reached a high level, creating a need for the joint use of maxillary prosthetic techniques at any time during the process of tumor treatment, to allow patients the earliest possible return to ordinary social life.

With this point of view, the author et al., in their experience for 20 years between 1981 and 2001 with 520 cases of maxillary defects, have focused on earlier starting of the production of maxillodental prostheses (MDP), shortening the number of days needed for its fabrication, and attempting to avoid complex procedures in the maxillofacial prosthetic treatment.

In the majority of the above cases (402 cases, fully documented primary cases), the timing of the start of MDP was decided through communication and discussion of postoperative conditions with the oncologic surgeons. Actually, the oncologists are responsible to select the starting time of allowing the patient to leave the hospital for the whole day. For seventeen cases out of 402 (4%) production of MDP started less than 2 weeks after surgery, 106 cases (26%) less than 3 weeks, and 203 cases (50%) less than 4 weeks (Fig. 1). In addition, the earliest start of production occurred in 4 cases, 7th postoperative day. Generally, it was most common for the fabrication of MDP to start as long as one year postoperatively. This delay in the start of prosthetics seems to be due to concerns about possible bleeding, infection, or delayed epithelialization of the surgical wound by the irritation of MDP treatment or early insertion of an MDP. When sound tissues such as the hard palate and the buccal mucosa are used as the main support for the MDP instead of using the scar tissue formed in the resected area or remaining nasal, para-nasal mucosa. There may be no concrete reasons for waiting for up to a year before starting prosthesis production.

The authors have designed techniques as described above without using defect wounds, targeting the earliest possible postoperative insertion of prosthesis from the viewpoint of improving patients' quality of life.

However, there were no incidents of bleeding, infection, or delayed epithelialization of surgical wounds when early insertion of MDP was done.

In some cases, it has been possible to give postoperative radiation therapy after inserting MDP; in such cases the dysfunctional period due to maxillary defect can be reduced if the MDP is inserted at an early date postoperatively. This contributes to bring the patient to normal feeding and verbal communication, and reduction of psychological stress, thus to earlier discharge from hospital and an advancement of their return to normal social life.

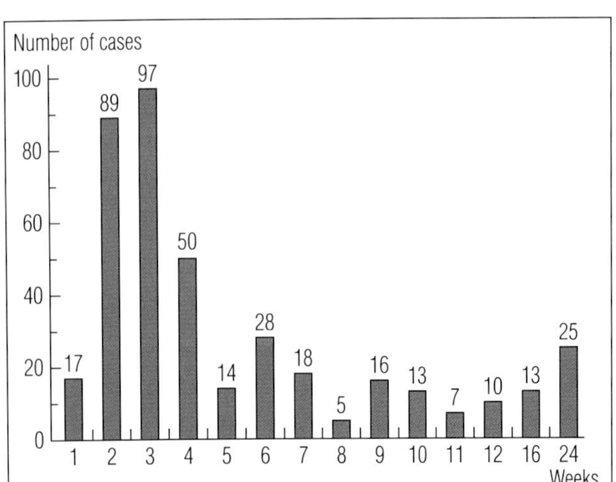

Fig. 1 Postoperative timing of start of maxillodental prosthesis (weeks).

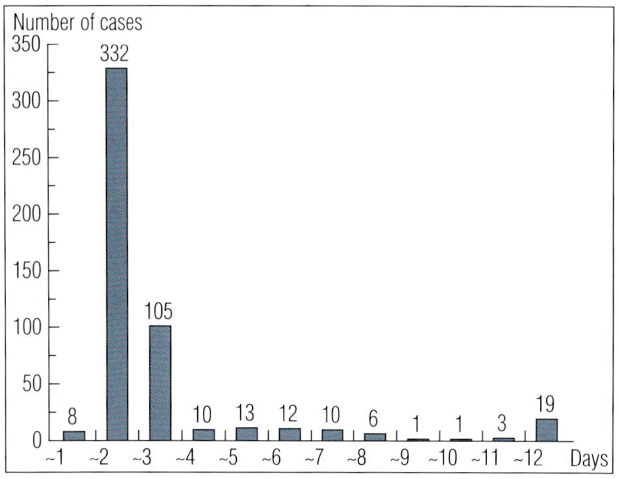

Fig. 2 Days from start of production of maxillodental prosthesis to insertion.

Early postsurgical production of maxillodental prosthesis

As previously mentioned, when the surgical oncologists have communicated with the maxillofacial prosthetic (MFP) department, this department and its technical laboratory prepare for MFP treatment. As long as no particular problem is found in initial examination, production of the MDP can start immediately. (Fig. 1)

In 8 cases, maxillofacial prostheses were produced on the day of the first visit to the MDP department. In 89% of all cases, prosthesis were inserted within 3 days after first visit (Fig. 2).

In an average case, 2 days are sufficient to produce an MDP, because the production processes can be simplified and unified, and those involved are familiar with and skilled in the production processes.

Standard processes for production of maxillodental prosthesis

[Clinical department] [first day]

10:00 1. Intraoral examination
10:30 2. Taking snap impression with stock tray
11:30 5. Taking final impression with custom tray
6. Bite taking with eugenol paste
12:50 13. Trial application of wax MDP
Arrangement of anterior artificial teeth and confirmation of marginal fitting

[Clinical department] [Second day]

11:00 23. Intraoral adjustment of MDP
12:00 24. Instruction about handling, and placement or removal of MDP
25. Instructions for functional training

[Dental technical department]

10:50 3. Production of cast for examination and cast for production of tray
4. Production of custom tray
7. Production of cast for preservation
Production of working cast for producing MDP
12:00 8. Determination of margins of denture base section and obturator part
Determination of direction for insertion and removal of MDP from undercut of maxillary defect
9. Mounting of cast on an articulator
10. Production of clasp(s) as retainer(s)
11. Production of bite plate on base plate
12. Arrangement of artificial teeth in anterior region
14. Completion of wax MDP following preparation of obturator
15:00 15. Flasking for wax replacement
16. Removal of wax
17. Injection of pour-type resin
18. Pressure-curing
19. Excavation of prosthesis from dental stone
16:10 20. Rough polishing
17:00 21. Final polishing
18:00 22. Elimination of excess weight from the prosthesis

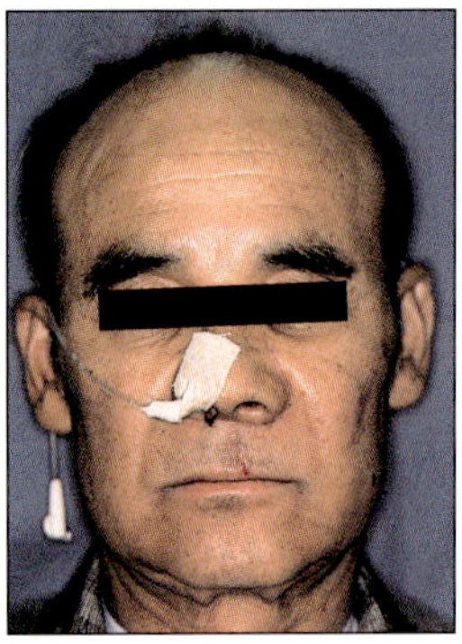

Fig. 3 62-year-old male with maxillary gingival cancer. Linac 20 Gy preoperative radiation. Partial maxillectomy was done. Facial appearance at first visit for MDP on seventh postoperative day on tube feeding.

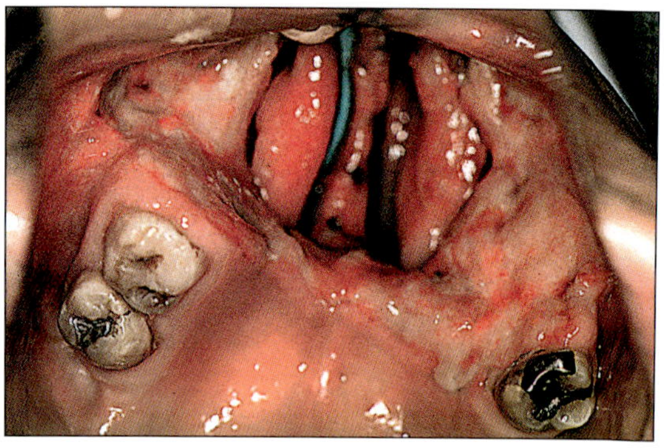

Fig. 4 Mouth opening range: 37mm. HS classification: $H_5S_0D_1T_2$ (#16, #45). 6-4 classification: 4/6-0/4 defect.
Residual teeth: #16, 17, 27 and #37, 45. Intraoral view at 7 days postoperatively. Wound is still unstable.

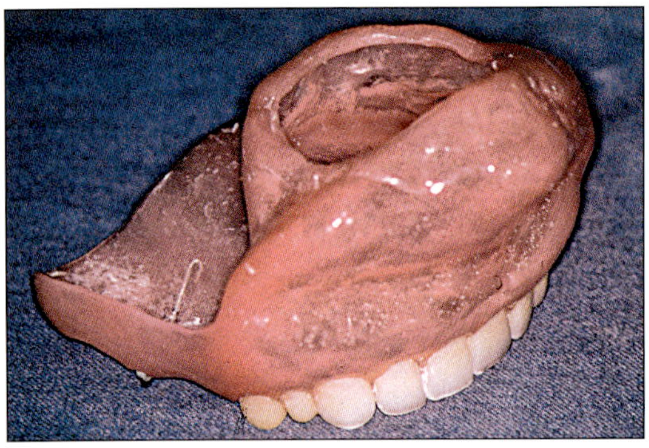

Fig. 5 Taking impression at 7 days postoperatively. Produced MDP. Partial-denture type hollow MDP without ceiling (weight: 9.3g). Ball clasps on #16, 17.

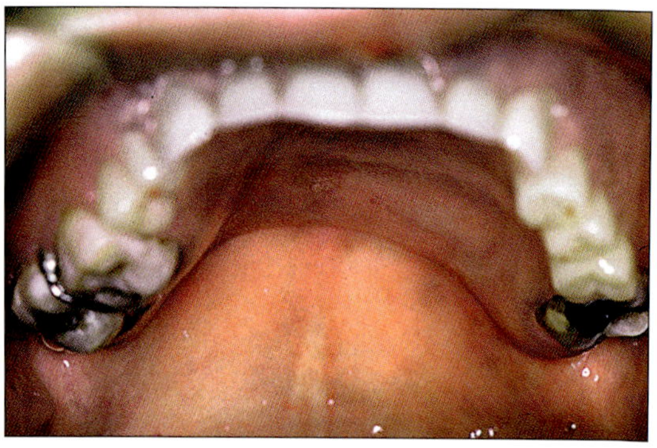

Fig. 6 Fabricating MDP at first visit and insertion on the following day.

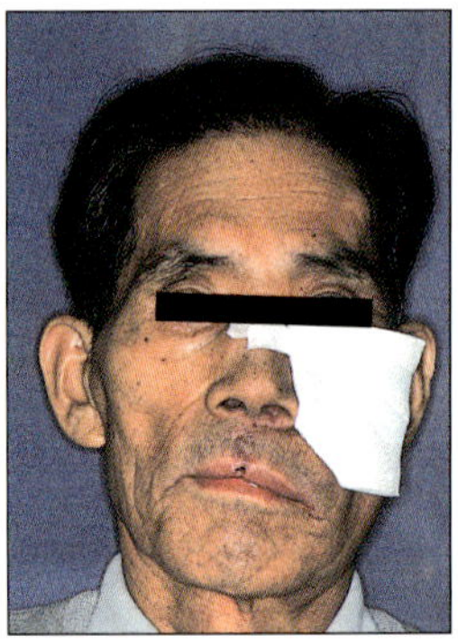

Fig. 7 66-year-old male with left maxillary sinus cancer. After preoperative chemo-radiotherapy. Facial appearance at first visit after total maxillectomy (11th postoperative day).

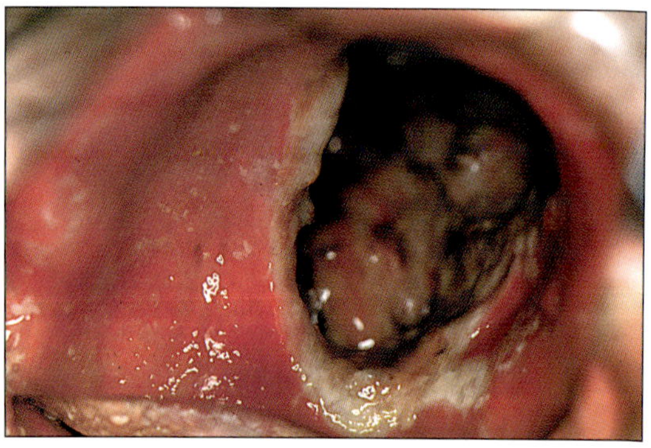

Fig. 8 HS classification: $H_4S_0D_2T_4$ (#13, #43). 6-4 classification: 3/6-0/4 defect. Mouth opening range: 21mm. No maxillary residual teeth (Only #33, 43 remain). The wound is not yet stable.

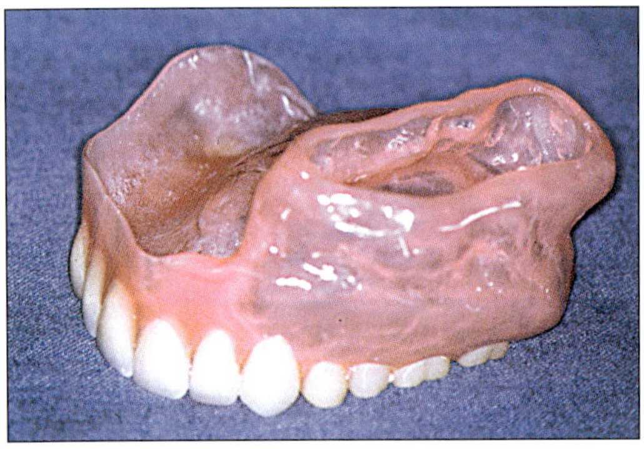

Fig. 9 MDP with open type obturator for totally edentulous patient (weight: 9.8g).

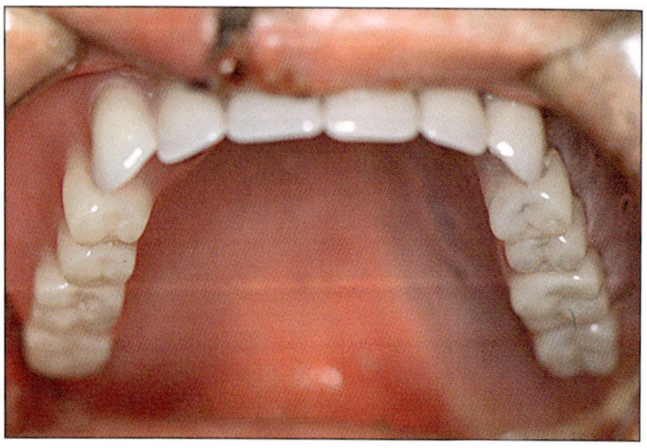

Fig. 10 Completion of maxillary prosthesis on the day after the first visit and maxillary prosthesis is inserted at 12 days postoperatively.

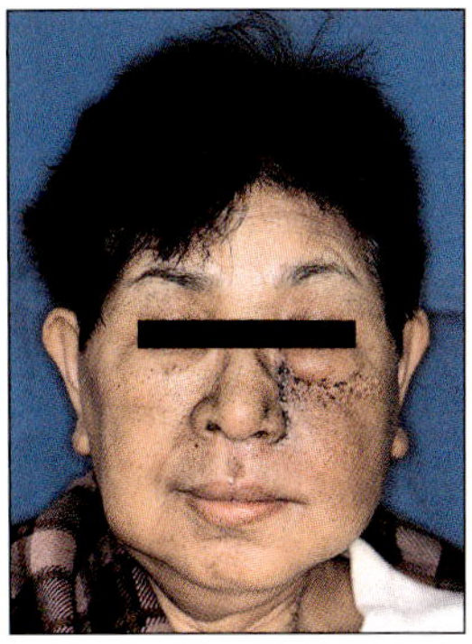

Fig. 11 66-year-old female with left maxillary sinus carcinoma. Facial appearance at first visit (17th day postoperatively). After left total maxillectomy and left neck dissection following radiotherapy.

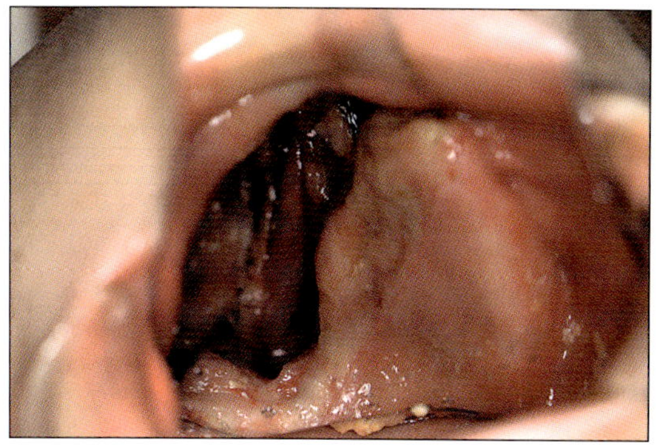

Fig. 12 HS classification: $H_3S_0D_2T_4$ (#13, #43). 6-4 classification: 3/6-0/4 defect. Mouth opening range: 24mm. No maxillary residual teeth (#34, 45 remain).

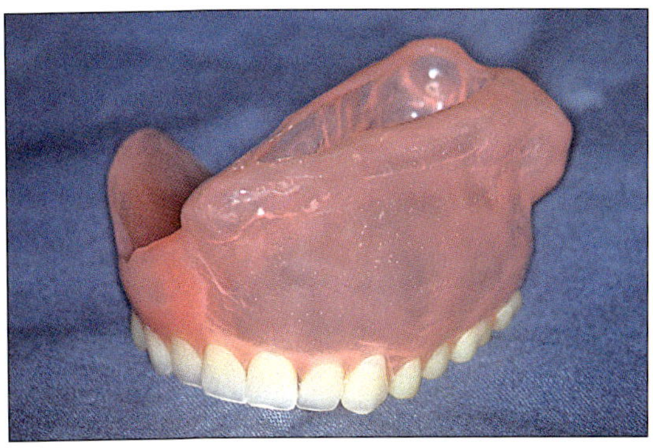

Fig. 13 MDP with open type obturator for totally edentulous patient (weight: 12.6g).

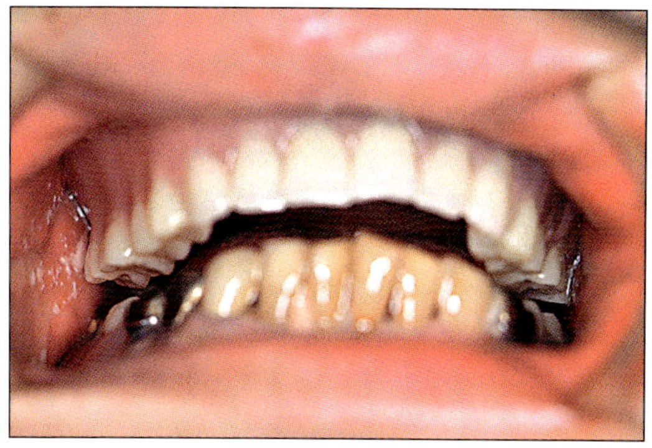

Fig. 14 Insertion of MDP on the day after the first visit (18 days postoperatively).

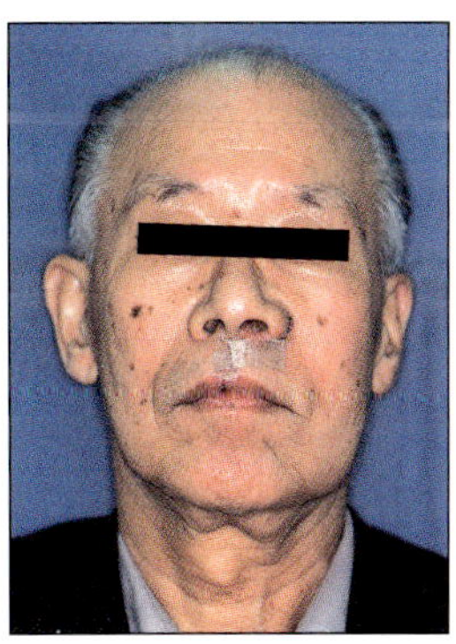

Fig. 15 70-year-old male with left maxillary gingival cancer. Facial appearance at first visit (7 days postoperatively).

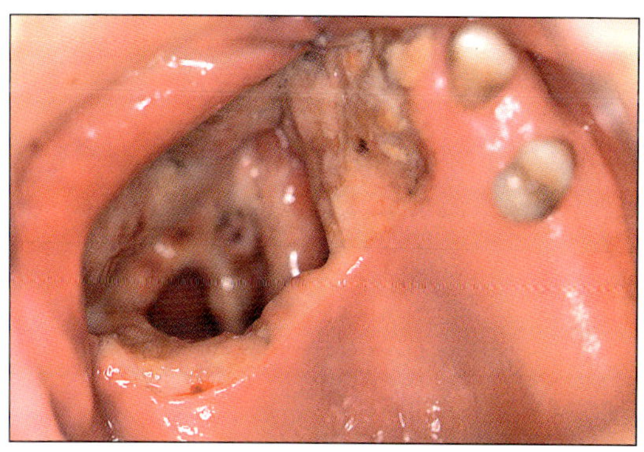

Fig. 16 Partial maxillectomy following preoperative radiation of 24 Gy. HS classification: $H_3S_0D_0T_3$ (#13, #23). 6-4 classification: 2/6-0/4 defect. Residual teeth: #13, 15 and #34, 37, 44. Mouth opening range: 51mm.

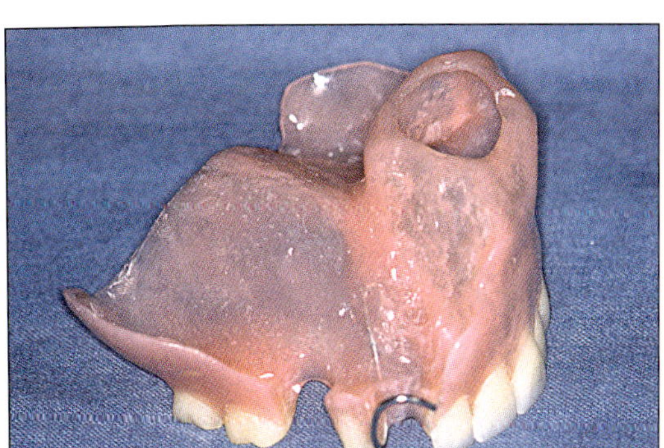

Fig. 17 MDP with open type obturator for partially edentulous patient (weight: 9.9g). Wire clasp used on #13.

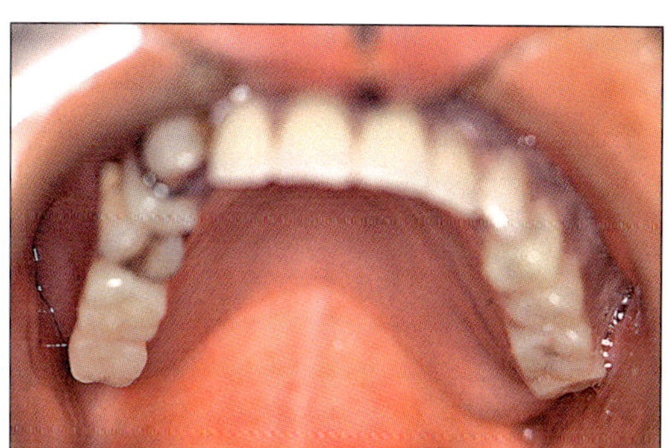

Fig. 18 Insertion of maxillary prosthesis on the day after the first visit (8 days postoperatively).

CHAPTER 12

Changes of maxillary defects

It is generally said that postoperative maxillary defect regions undergo dynamic change following the immediate aftermath of surgery and that it takes about 3 months till visible changes become settled. Then subsequently only gradual changes may follow, as seen in photographs. Also, changes of maxillary defects do not always occur at a fixed rate. Particularly following the resection of gingival primary tumors, dynamic changes occur for rather short periods of time. These changes may cause the maxillodental prosthesis (MDP) to tend to be easily displaced or to become impossible to insert.

These changes over time, including changes on the unaffected side, result in poor fitting of MDP defects becoming filthy, or food leakage, to the nasal cavity. Therefore, it is necessary to do observations over a certain period of time and to adjust MDP.

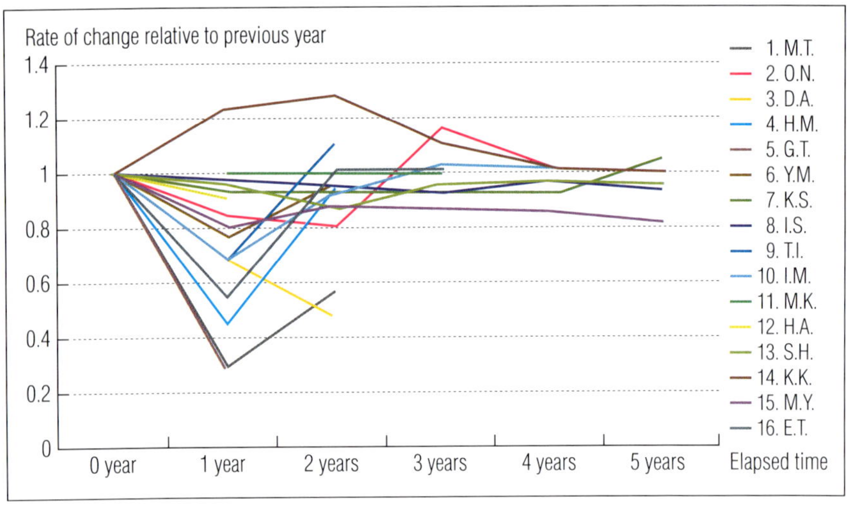

Fig. 1 Changes of maxillary defect regions over time after resection of maxillary gingival cancer, and variations relative to previous year's models.

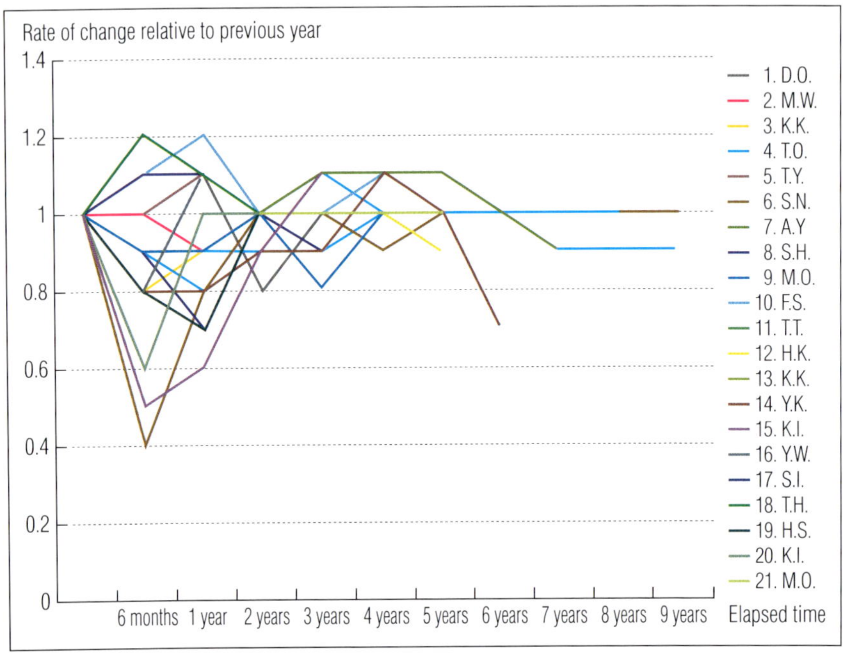

Fig. 2 Changes of maxillary defect regions over time after resection of maxillary sinus cancer, and variations relative to previous year's models.

Changes of maxillary defect regions

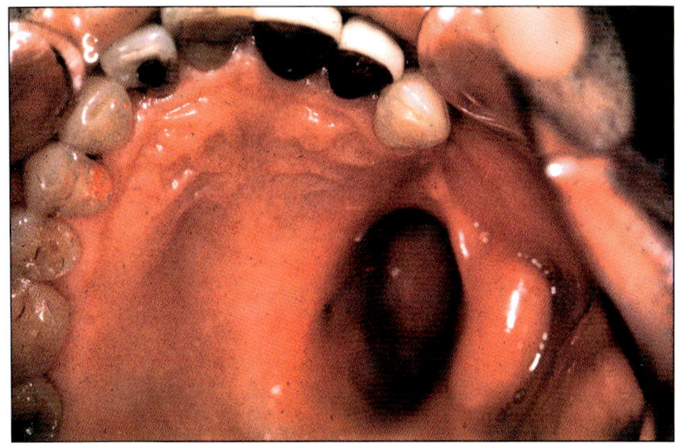

Fig. 3 52-year-old male at 60th postoperative day. Right partial maxillectomy due to malignant pleomorphic adenoma of hard palatal. HS classification: $H_3S_0D_0T_0$ (#11, #41). 6-4 classification: 2/6 - 0/4 defect. Maxillary defect in the region corresponding to #14–17, alveolar process remaining on the buccal side of #17, mouth opening range 45mm. Residual teeth are #13, 27 and #37, 47.

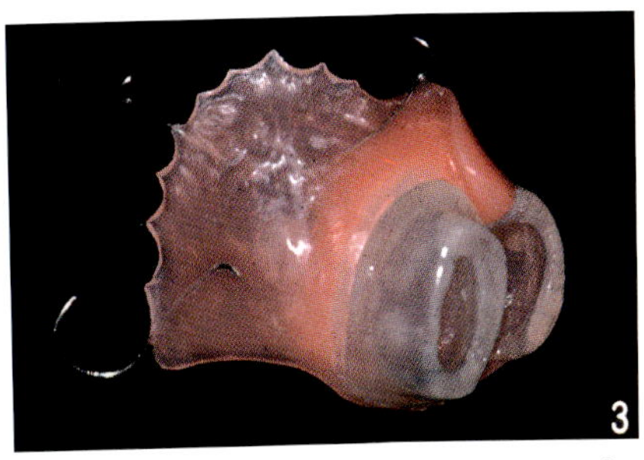

Fig. 4 MDP with open type obturator for partially edentulous patient (weight: 10.5g). Silicon resin is used partly for the obturator. Wire clasps on #13, 16, 27. Inserted 72 days postoperatively (silicone: Orthocon®, Sankin Co. Ltd., resin for plate: Pradon65®, Kulzer Co. Ltd).

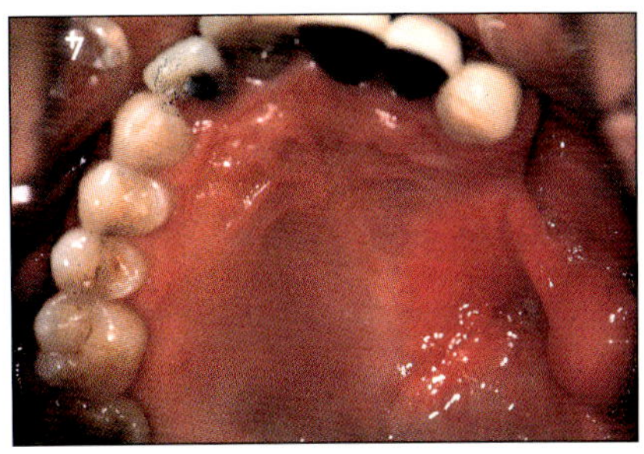

Fig. 5 Four months after first visit. Size of maxillary defect region has shrunk to about 2mm in diameter. The residual alveolar process has changed to become spherical.

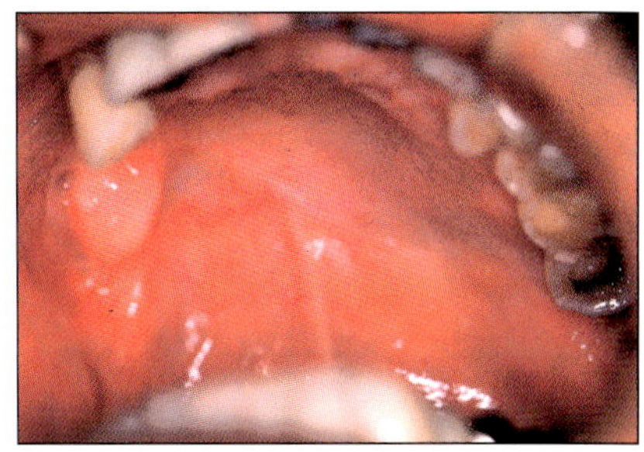

Fig. 6 About 5 years after first visit. Oronasal fistula of the maxillary defect has closed. The alveolar process has become more spherical.

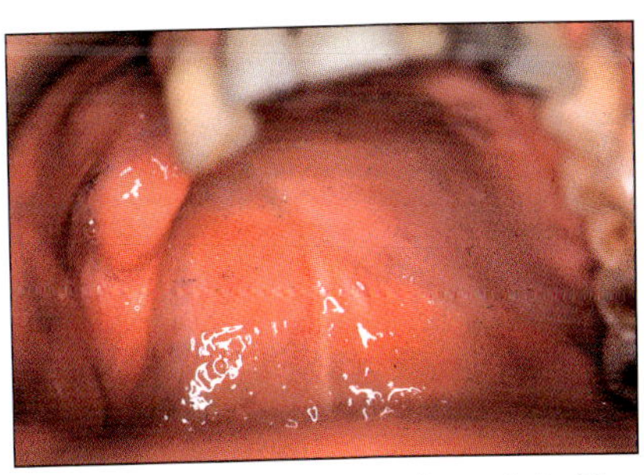

Fig. 7 Nine years after first visit. The residual alveolar process has become well-rounded and no alveolar ridge is found.

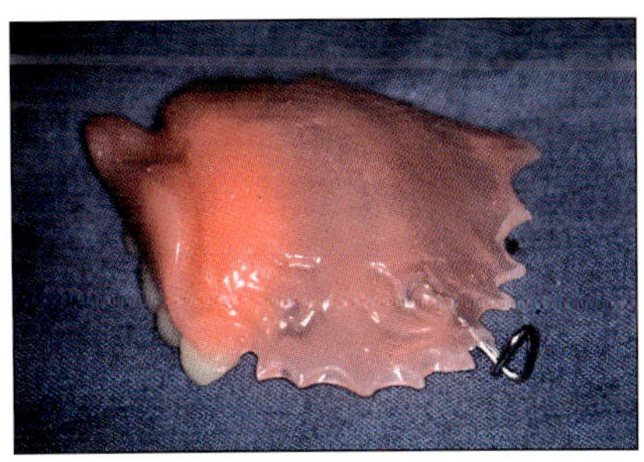

Fig. 8 Maxillary prosthesis fabricated after 9 years (weight: 8.3g). MDP for partially edentulous patient with a clasp on #23. The shape of the obturator part is very different from that of the maxillofacial prosthesis made at the time of the first visit.

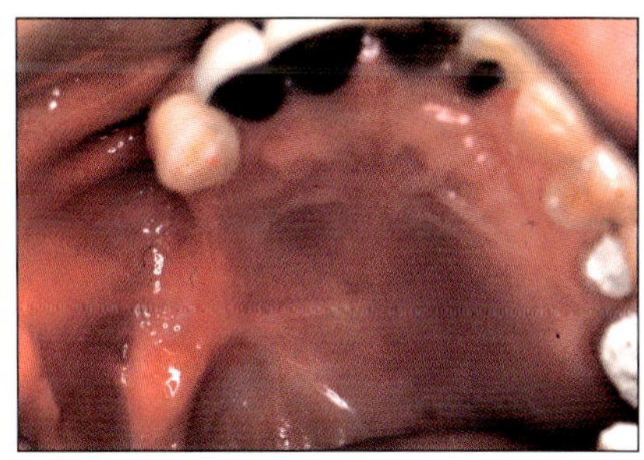

Fig. 9 Note the difference between the intraoral view after 12 years and that at the first visit.

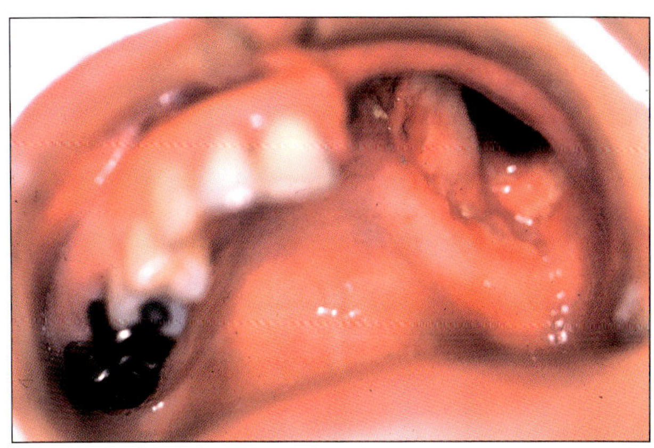

Fig. 10 52-year-old female with left maxillary gingival cancer. Twenty-one days after partial maxillectomy; mouth opening range is 44mm. HS classification: $H_3S_0D_0T_0$ (#11, #41). 6-4 classification: 2/6 - 0/4 defect and maxillary defect at #21–27 region. Residual teeth are #11–17 and #37, 47.

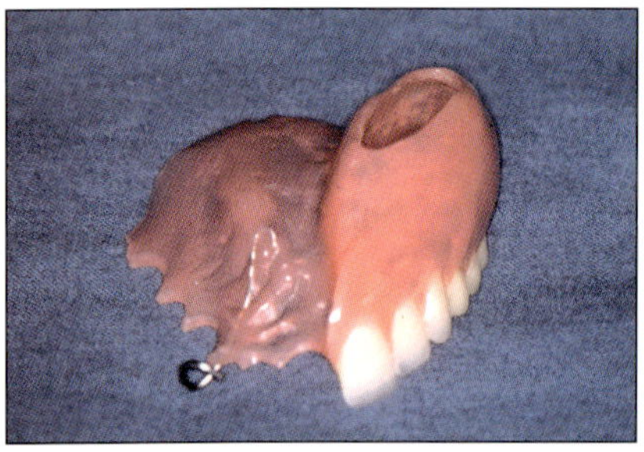

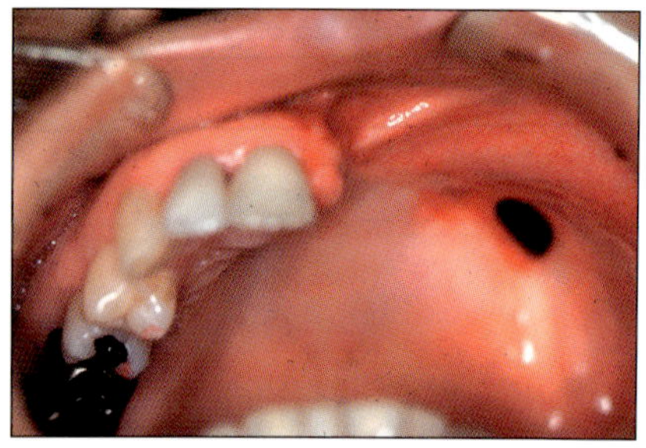

Fig. 11 *(left)* MDP with open type obturator for partially edentulous patient was inserted at 22 days postoperatively. (weight: 7.2g). Wire clasp on #13.
Fig. 12 *(right)* Nine months after first visit. Some changes were seen in the small anterior defect and in the fairly large posterior defect (10 × 5 mm).

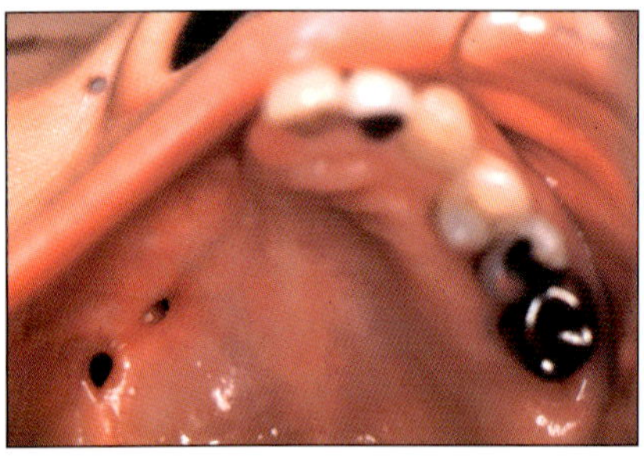

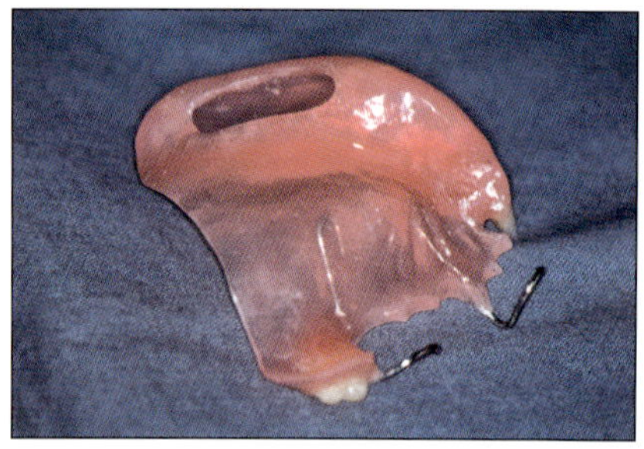

Fig. 13 *(left)* Five years after first visit. Anterior defect of 1 × 1mm and posterior defect of 2 × 2mm. Note that impression materials may enter the nasal cavity or maxillary sinus during the impression taking.
Fig. 14 *(right)* Five years since the first visit. MDP with open type obturator for partially edentulous patient (weight: 7.5g). Wire clasps were used on #13, 17.

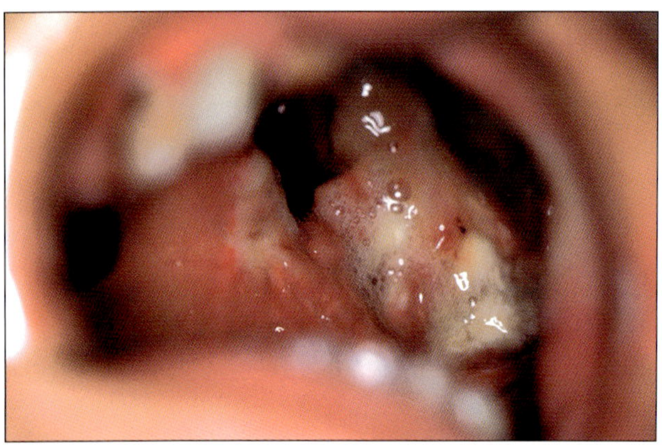

Fig. 15 58-year-old female with cancer of left maxillary sinus. Fourteen days after extensive total maxillectomy with total exenteration of the orbit following chemotherapy and preoperative radiotherapy. Mouth opening range 18mm. HS classification: $H_6S_0D_3T_2$ (#12, #43). 6-4 classification: 3/6 - 1/4 defect. Residual teeth are #12, 13, 16, 17 and #33, 34, 36.

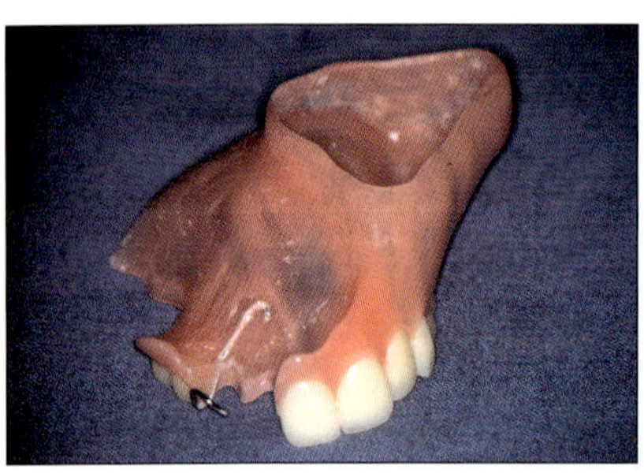

Fig. 16 Fifteen days postoperatively. MDP with open type obturator for partially edentulous patient with a wire clasp used on #18 (weight: 9.4g).

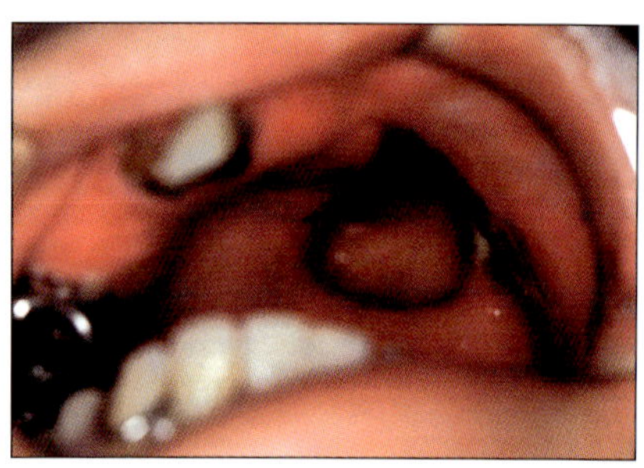

Fig. 17 The wound is healed at 7 months after the first visit. No changes in the defect are found.

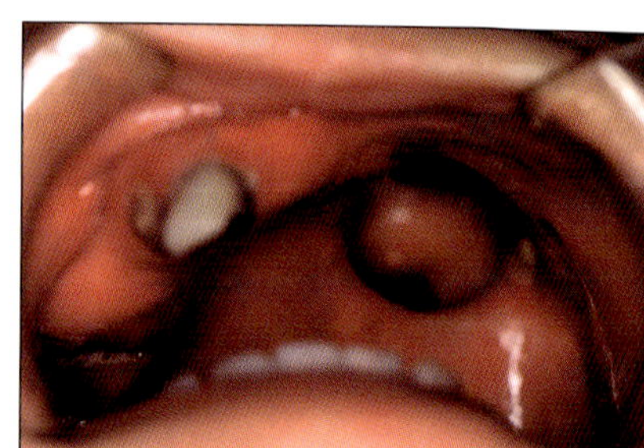

Fig. 18 One year since the first visit. The defect shows an almost circular contour, because of the scar bundle.

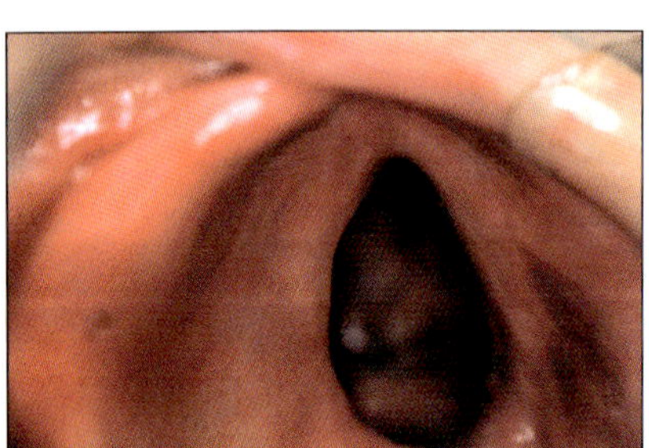

Fig. 19 Nine years following the first visit. The defect shape has become guttate due to the scar bundle. All teeth have been lost.

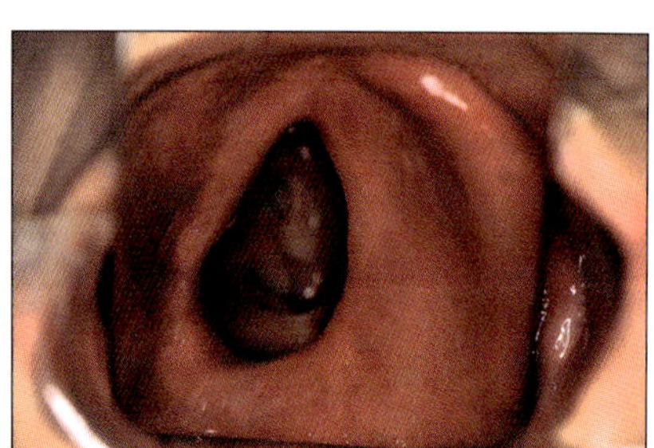

Fig. 20 10 years since first visit. The guttate defect has become smaller.

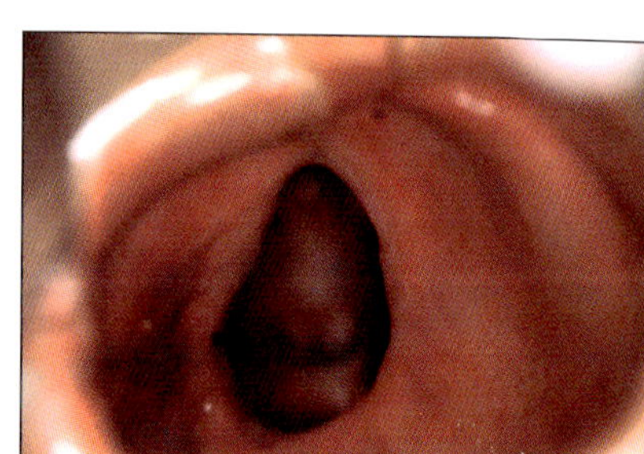

Fig. 21 12 years since first visit. Scar bundle has become larger.

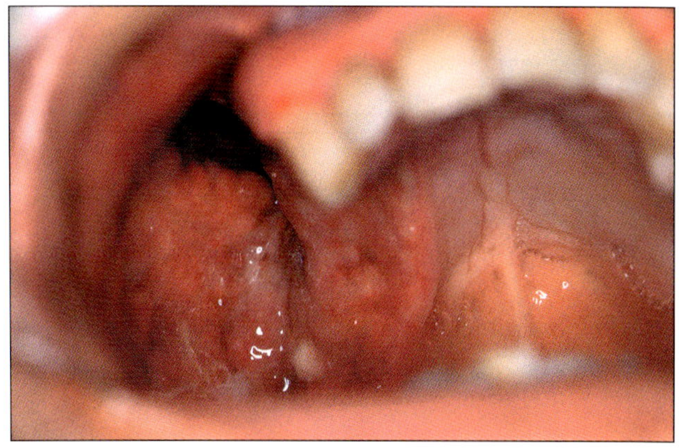

Fig. 22 61-year-old male with right maxillary gingival cancer. The wound is not yet stable at 9 days after partial maxillectomy. HS classification: $H_3S_0D_2T_0$ (#11, #41). 6-4 classification: 2/6 - 0/4 defect. #14–17 maxillary defect, mouth opening range 22mm. Residual teeth are #13, 28 and #38, 45.

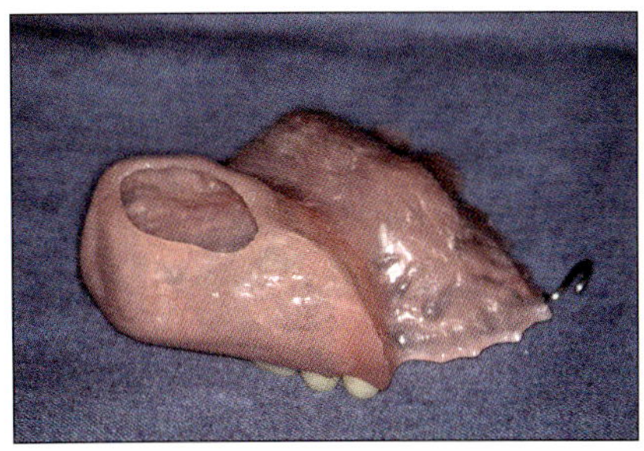

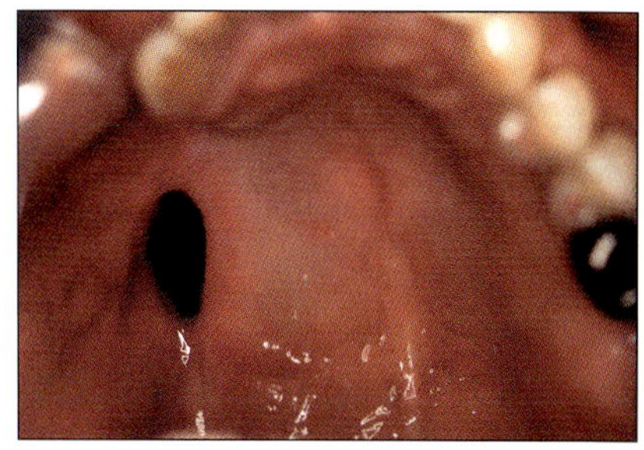

Fig. 23 *(left)* Inserted at 10 days postoperatively (weight: 9.8g). MDP with open type obturator for partially edentulous patient with a clasp on #13.

Fig. 24 *(right)* Five months since first visit. The maxillary defect has been reduced to about 10 × 20mm.

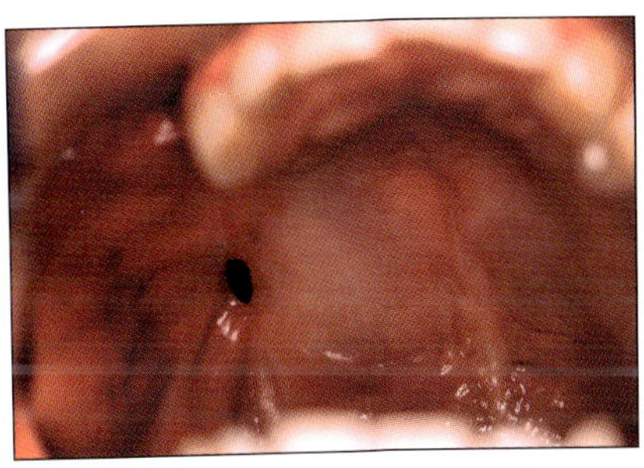

Fig. 25 Two years since first visit. The maxillary defect has been further reduced (5 x 4mm).

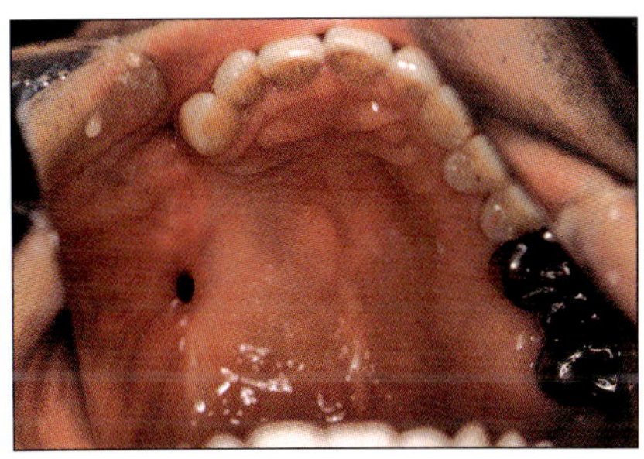

Fig. 26 Two and half years since first visit. The maxillary defect has been reduced to 4 x 3mm.

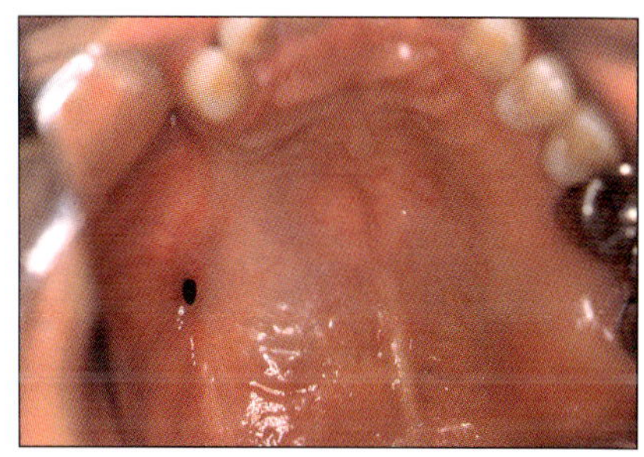

Fig. 27 Four years since first visit. The maxillary defect has changed to 3 × 2 mm.

Re-fitting of maxillodental prosthesis to maxillary defect

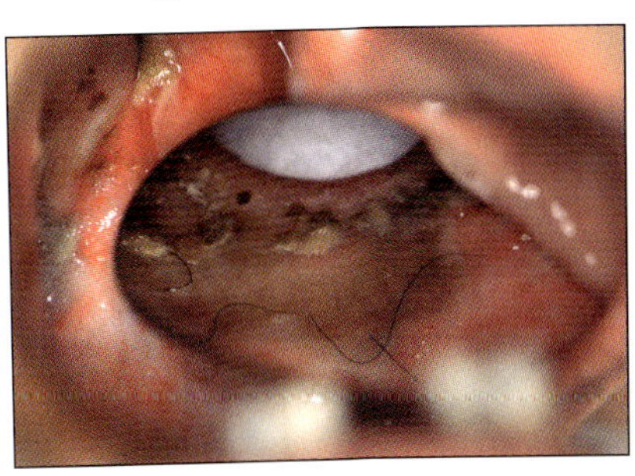

Fig. 28 The patient had not realized that there was poor fitting of the MDP, therefore had not come for follow up for MFP. The nasal cavity become seriously contaminated.

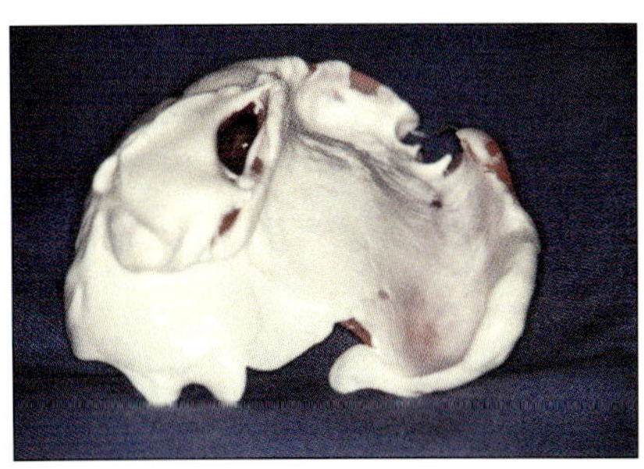

Fig. 29 To check the fit of the MDP to the maxillary defect region in another case, an impression was taken with silicone impression material. Depending on how poorly fitted a prosthesis is, it may be faster to make a new prosthesis than to adjust the old one.

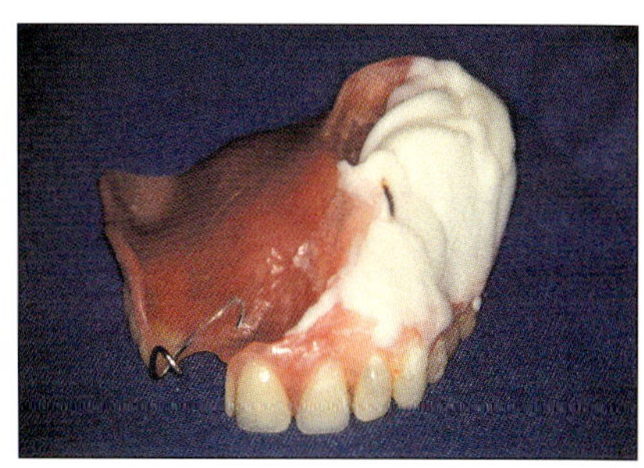

Fig. 30 In the same case as in Fig. 29. Another impression is taken only in the maxillary defect region.

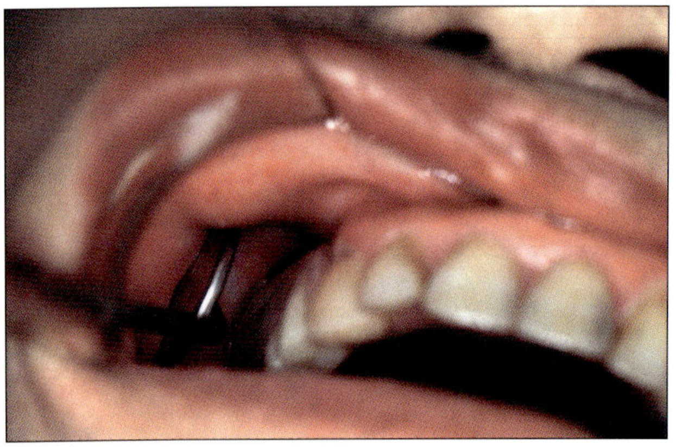

Fig. 31 Because the buccal scar has softened a space is left between the MDP and the buccal region.

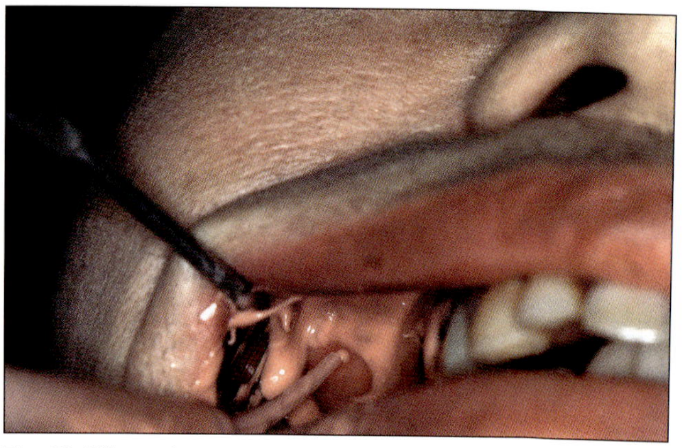

Fig. 32 Silicone impression material is applied to the buccal surface of the MDP, which is inserted into the oral cavity. Then additional impression material is poured into the remaining gap.

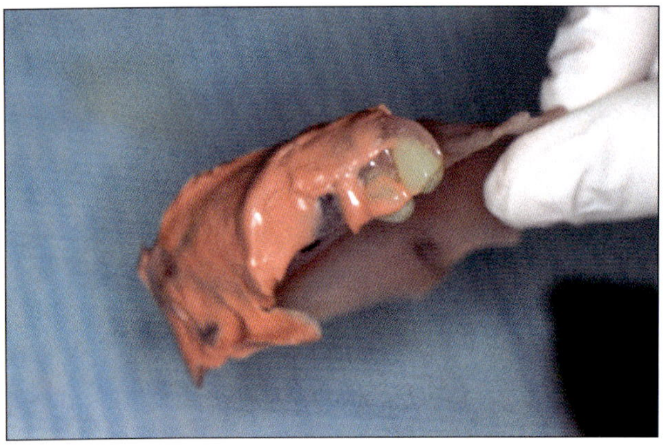

Fig. 33 A plaster core is made from this impression.

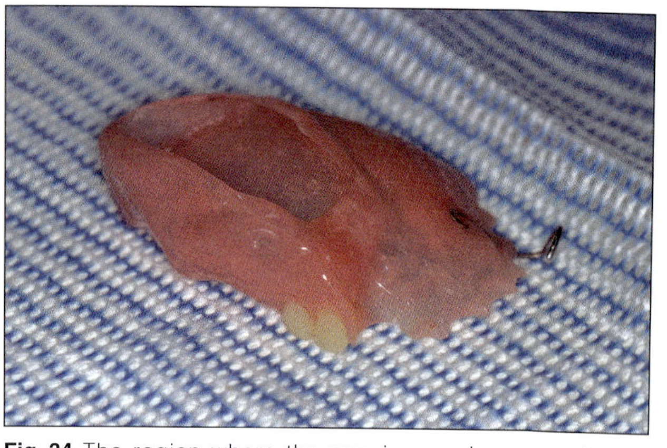

Fig. 34 The region where the new impression was taken is replaced by denture plate resin.

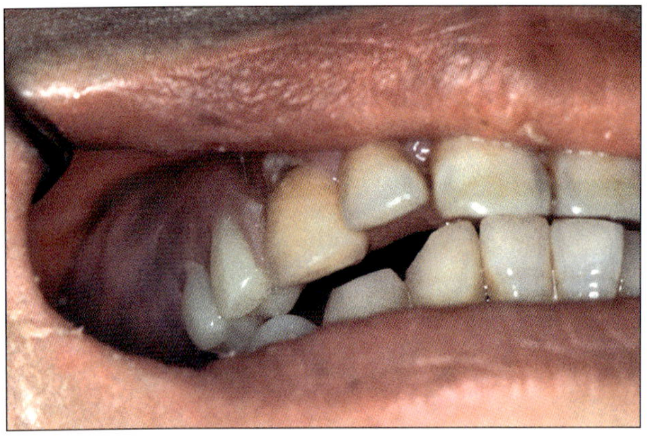

Fig. 35 This repair of the MDP has closed the gap at its buccal area.

SECTION 3

Defects of Palate and Oropharyngeus

CHAPTER 13

Soft palate defect prostheses

Excision of oropharyngeal tumors, and congenital malformations such as cleft plate, cause soft palate defects that result in disturbance or loss of functional separation of the oral, nasal, and pharynx.

Surgical reconstruction by skin flap after tumor resection on photoplasty is often used to improve articulatory disorders and deglutition disorders caused by the above-mentioned defects. On the other hand, it is not always possible to achieve compensation or reconstruction of the function of the soft palate fauces region perfectly. In such cases, a prosthesis is often needed to assist the function of the oropharynx itself, and also for aiding masticatory function.

In particular, if improvement of function can be achieved by prosthetic method for a soft palate defect, a more convenient method is to apply a maxillary prosthesis first without carrying out any flap reconstruction for the defect in this region.

This prosthetic functional "reconstruction" method places fewer physical burdens on the patient, and is connected to shortening of the time needed for such surgery as tumor resection; it can also be an important factor in minimally-invasive treatment if the use of this method commencing in the early period after surgery is taken in account.

In addition, by minute adjustments and reproduction of prostheses, the condition of improvement of function to quite a high level can be maintained without using the patient's physical resources.

This is the same as for alveolar process-hard palate defects.

Defect forms and classification (Re-insertion)

Defect forms are classified according to the ratio determined by comparing the area of the soft palate with the scope of the soft palate defect. Basically, soft palate defects are indicated together with alveolar process-hard palate defects. This area is indicated by 6, and a soft palate defect area is indicated by 4. Each such defect is indicated by using 6 or 4 as the denominator; this is called "6-4 classification" (Fig. 1).

This defect classification is used as follows; A case where there is no defect of the soft palate part is described as a 0/4 defect (Fig. 2), and a defect of the frontal edge of the soft palate part is called a 1/4

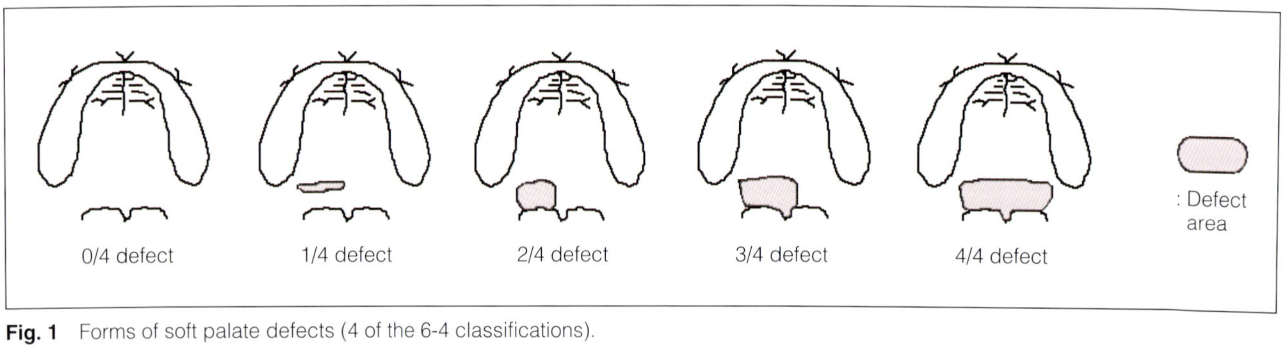

Fig. 1 Forms of soft palate defects (4 of the 6-4 classifications).

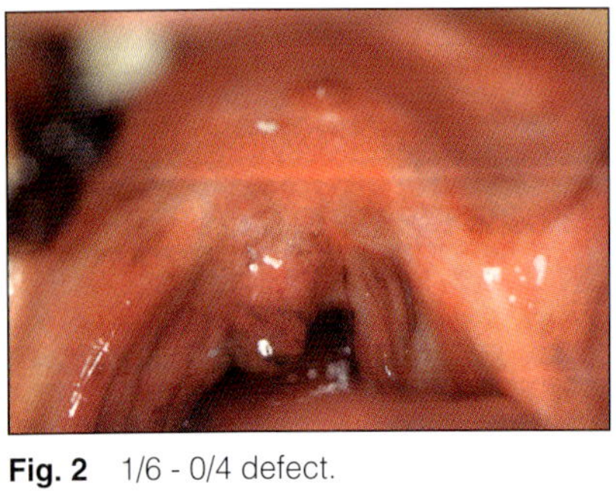

Fig. 2 1/6 - 0/4 defect.

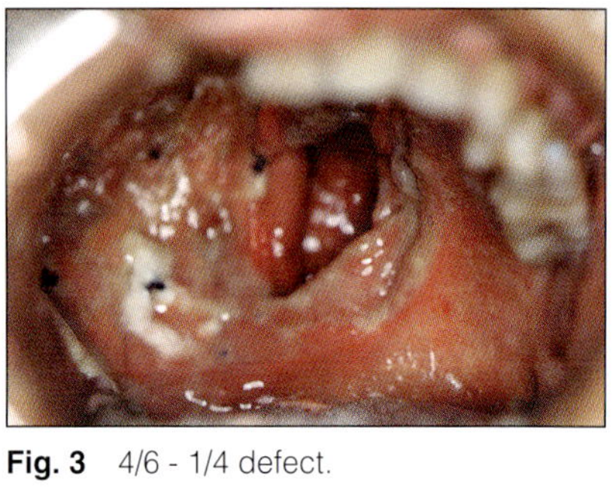

Fig. 3 4/6 - 1/4 defect.

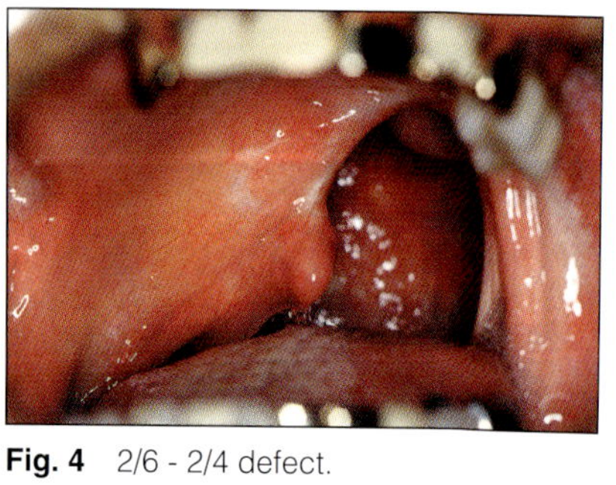

Fig. 4 2/6 - 2/4 defect.

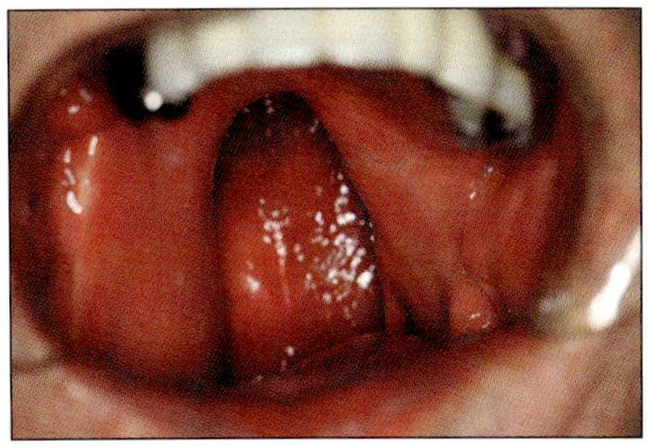
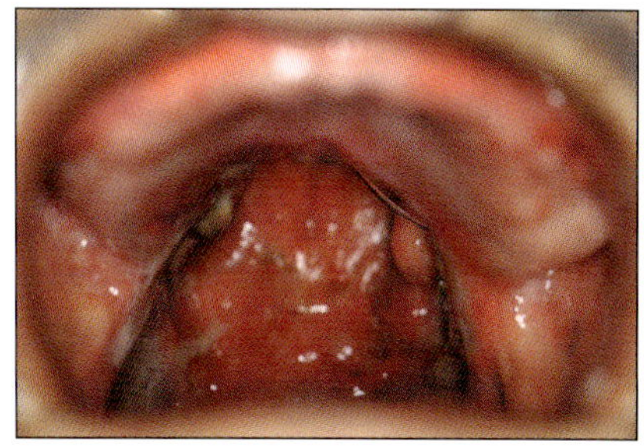

Fig. 5 *(left)* 1/6 - 2/4 defect (skin flap reconstruction to the lateral wall).
Fig. 6 *(right)* 1/6 - 3/4 defect.

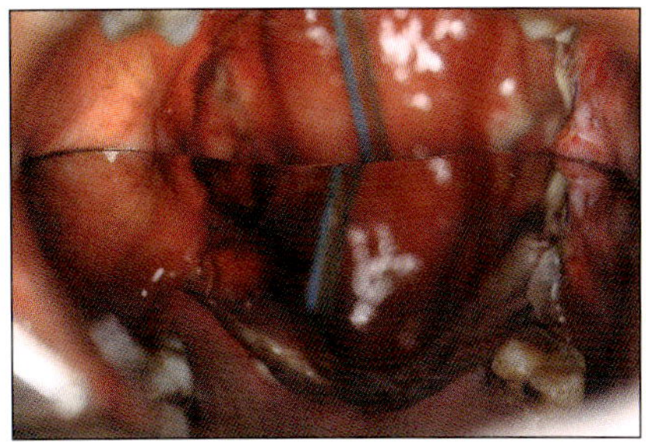
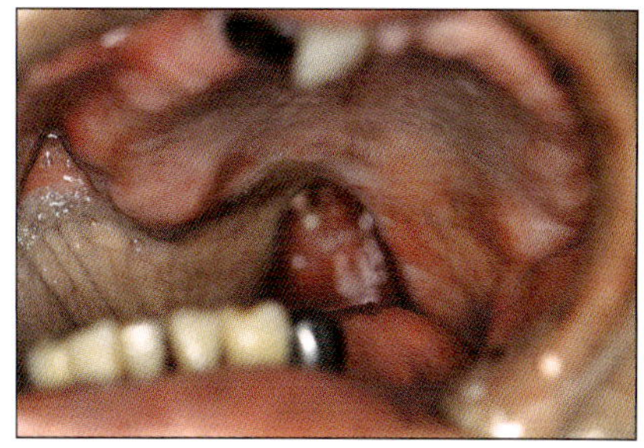

Fig. 7 *(left)* 0/6 - 4/4 defect (mirror image).
Fig. 8 *(right)* 0/6 - 4/4 defect (lateral wall reconstructed with skin flap).

defect (Fig. 3). When the uvula is set as the standard, a defect which reaches the rear edge of soft palate, and which does not include the uvula, is called a 2/4 defect (Figs. 4 and 5). Skin flap reconstruction for the pharyngeal lateral wall is done in some 2/4 defect cases; Fig. 4 shows a case of excision only, and Fig. 5 shows a case with skin flap reconstruction. A defect reaching the rear edge of the soft palate, including the uvula, is called a 3/4 defect (Fig. 6). A defect of the whole soft palate is called a 4/4 defect (Figs. 7 and 8). Fig. 8 shows a case in which skin flap reconstruction was done on the pharyngeal lateral wall.

Clinical procedure of soft palate defect prosthesis

Impression-taking is one of the most important operations in clinical prosthetic treatment. The operator must understand which regions are functionally important, and which regions are important from the viewpoint of follow up for recurrence, and must take precise impressions of each region.

In cases of soft palate defects, impression-taking of the entire circumference of the oropharyngeal region is essential. It is necessary to reproduce the functional structure of Passavant's cushion, if present. When selecting impression materials and impression procedures, it is necessary to keep in mind that the hardness and properties of the masticatory mucous membrane of the alveolar part and those of the peripheral mucous membrane in this region are completely different. In addition it is most important to note that the impression of the soft palate area cannot be taken without once occluding the primary respiratory tract.

Any kind of impression material can be used as long as the operator has full knowledge of the distinctive characteristics of it, although it must be material that is not likely to sag and a short curing time is desirable. The author uses alginate-based impression material for which adjustment of hardness can easily be done by altering the water temperature and water/powder ratio. Ideally, the best materials and devices to be employed are those to which the operator is accustomed.

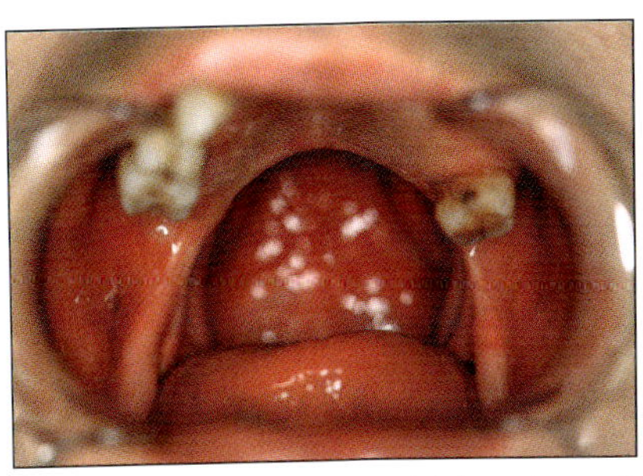

Fig. 9 Case 1. 71-year-old female, soft palate tumor. Complete defect of soft palate after ablative surgery. HS classification: H0S4D0T2 (#13, 43) 6-4 classification: 0/6, 4/4 defect. Mouth opening: 42mm. Residual teeth: #13, 15, 16, 24, 27 and #32, 33, 43, 44.

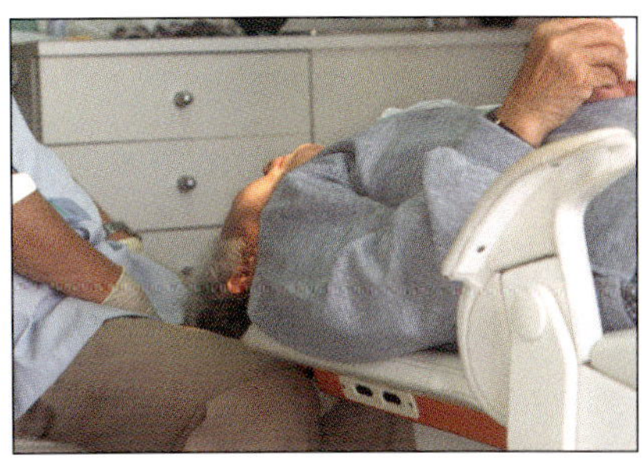

Fig. 10 During impression-taking, the body position of the patient is set so that the pharyngeal back wall is angled slightly downward from the horizontal plane in the parietal direction, in order to prevent sagging-in of the impression material into the lower pharyngeal cavity.

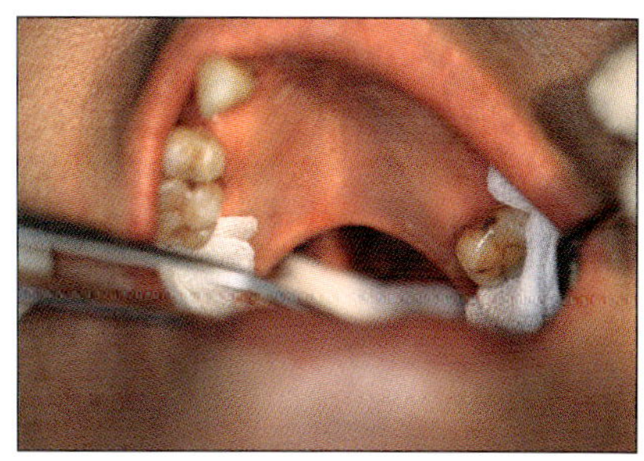

Fig. 11 Saliva in the oral cavity and pharynx must be thoroughly suctioned and wiped off by sponge, to dry these areas so that the impression materials will adhere well to the mucosa.

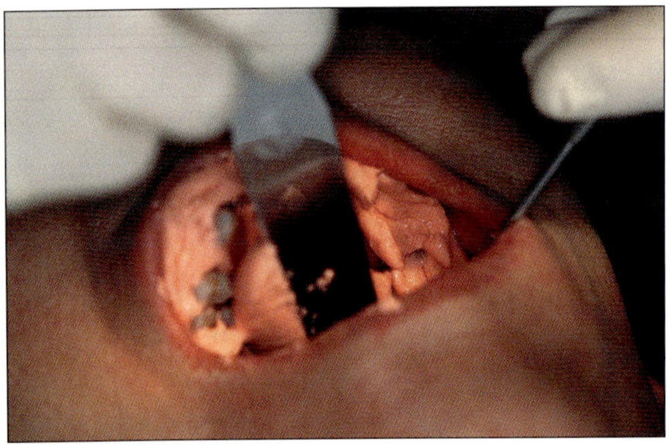

Fig. 12 Impression material is heaped on a ready-made tray, and simultaneously the hard palate defect part and remaining teeth are coated with impression material. Impression material is mixed by 2 persons. One mixes the portion of impression material for the ready-made tray, and the other person mixes one for coating the oral cavity. The mixing of the impression material for coating the inside of the oral cavity should be started slightly later than the mixing of one for the tray.

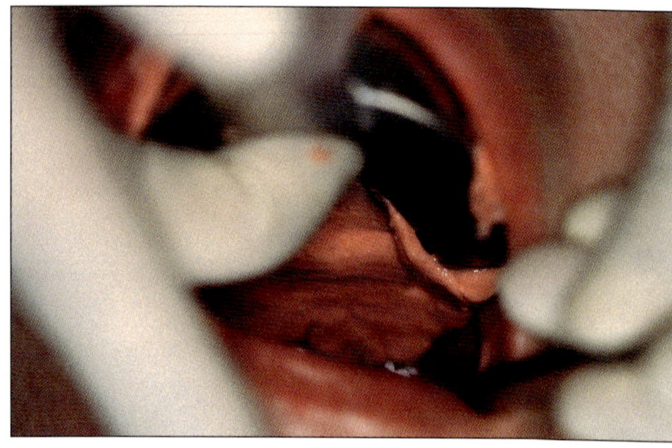

Fig. 13 The prepared tray is inserted into the patient's oral cavity. The impression material is pushed antero-posteriorly to the pharyngeal posterior wall of which the impression is most important.

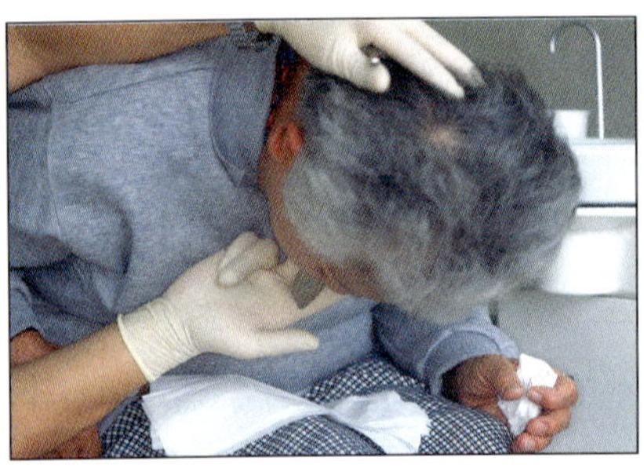

Fig. 14 The patient is instructed to bend the head forward until the impression material has cured, and to rotate the head to left and right with the chin pulled in toward the neck.

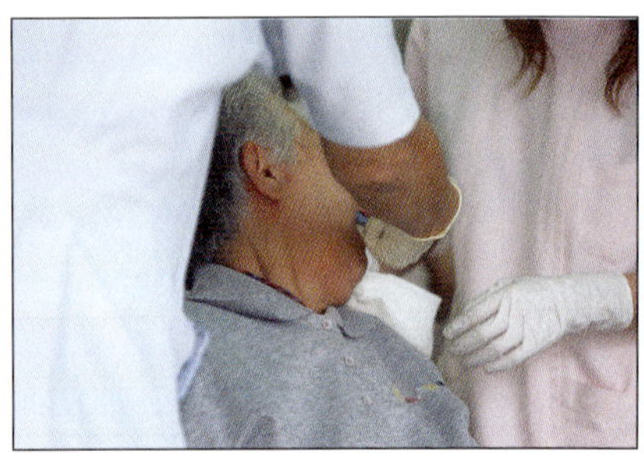

Fig. 15 This is the most important part of the procedure, equivalent to "muscle trimming" for the pharyngeal lateral and posterior walls. The patient is told to pronounce the short "a" sound in a loud voice repeatedly, to take the impression of Passavant's cushion or pharyngeal constrictor muscle.

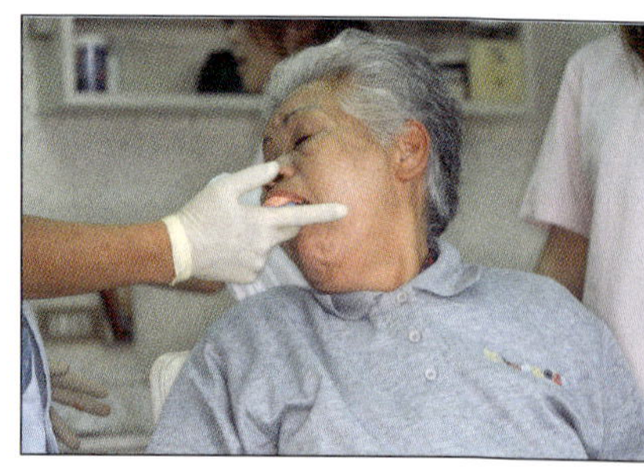

Fig. 16 These processes are important for a good functional impression of the oropharyngeal region. The patient should practice this movement before the final impression-taking.

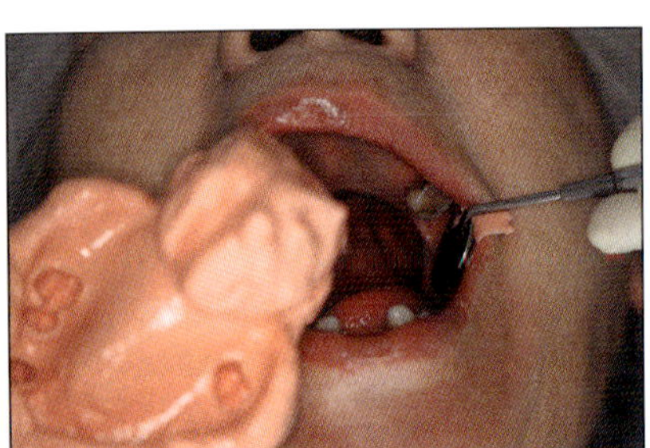

Fig. 17 To take out the preliminary impression, first float up the pharyngeal part, then detach anterior to posterior tooth part. This is necessary because the impression corresponding to the front edge of the oropharyngeal defect site often becomes hooked on the rear edge of the remaining hard palate.

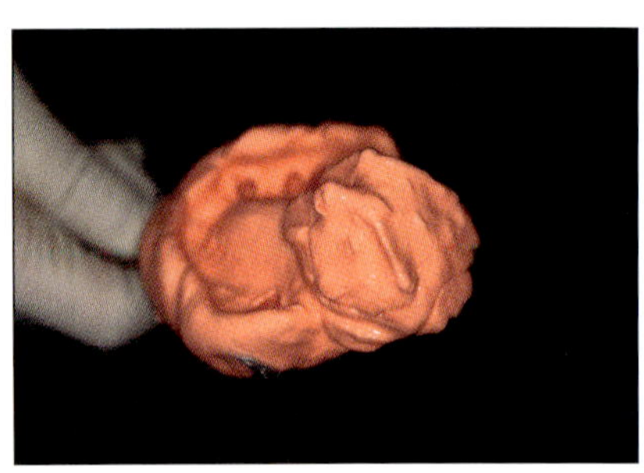

Fig. 18 After the preliminary impression has been taken, carefully confirm that the impression of the lateral and posterior pharyngeal wall has been taken accurately.

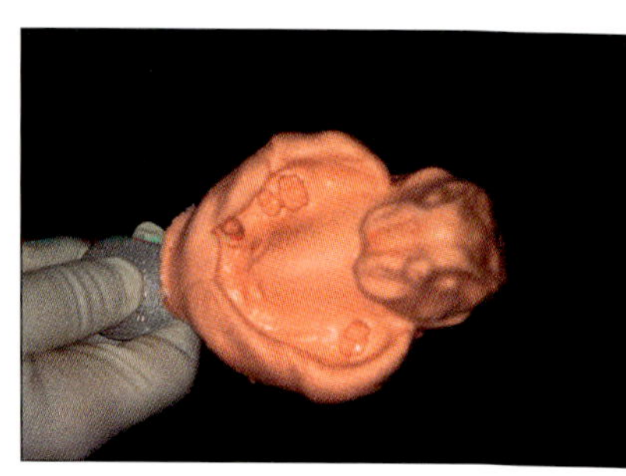

Fig. 19 The impression of the pharynx is most important.

Impression-taking for working model

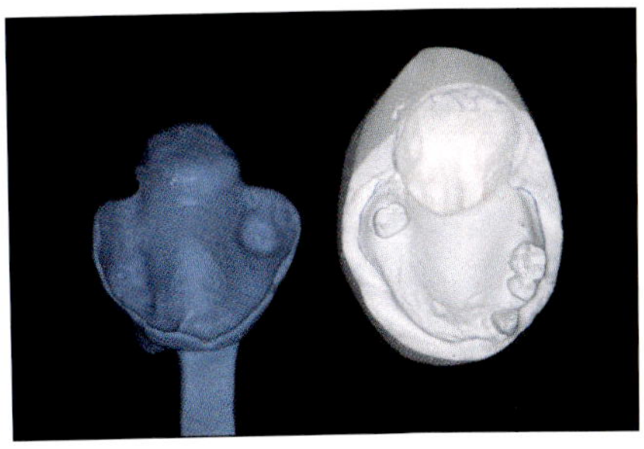

Fig. 20 A custom tray and a study model are produced using the preliminary impression model. The photo shows the custom tray on the study model.

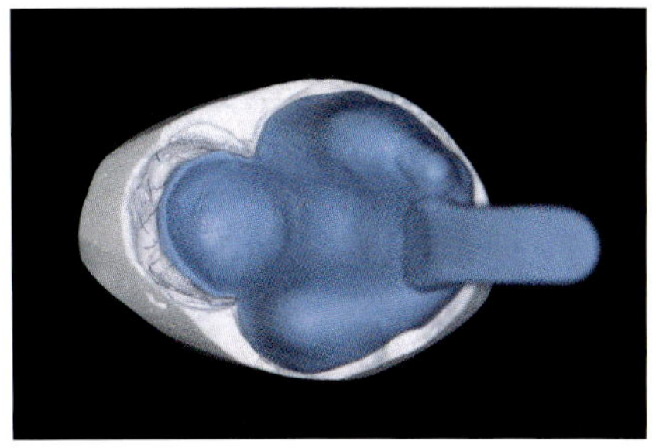

Fig. 21 A gap of about 10mm is left between the tray and the pharyngeal posterior wall. This is because a large space for impression material is needed in order to take the functional impression of the pharynx, which is quite soft and has a wide range of movement.

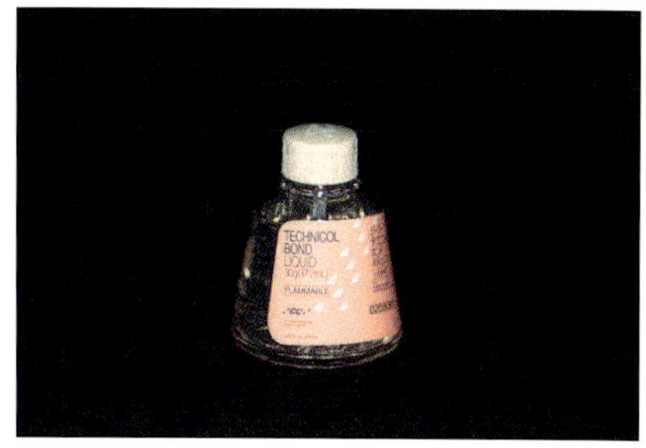

Fig. 22 This custom tray is coated with the adhesive agent for the alginate-based impression material, then dried. Impression material adhesive agent: TECHNICOL BOND® (GC Corp.)

Fig. 23 *(left)* The final impression-taking procedure is almost the same as the preliminary impression-taking procedure.
Fig. 24 *(right)* The final impression is left in the mouth a bit longer than for an ordinary denture impression. The final impression should be removed when the surface of the impression has started to dry.

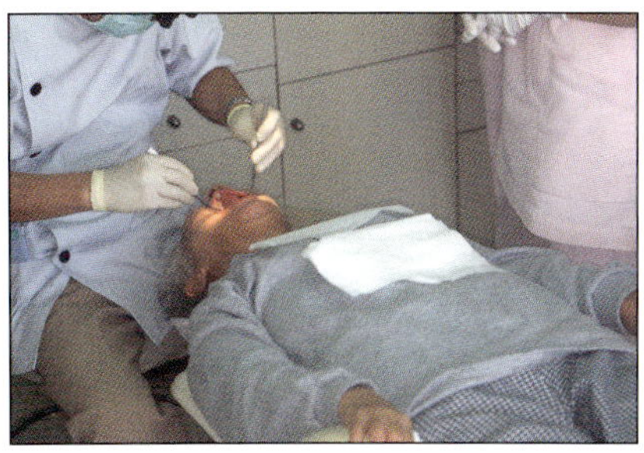

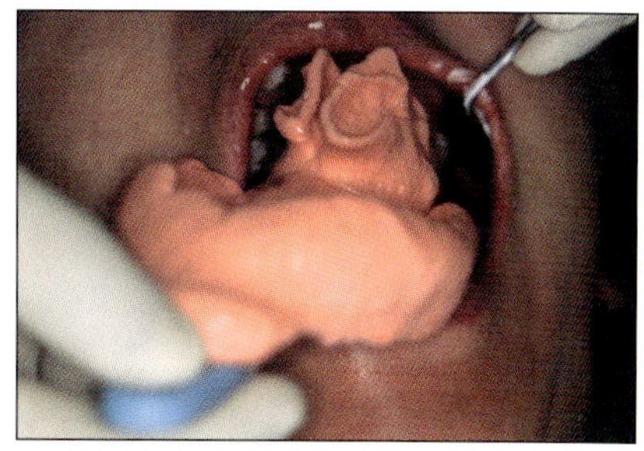

Fig. 25 *(left)* Confirm the final impression of the oral and oropharyngeal region. Prepare a working model from this working impression.
Fig. 26 *(right)* The following procesure is the same processes for ordinary denture production.

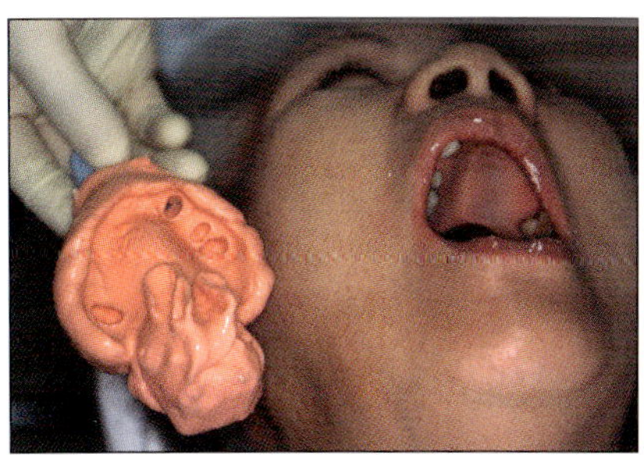

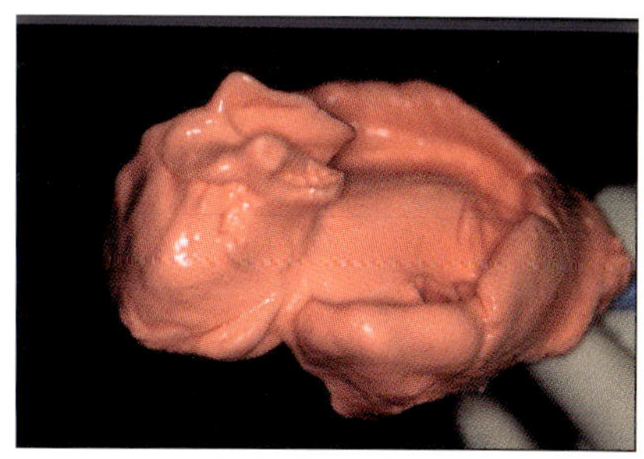

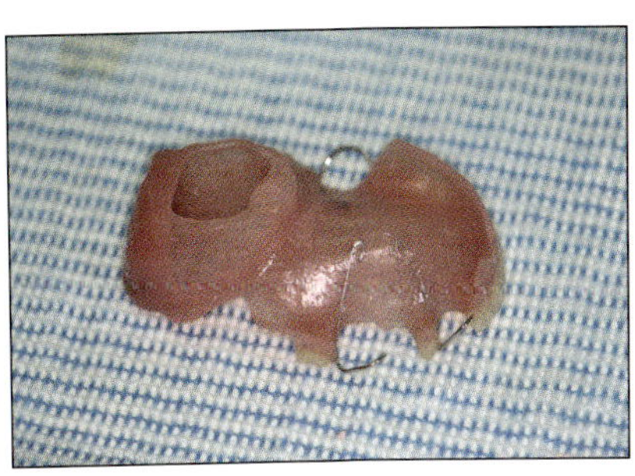

Fig. 27 After polymerization, processing for tho pharyngeal obturator part is stopped before final polishing. Maintain sufficient thickness of the part corresponding to the pharyngeal posterior wall to make it possible to adjustment and reduce the thickness later.

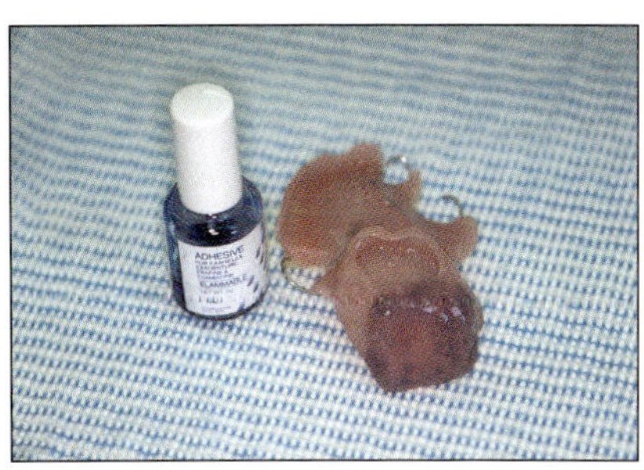

Fig. 28 Silicone adhesive agent (blue) for FIT CHECKER® is convenient to use to achieve precise compatibility for pharyngeal function. Use this agent to coat the part corresponding to the pharyngeal posterior wall (ADHESIVE®, GC Co.).

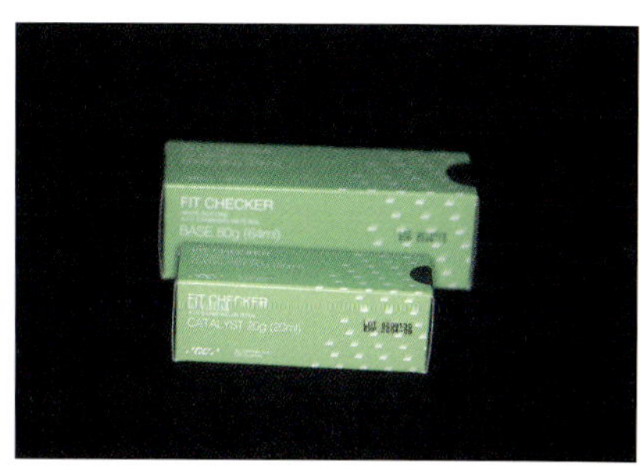

Fig. 29 (FIT CHECKER®, GC Co.)

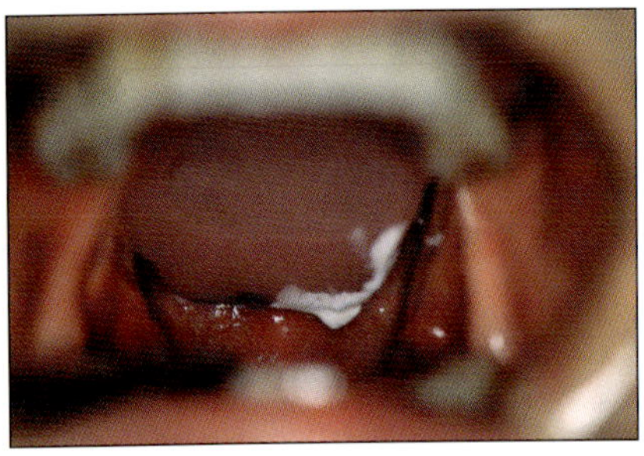

Fig. 30 Mix the retarder and softener with about 1cm of FIT CHECKER®, and apply a thin coat of this mixture to the part of the prosthesis that corresponds to the pharyngeal posterior wall, then put the prosthesis in place and have the patient make pharyngeal movements.

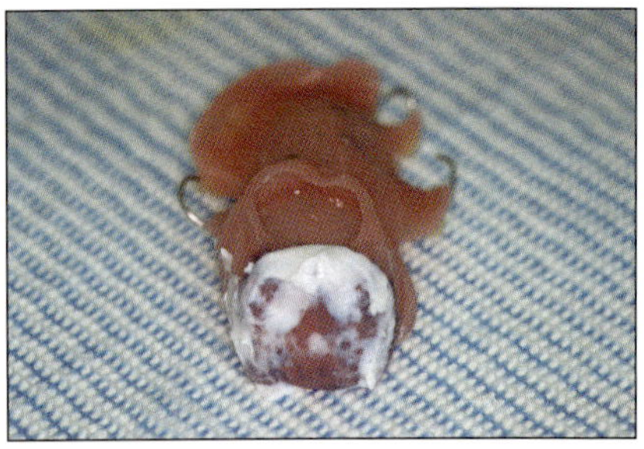

Fig. 31 After the FIT CHECKER® has cured, the prosthesis is detached. Coated area shows blue, white and pink in color. Pink means that the denture-base resin is exposed; therefore this part needs to be ground out more. Blue is the color of the adhesive agent, and blue part means that there is almost no gap, so this part is ground slightly.

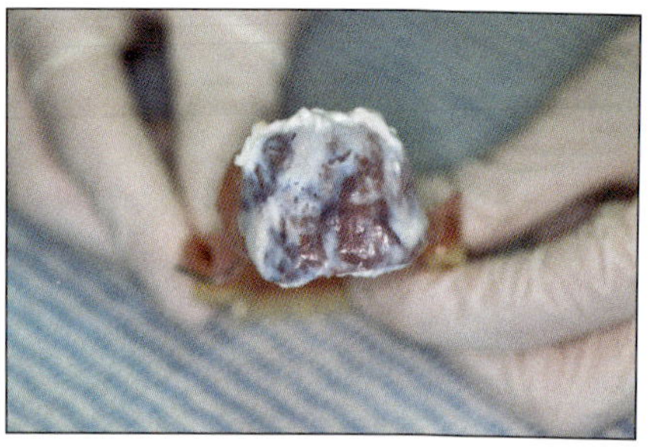

Fig. 32 White is the color of the FIT CHECKER® itself, and appearance of this part means that there is some gap, so this part is not touched. This procedure is repeated a few times until the thickness of the white part has become 0.5–1mm and adjustment is completed.

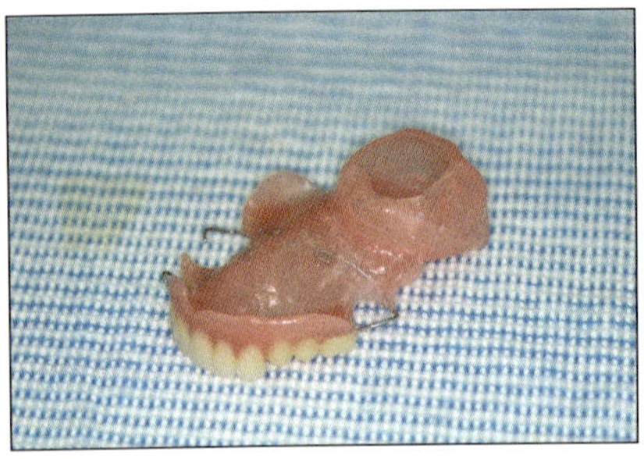

Fig. 33 To achieve good balance of the prosthesis, reduce the weight of the pharyngeal obturator by grinding out its inner surface so to be as light as the denture part. If the pharyngeal part is heavy, it can be easily become detached.

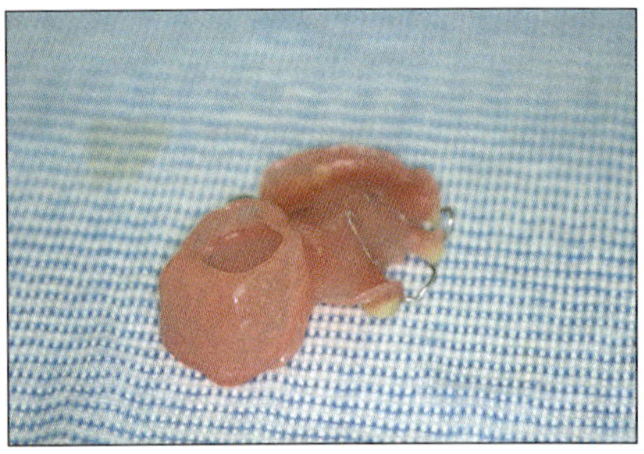

Fig. 34 This is the completed maxillodental prosthesis with open type obturator for partially edentulous patient (weight: 13.4g). Wire clasps were used for #13, 16, 27.

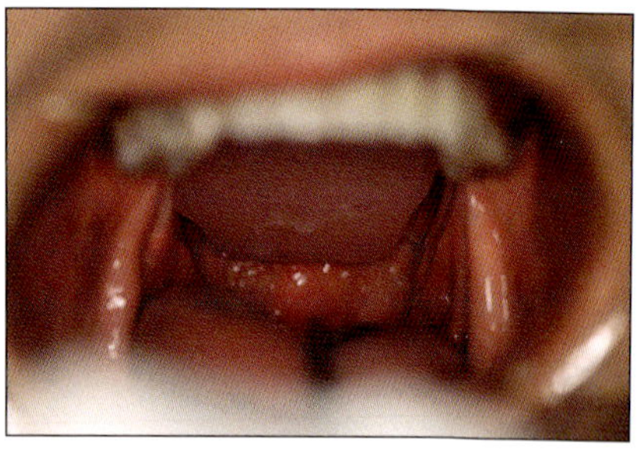

Fig. 35 View showing maxillopharyngeal prosthesis placed in position.

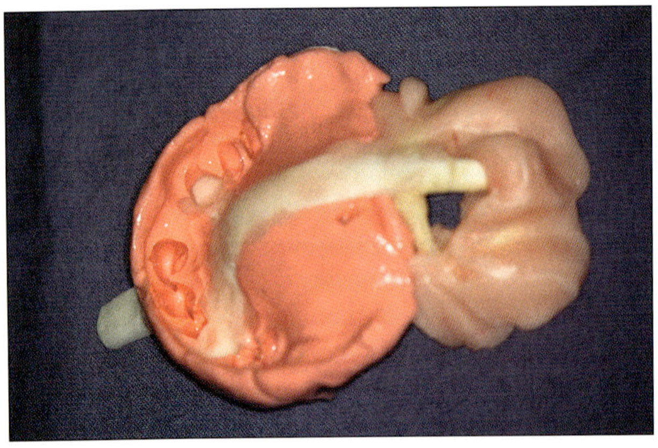

Fig. 36 Case 2. The soft palate was surgically resected with neck dissection. After 40 Gy of preoperative irradiation, followed by another 40 Gy of radiation. After the failure of secondary soft palate reconstruction with a retropharyngeal flap, prosthetic reconstruction was attempted for this case. When the patient's pharyngeal region cannot be observed well because of the limited mouth-opening or of interference by the tongue, etc., and impression-taking by the one-step method is difficult, double impression-taking is sometimes appropriate for such case.

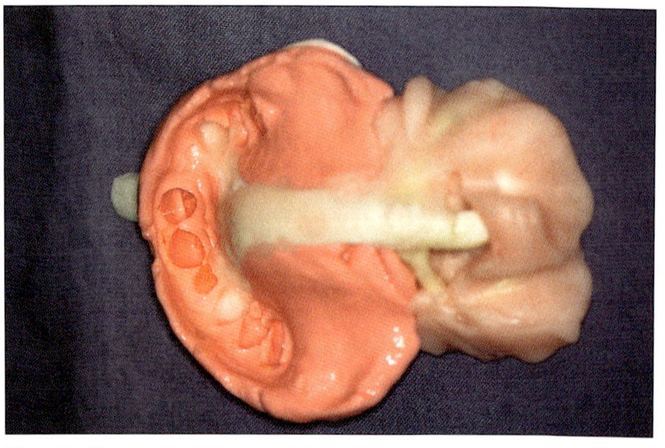

Fig. 37 First, a tray that reaches the posterior pharyngeal wall, regulated by the remaining maxillary teeth, is prepared using self-curing resin. Next, a tray for taking an impression of maxillary hard palate with dentition, is prepared by the direct method, on the tray prepared just previously. After the impression of the pharyngeal region has been taken using a non-sagging impression material, the impression of maxillary dentition and the hard palate is taken using alginate-based impression material over the impression previously taken.

Case of velopharyngeal incompetence

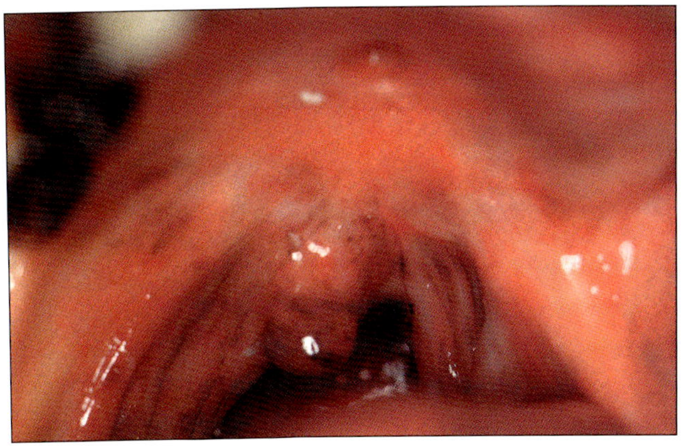

Fig. 38 Case 3. Partial excision of hard and soft palate was performed due to malignant melanoma of the palate. The first examination for the maxillary prosthesis was done on the 74th day after the operation. The soft palate has actually no tissue defect, so this is classified as a 1/6 - 0/4 defect according to the 6-4 classification.

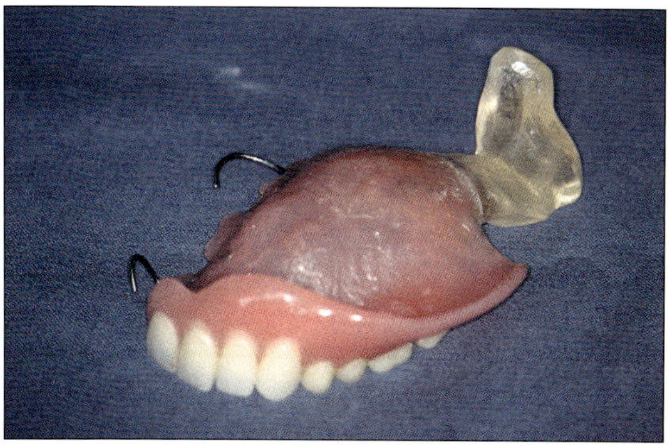

Fig. 39 There is a velopharyngeal incompetence due to dyskinesia of the soft palate. Non-chambered type maxillary defect prosthesis based on partial-denture type, or speech aid (weight: 12.7g).

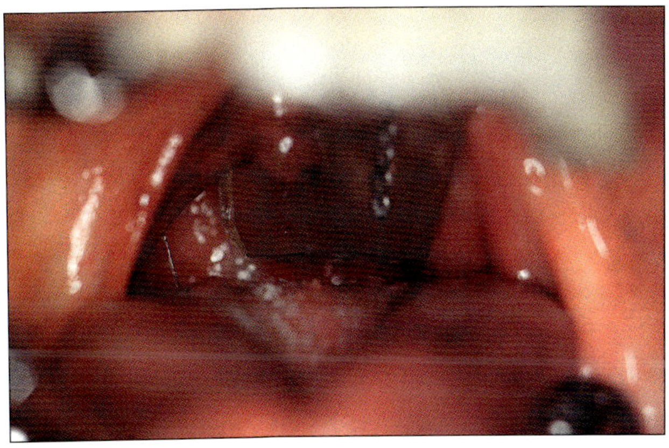

Fig. 40 View of device in place. Articulation function is well-recovered.

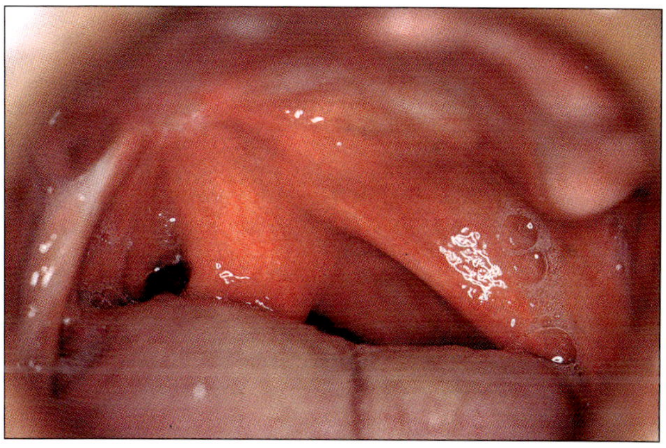

Fig. 41 Case 4. View after resection of the soft palate due to carcinoma. A round post-operative defect was spontaneously closed by scar contracture more than a year after surgery. According to the 6-4 classification, this is a 0/6 - 1/4 defect.

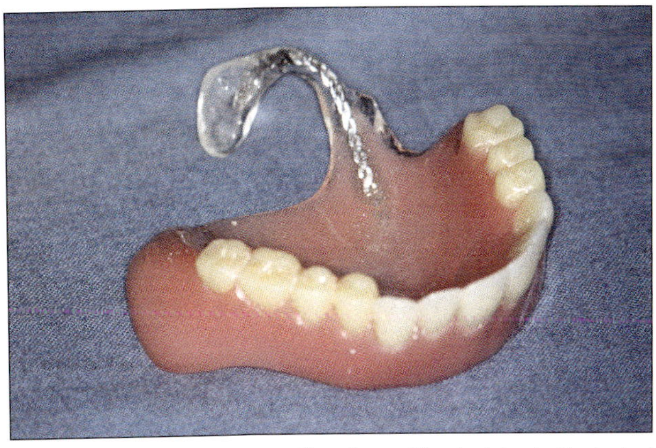

Fig. 42 This case shows malfunction without defect. Illustrated prosthesis with soft palate obturator, based on a full-denture type denture, or speech aid (weight: 15.5g).

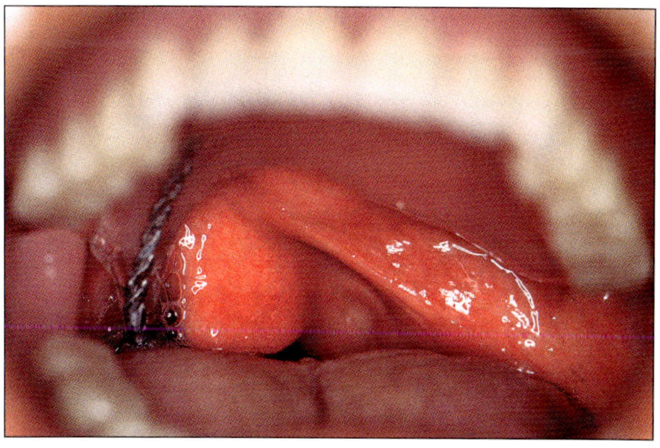

Fig. 43 View of prosthesis in place. Good recovery of function was obtained.

CHAPTER 14

Appliances for cleft lip and palate

1. Obturator feeding aid (Part 1)

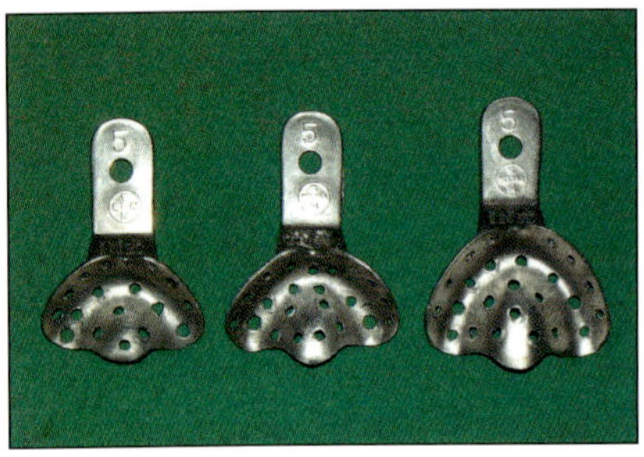

Fig. 1 A special tray must be prepared for taking the impression of the cleft palate of an infant patient shortly after birth, because ready-made trays are too large.

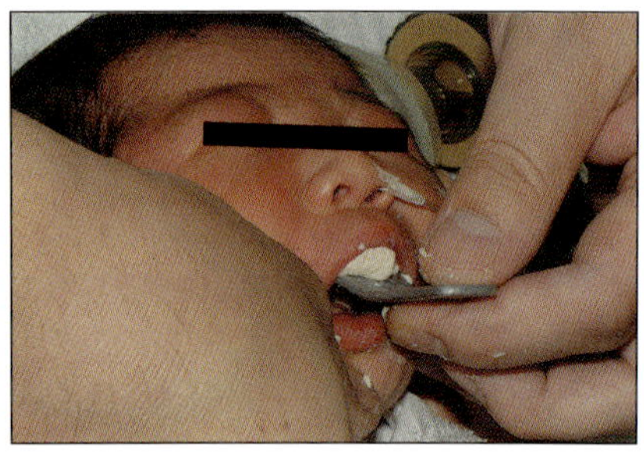

Fig. 2 Taking the impression with alginate impression material, using a tray that fits inside the patient's oral cavity

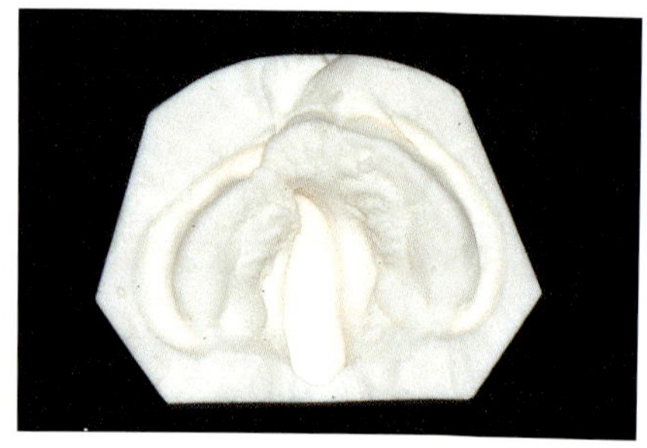

Fig. 3 Plaster model of patient's oral cavity.

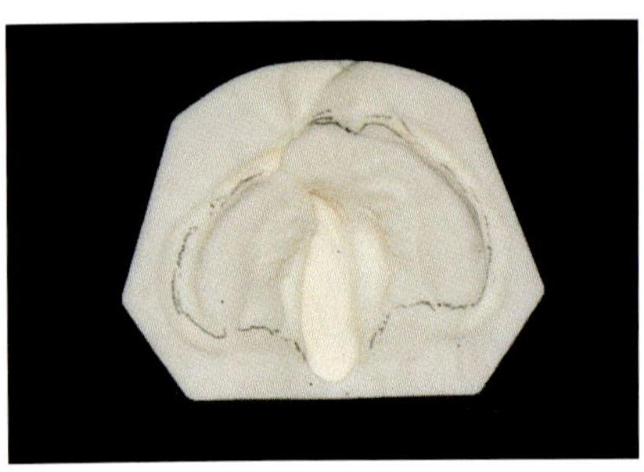

Fig. 4 Draw the outline of the palatal plate.

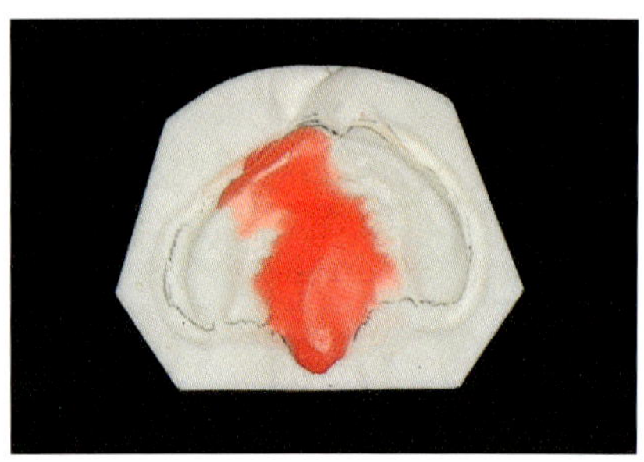

Fig. 5 Using wax, restore the parenchymal defect region such as the hard palate and cleft palate region to an ideal upper-jaw form.

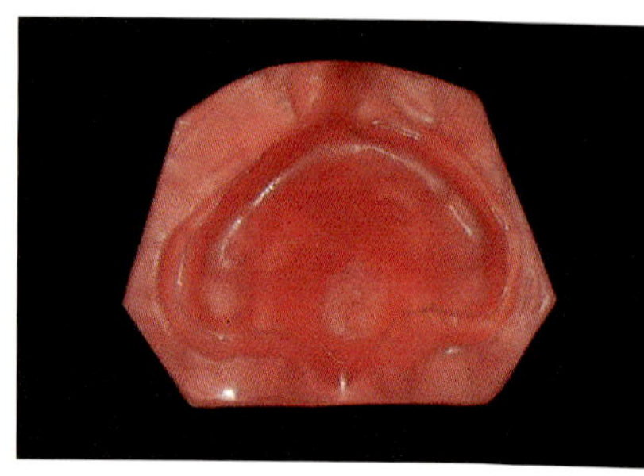

Fig. 6 After the recovery of ideal upper jaw mucous membrane form has been completed, do relief of the entire surface using 1 sheet of paraffin wax, take the impression, and prepare a duplicated model.

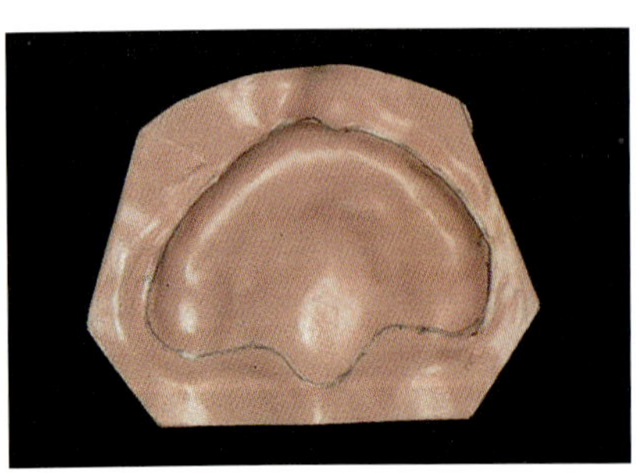

Fig. 7 Draw the bed outline on the duplicated model.

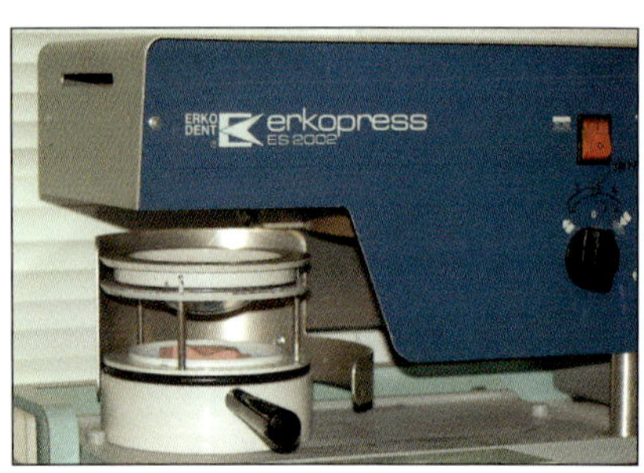

Fig. 8 Place 2mm of ERKODUR on the duplicate model, and press it using an Erkopress (ERKODENT).

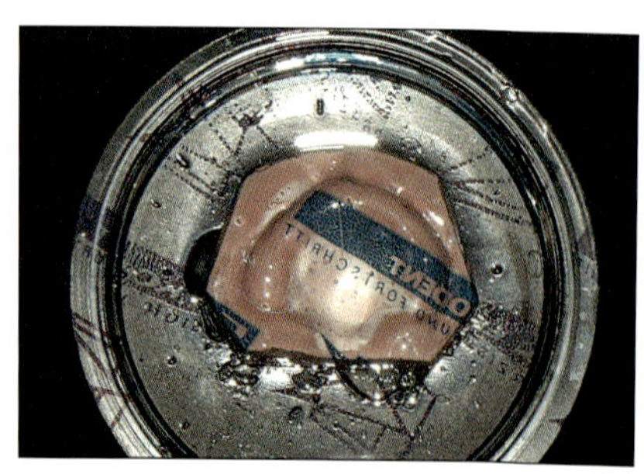

Fig. 9 The ERKODUR has been pressure-bonded to the duplicate model.

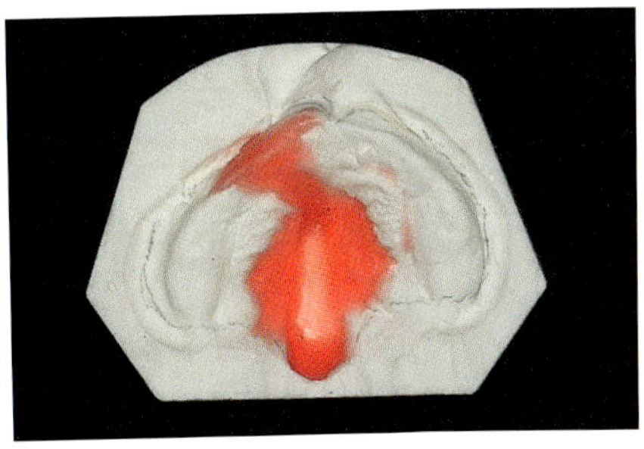

Fig. 10 On the original model, use wax to restore the form of the section where growth of the cleft palate is to be stimulated.

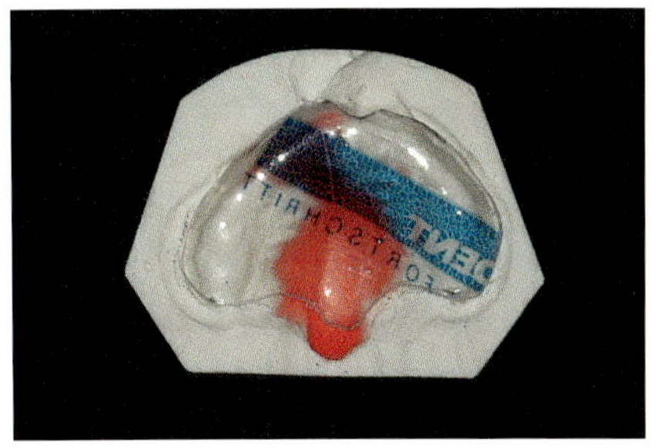

Fig. 11 Do trial fitting on the original model using ERKODUR cut to a form about 2mm smaller than the bed outline of the duplicate model.

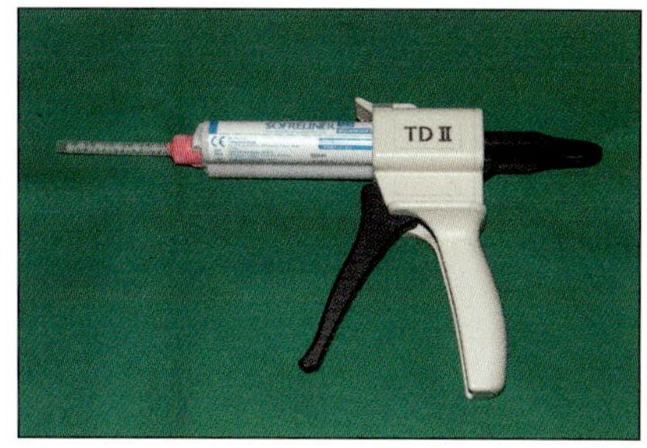

Fig. 12 Soft lining material (SOFRELINER, Tokuso) used for the inner surface of the obturator feeding aid.

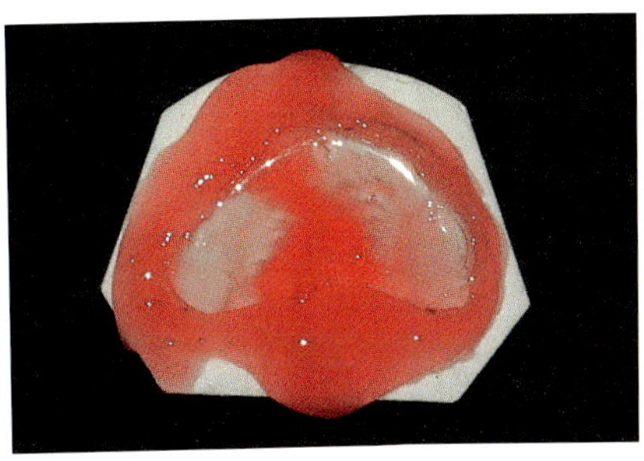

Fig. 13 The soft lining material has been attached to the inner surface of the ERKODUR and pressure-bonded.

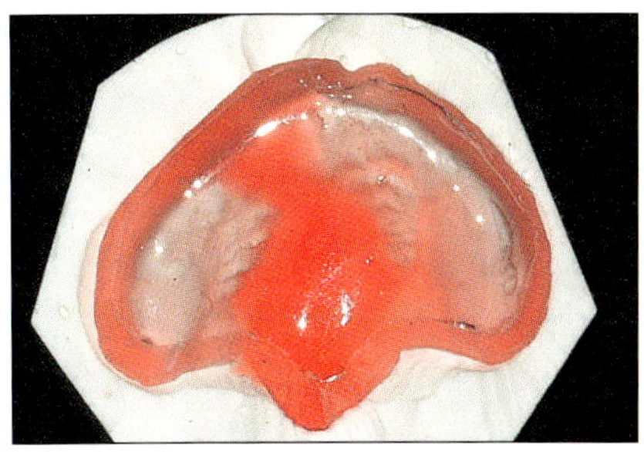

Fig. 14 After the soft lining material has cured, trim the obturator feeding aid using scissors and a cutter.

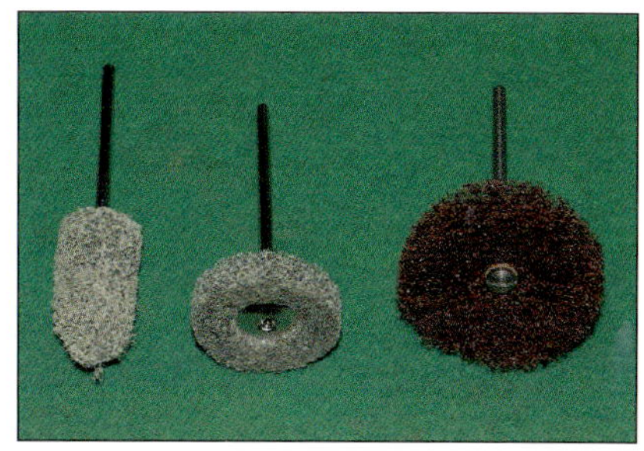

Fig. 15 Drill bits used to polish the surface of the soft lining material after cutting by scissors, etc.

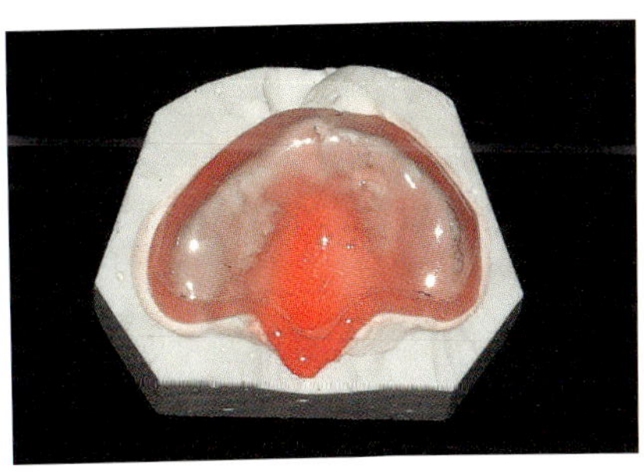

Fig. 16 The margin has been coated following polishing of the trimmed surface.

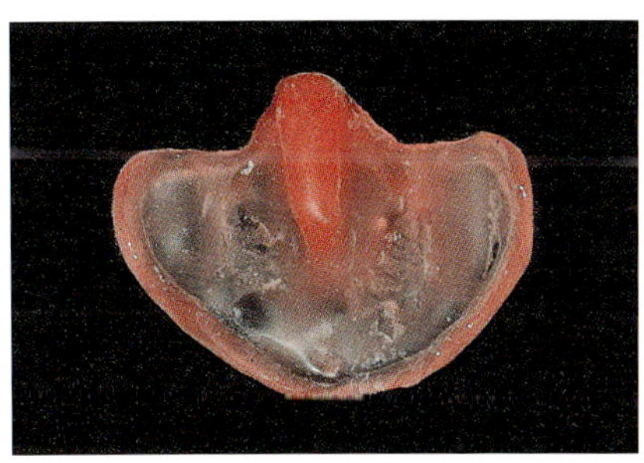

Fig. 17 There is a space in the inner section to stimulate the growth of the cleft palate section.

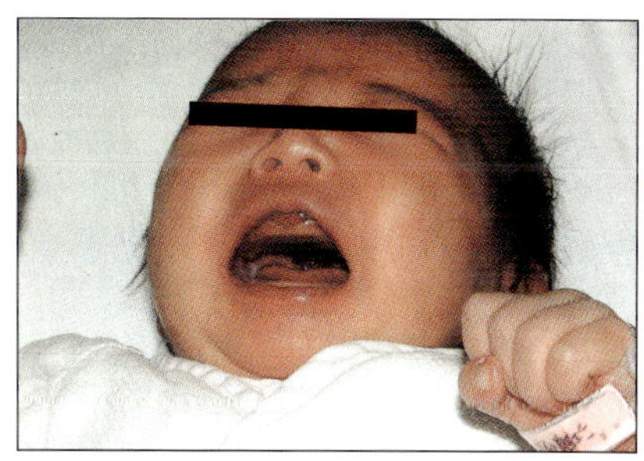

Fig. 18 The obturator feeding aid has been placed in position.

2. Obturator feeding aids (Part 2), Hotz bed

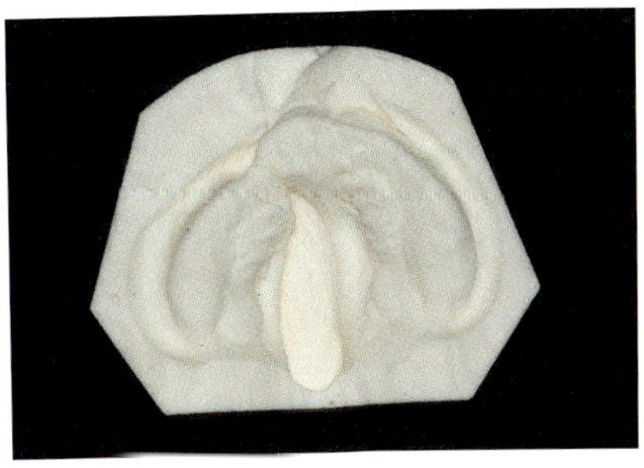

Fig. 19 Take an impression of the upper jaw of the cleft palate infant using alginate impression material, and make a plaster model.

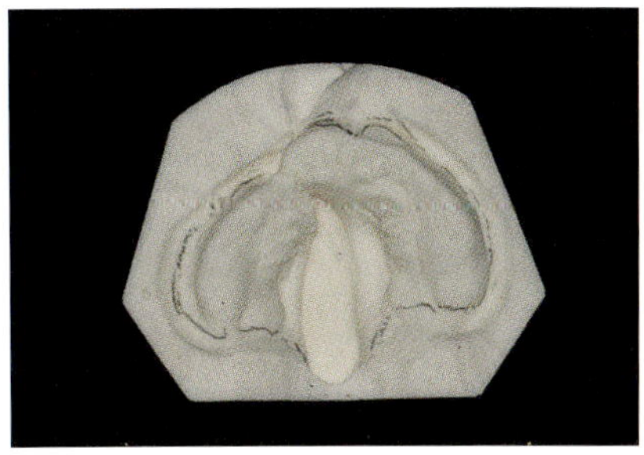

Fig. 20 Mark the outline of the obturator feeding aids for the Hotz bed.

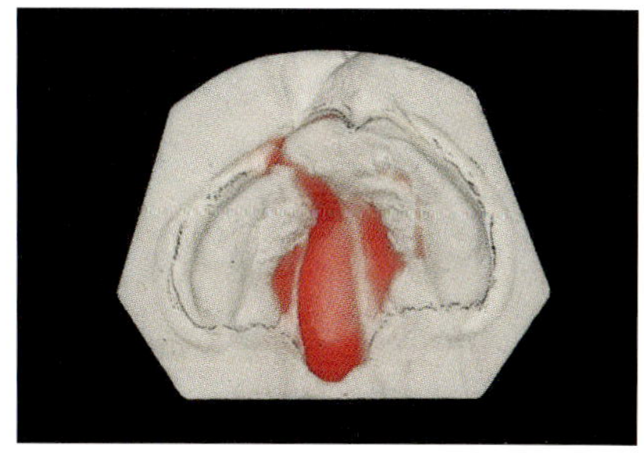

Fig. 21 Define the undercutting region of the cleft palate relief region, and make a duplicate impression of the plaster model.

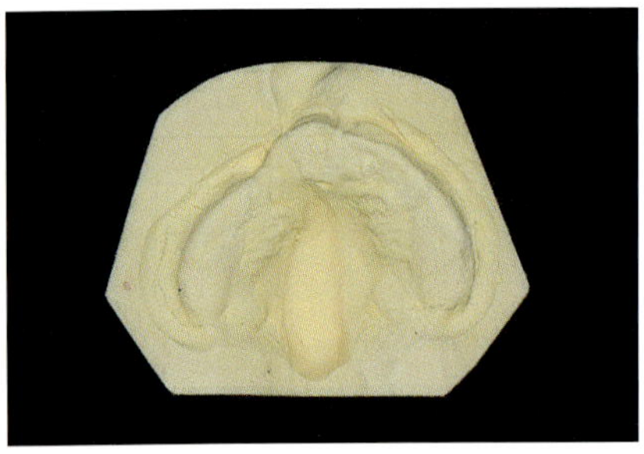

Fig. 22 Duplicate the model after doing relief of undercutting of the cleft palate.

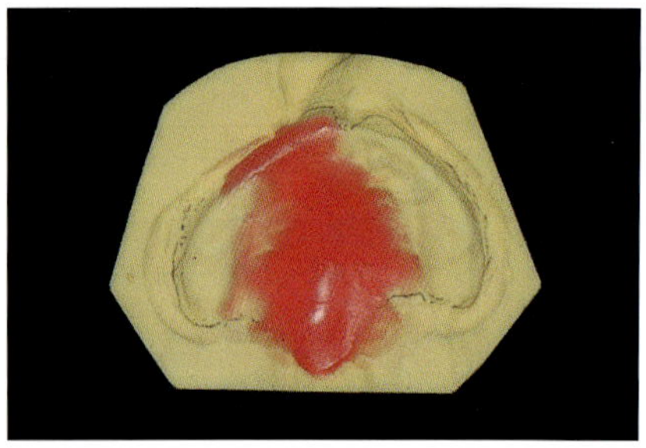

Fig. 23 After the outline of the palate has been marked on the duplicated stone cast, modify the palate form using wax to create an ideal form.

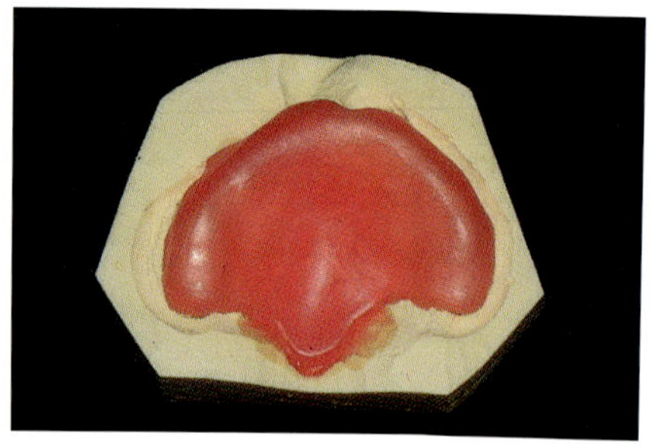

Fig. 24 Wax up the palatal plate using a sheet of paraffin wax or wax sheet about 2 mm thick. At this time, adjust the form of the wax on the edge of the plate to make it slightly rounded.

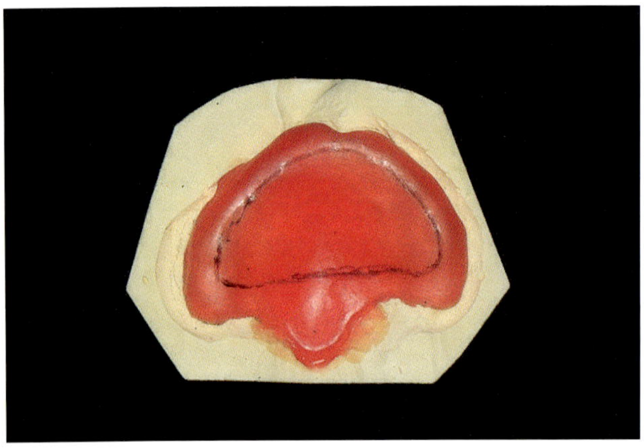

Fig. 25

(1) Draw the outline of the hard resin using an oil-based marker, with the alveolar crest as a guide.
(2) Apply a coating of Vaseline on the surface of the paraffin wax as a separating agent, to 2 – 3mm outside of the outline of the hard resin.
(3) Using double layers (thickness: approx. 0.9mm) of #26 sheet wax, press so that the sheet wax layers contact the outline of the plate, then fuse the periphery and adjust the form as needed.
(4) Finish the soft palate and hard palate region as a gently sloping form.

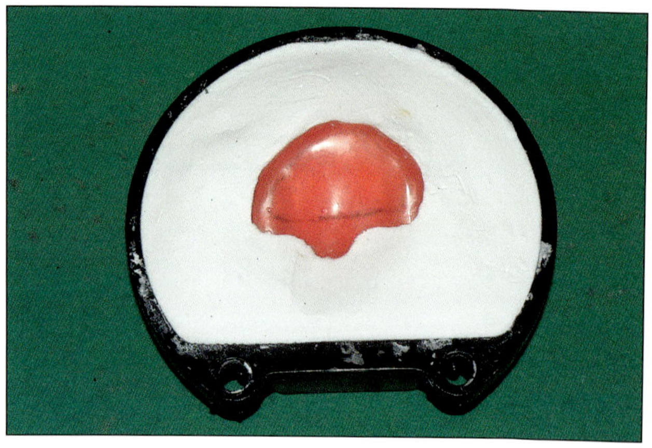

Fig. 26

(1) Soak the model so it absorbs sufficient water, and embed it in the bottom flask. At this time, sink the periphery of the wax pattern about 1 mm into the plaster.
(2) After the plaster has cured, coat the surface with separating agent, and set up the top flask to complete the embedding of the model.

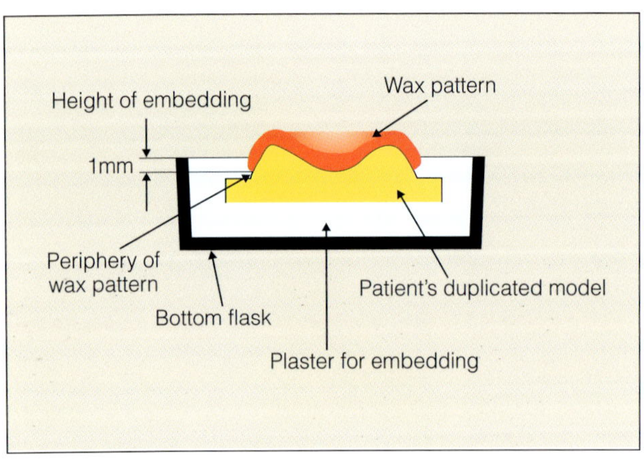

Fig. 27 Embedding in bottom flask.

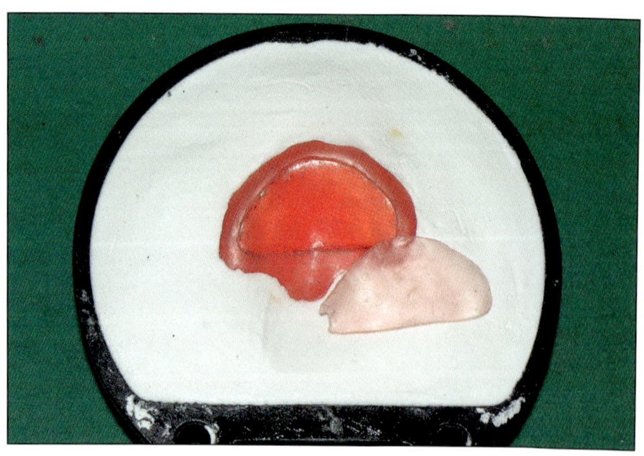

Fig. 28

(1) After the plaster has cured, separate the flasks without heating them, in order to prevent deformation of the wax.
(2) Make a cut with a knife along the outline drawn on the palatal region of wax remaining in the bottom flask, and cut out the sheet wax.

Fig. 29
(1) Apply a coat of resin-separating agent on sections other than the palatal center region in the top flask. In order for the thermopolymerizing resin to adhere, the resin-separating agent is not applied to the palatal center region.
(2) Fill the cavity of the wax palatal region in the bottom flask with clear thermopolymerizing resin via a polyethylene film, and remove burrs at least twice.
(3) Press the filled clear thermopolymerized resin at ordinary temperature for about 15 minutes.
(4) Separate top and bottom flasks, and eliminate the wax of the bottom flask. Hard resin adheres to the palatal region in the top flask.
(5) After coating the bottom flask with resin-separating agent, fill with soft rebase material.
(6) Polymerization requires 1 hour in the range from room temperature to 70°C, and a further 1 hour at 100°C.

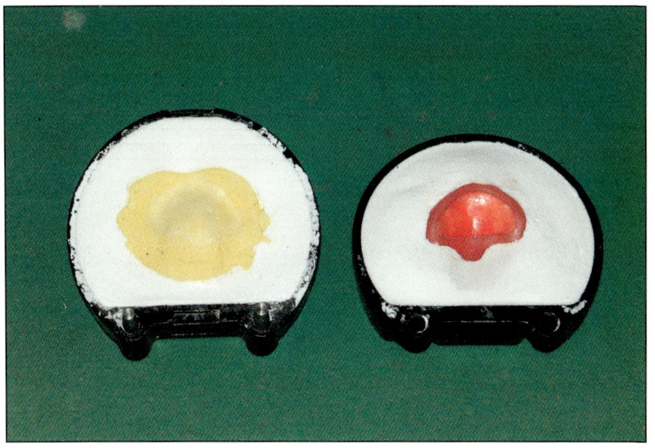

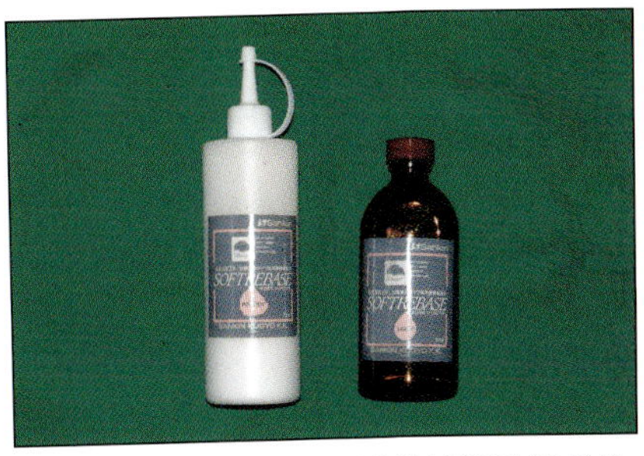

Fig. 30 Soft rebase (SANKIN KOGYO K.K., Japan) is used for the palatal mucous membrane surface of the Hotz plate.

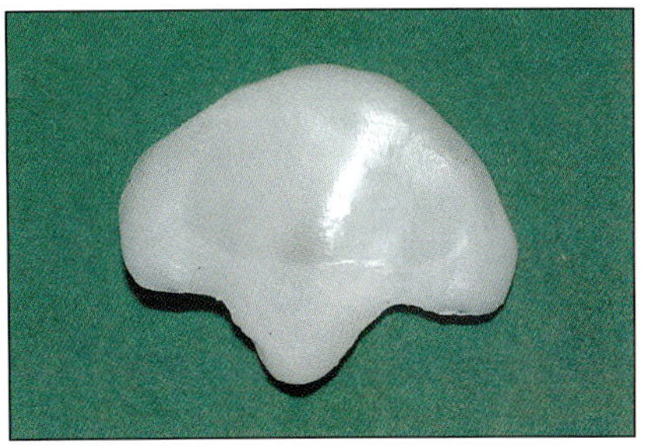

Fig. 31 After polymerization is complete, polish the soft rebase material to finish it. Clear hard resin is adhered to the soft rebase material at the center of the palatal region.

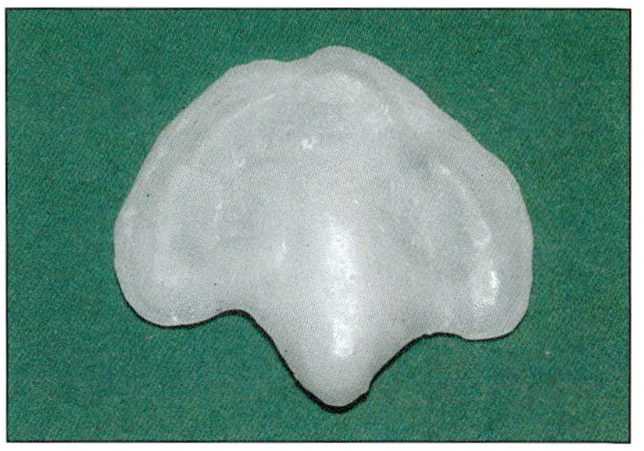

Fig. 32 The entire surface in contact with mucous membrane is soft rebase material.

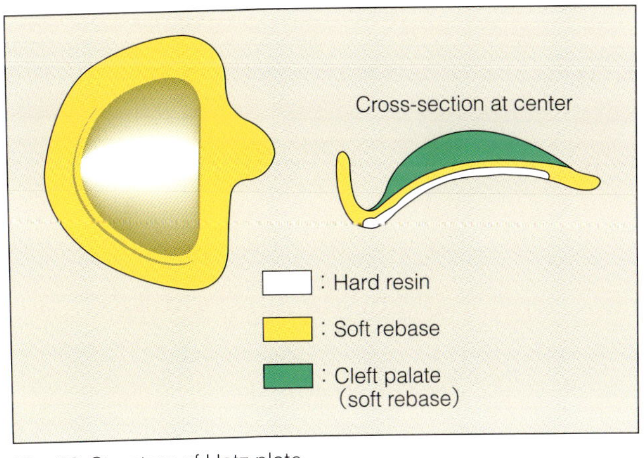

Fig. 33 Structure of Hotz plate.

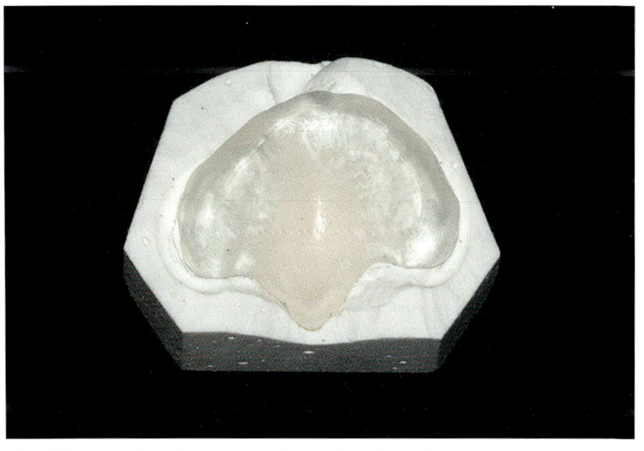

Fig. 34 The plate is set into the patient's oral cavity.

SECTION 4

Mandibular Defects

CHAPTER 15

Classifications of mandibular defects and treatment planning

Classification

The following shows classifications of mandibular defects proposed to date. However, many of these are not directly related to the actual work of prosthesis production.

The purposes of classification must be clarified prior to adopting a classification. When classifying mandibular defects for reference to treatment, the degree of disability due to each defect, and possible treatment methods, must be considered. When the classification is for the purpose of presenting the results of research to an academic society, a widely accepted classification is desirable.

Some classifications have already been attempted, but these were made on the basis of the prosthetic techniques of those times; therefore under present circumstances in which implants are extensively used, treatments and classifications do not match with such obsolete classifications in some aspects.

1) Classification by Conter [1] (Fig. 1)

Conter et al. designed classifications of I – V for the study of edentulous-jaw patients and the evaluation of jaw prosthetic methods at the time. This classification is based on a concept of prosthetics used in the past.

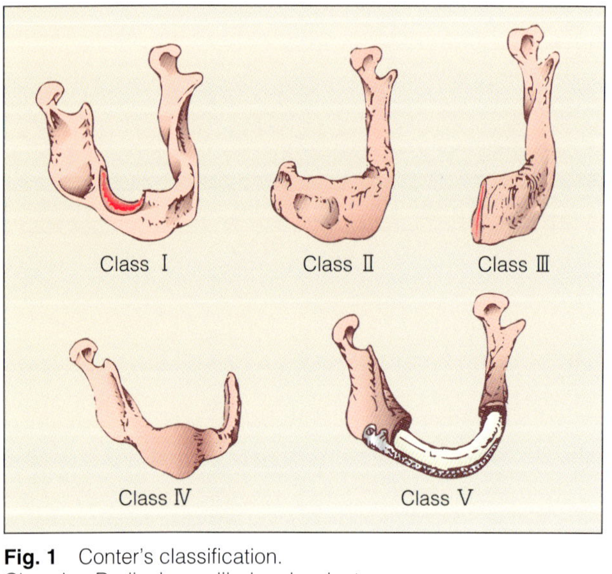

Fig. 1 Conter's classification.
Class I : Radical mandibular alveolectomy.
Class II : Lateral mandibular resection.
Class III : Lateral mandibular resection. (A) without hemiglossectomy, and (B) in conjunction with hemiglossectomy.
Class IV : Lateral bone and split-thickness skin graft.
Class V : Anterior bone and split-thickness skin graft.

2) Classification by Kobayashi [2]

Kobayashi classified mandibular defects with consideration of mandibular continuity and temporomandibular joints, with the aim of understanding the degree of difficulty of treatment in each case.

3) Classification by Matsuura [3]

Matsuura's classification was made with consideration of the degree of difficulty of oral and maxillofacial prosthetic treatment. This classification includes facial defects, maxillary defects and mandibular defects. Therefore, the pathological status of such a variety of defects is clearly expressed. The severity of such defects is precisely reflected. As a result, easy evaluation of treatment is to be expected.

4) Classification by Furuta [4] (Fig. 2)

Pathological conditions of defects are expected to be clearly classified for understanding by other clinicians. Mandibular defects and results of various treatments can easily be compared using this classification, allowing information about such defects to be used for reference in treatment by other clinicians.

Matters requiring special attention for jaw prosthetics

The basic diseases that have caused mandibular defects, such as malignant tumors, must be thoroughly understood. Depending on the disease that has caused a defect, there is a possibility of some limitations in prosthetic treatment. In the case of a malignant tumor, we must always assume that there is a possibility of recurrence of the malignancy. Malignant tumors sometimes reoccur during prosthetic treatment. When the compatibility of a prosthesis has suddenly become poor, and when reddening and a new tumor occur quickly, this must be reported to the oral surgeon, with consideration of the possibility of recurrence of the malignant tumor. In malignant tumor cases, there must be thorough communication with the oral surgeon and radiologist, and the medical information must be understood before creating maxillary prosthetics. It is also necessary to thoroughly understand how well the patient and the patient's family comprehend the pathological condition. It is because explanation of a disease to a patient with a malignant tumor and to the family is always delicate.

Table 1 MR classification. Note) No application of M3a

M factor (mandibular defect form)	Mark
1. Alveolar process defect	M1
a. Anterior tooth part	M1a
b. Posterior tooth part	M1b
c. Extensive part	M1c
2. Partial defect of mandible	M2
a. Anterior tooth part	M2a
b. Posterior tooth part	M2b
c. Extensive part	M2c
3. Defect of one side of mandible	M3
b. Dissected part is posterior tooth part	M3b
c. Dissected parts are anterior tooth part/ posterior tooth part on opposite sides	M3c
R factor (Existence of reconstruction)	
Yes	R0
No	R1

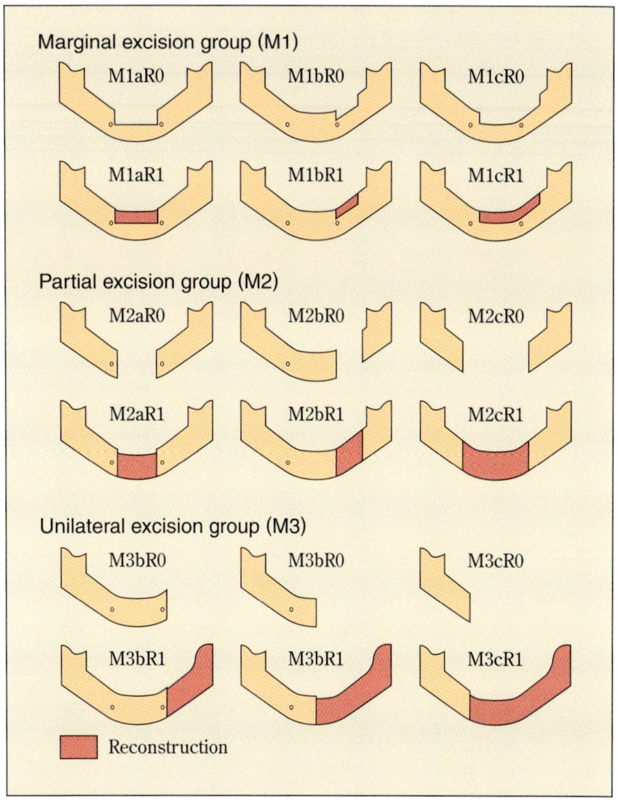

Fig. 2 MR classification of mandibular defects.

Items to be examined for planning of treatment

The following matters should be examined prior to planning treatment for cases in which there are accompanying mandibular defects. The treatment plan should be considered on the basis of these items.

1) Disabilities caused by defects

Before treatment it is necessary to thoroughly consider which matters should be assigned the greatest importance, and also how to conquer the disability. It is necessary to thoroughly understand the patient's requests before treatment. Disabilities caused by defects include masticatory disturbances, speech disturbances, and swallowing disorder. Imperfect closure of lips, poor saliva control, and esthetic disabilities are also important elements from the viewpoint of social life.

In examination of the mandibular defect region, further mandiblular elements are the presence of an alveolar ridge, the number of remaining teeth, existence of masticatory muscles and lateral displacement by muscles. Additional important elements are maxillary defects, opposing teeth, positional relationship between the maxillary alveolar ridge and mandibular alveolar ridge, and of mouth opening range.

2) Applicable treatments

It is important to consider and secure the staff, techniques, and equipment that can be used in the concerned medical institution. The levels of ordinary dental treatment, reconstructive techniques such as various attachments, implants and bone grafts, and hyperbaric oxygen treatment, must be carefully examined and confirmed.

3) Cases in which the mandible is not reconstructed

In some cases, oral function can be recovered to a certain degree using a maxillodental prosthesis even without reconstructing the mandible. When reconstruction of the mandible is judged to be necessary, bone graft is done, and the reconstructed mandible should be re-evaluated regarding its position, height, width and degree of absorption before initiating prosthetic treatment.

4) Cases in which mandible has been reconstructed

When the mandible has already been reconstructed, the variety of mandibular used for reconstruction, condition of reconstruction of mandibular body and alveolar part, and, sometimes, whether the soft tissue covering the alveolar ridge is mucous membrane or skin, are evaluated.

5) Formulation of final plan

Prior to determining the form of prosthesis, it is necessary to consider whether it is possible to use an ordinary maxillodental prosthesis or an implant denture, then to consider the design of the prosthesis and the occlusal relationship, etc.

References

1) Robert Conter & Thomas A, Curtis: Prosthetic management of edentulous mandibulectomy patient. Part I. anatomic, physiologic, and psychologic consideration. J.Prosth.Dent 25:446-4571971.
2) Shunzou Kobayashi: Maxillary & Mandibular Prosthetics. J Jap Dent Assoc. 31:1207-1215, 1979. (in Japanese)
3) Masaro Matsuura: Forms and classifications of maxillofacial prosthetics. (Maxillofacial prosthetics) The Dental. 2:333-344, 1984 (in Japanese)
4) Isao Furuta, Masayuki Iwai. The forms and classification of mandibular defect. -Study of MR classifications-. Dental Journal 38(4):485-489, 1993. (in Japanese)

CHAPTER 16

Fabrication method for mandibular prostheses – from impression taking to placement –

1. Production method for mandibular prostheses

The mandible can be considered one of the central elements of oral and maxillofacial function because the mandible itself moves and, in the same time, provides support for surrounding soft tissue.

Cases for which mandibular prostheses are used show a very wide range of postoperative forms including reconstruction of the mandibular arch and reconstruction of soft tissue defects by various skin flaps, in addition to cases in which no reconstruction has been done following marginal mandiblectomy and segmental resection of the mandible. There are also many cases for mandibular prostheses, in which the main defect is a buccal defect or defect of the tongue and oral floor, accompanied by a mandibular defect.

Due to the mandibular complex functions, there are many cases in which improvement of all problems cannot be expected simultaneously at the time of improvement of one main problem caused by mandibular defect. We should consider various matters such as, "What can be done by the mandibular prosthesis? Can the improvement of ingestion and swallowing disorders be achieved? Can the improvement of disarticulation or esthetic disorders be achieved? Or is such improvement impossible to achieve?"

Taking of actual impression

Actual impression taking for maxillofacial prosthetics, just as for prosthetics for other regions, it is important to use procedures and materials which the operator has been employing daily and has become skilled in using.

There are no drastic differences between the taking of impressions for mandibular prostheses and for ordinary prostheses, because of the danger of aspiration is relatively small due to the characteristics of this region while a large quantity of impression material is needed at one time. It is necessary to become practiced in the method of achieving proper timing of the mixing of impression material. In particular, insertion of the tray to the area and muscle trimming demand great skill. It is no exaggeration to say that the form of prosthesis on the regions other than masticatory mucosa is determined by impression taking. A total of 3 persons, 1 operator and 2 assistants, is needed for the impression taking of prostheses. The operator directs the mixing of impression material while removing saliva from the region where the impression will be taken, keeping the region in appropriate condition. The 2 assistants start mixing impression material almost simultaneously.

When the mixing of impression material is complete, one assistant heaps up the impression material on a ready-made tray. Another assistant passes the mixed impression material to the operator. The operator quickly spreads the impression material on the dried region to take the impression, using a spatula. Next, the operator inserts the tray with enough impression material into the patient's oral cavity.

After that, the patient is asked to do a check of tongue and lip movements for muscle trimming just as for an ordinary dental prosthesis, and waits for curing of the impression material.

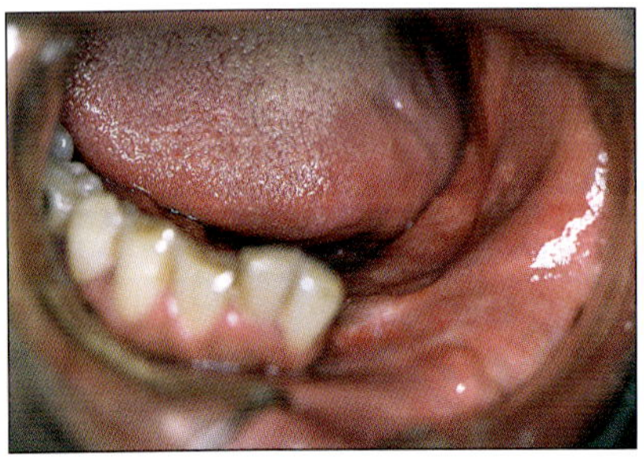

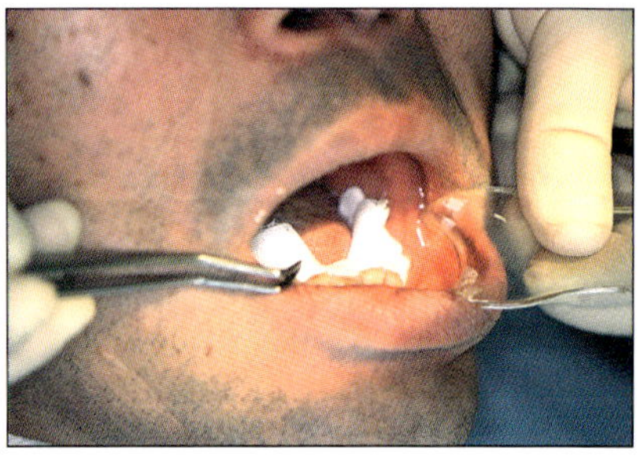

Fig. 1 *(left)* 50-year-old male, left side mandibular gingival cancer. Subsequent to the left side segmental resection of mandible and bridging of the defect. Mandibular defect in #32–37 region, with hyper mobility of the soft tissue of the defect area. Residual teeth are #17–27, #31–46.

Fig. 2 *(right)* Place the patient in Semi-Fowler position. After try-in of the ready-made tray, wait for the mixing of impression material, while wiping off saliva with gauze-sponges.

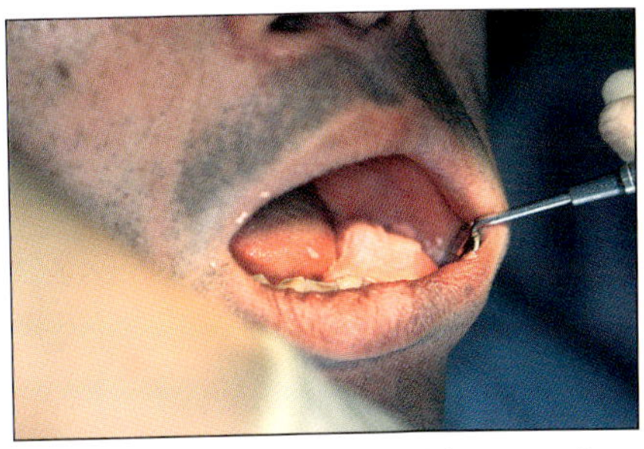

Fig. 3 Impression material is spread on the region where the impression taking is to be done.

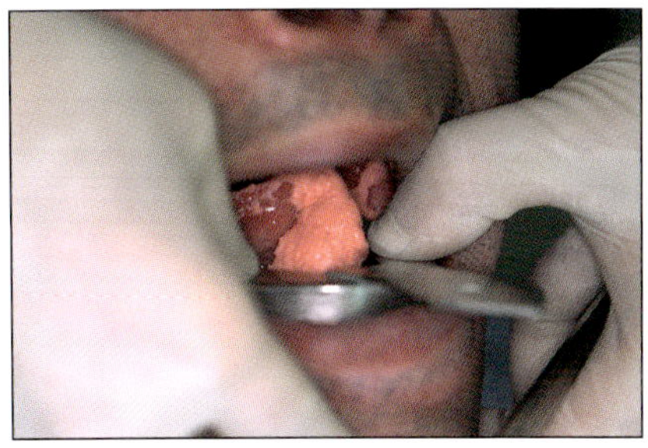

Fig. 4 Impression material is heaped up on a ready-made tray in the same way as for ordinary preliminary impression taking, and the impression material on the tray is pushed onto the top of the impression material previously spread on the impression region.

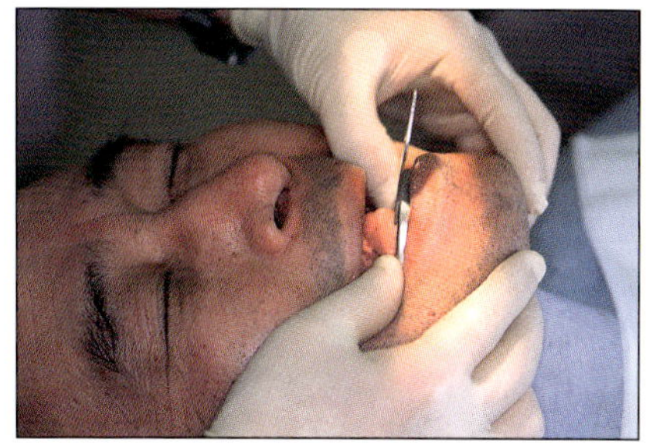

Fig. 5 Have the patient move the tongue and buccal region and then carry out muscle trimming. Waiting for curing of the impression material while holding the tray.

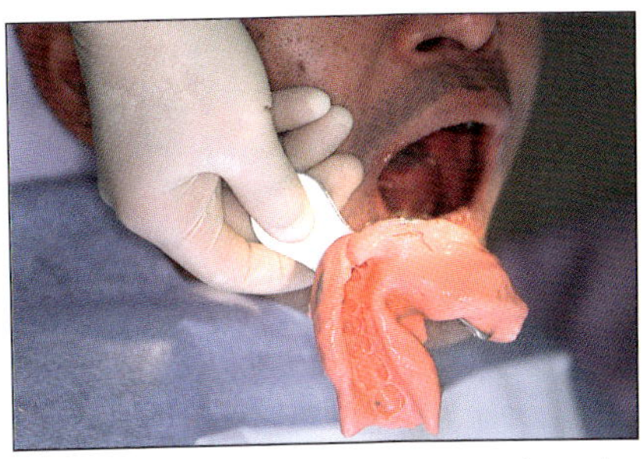

Fig. 6 The tray is taken out after the impression material has cured. The custom tray is prepared immediately.

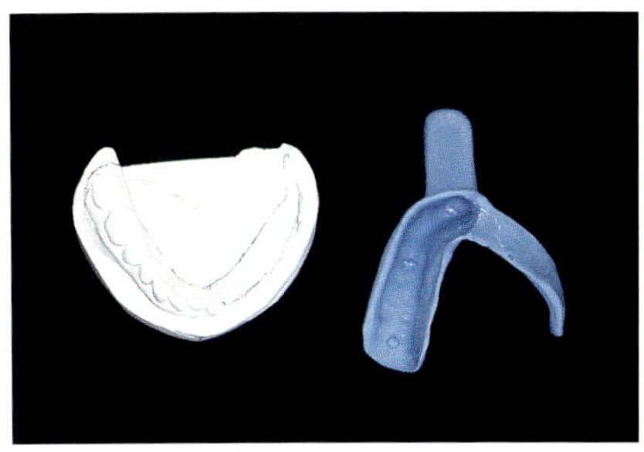

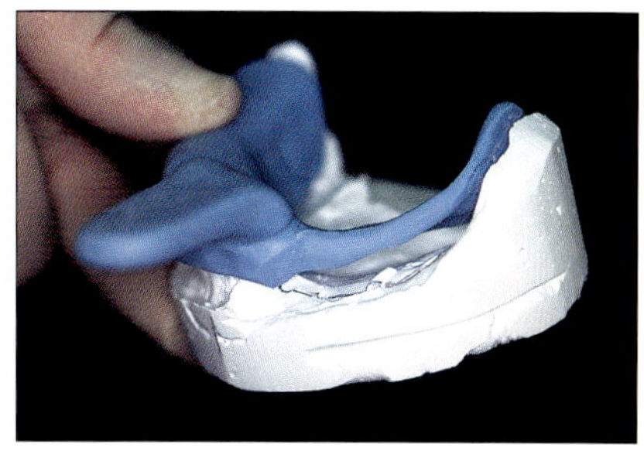

Figs. 7 and 8 Prepare a preliminary model using dental stone and examine it to determine the range for final impression taking, and prepare the custom tray. The thickness of the impression material at the time of final impression taking is adjusted by paraffin wax in accordance with the mobility of the soft tissue. One sheet of paraffin wax is used for the healthy side and 3 – 4 sheets are used for the defect side. Estimated thickness of impression material on the defect side in this case was approximately 7mm.

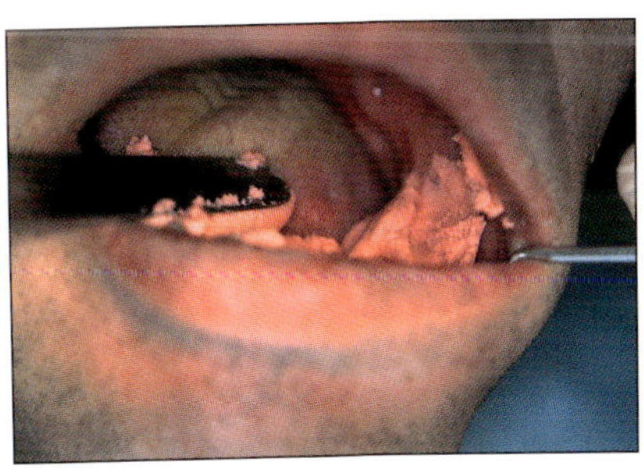

Fig. 9 The final impression-taking procedure is the same as the preliminary impression-taking procedure. Dry the inside of the oral cavity, and carefully apply a coating of impression material, mainly on the mandibular defect side. The impression material is mixed so it is slightly softer than that used for preliminary impression-taking to improve its flow.

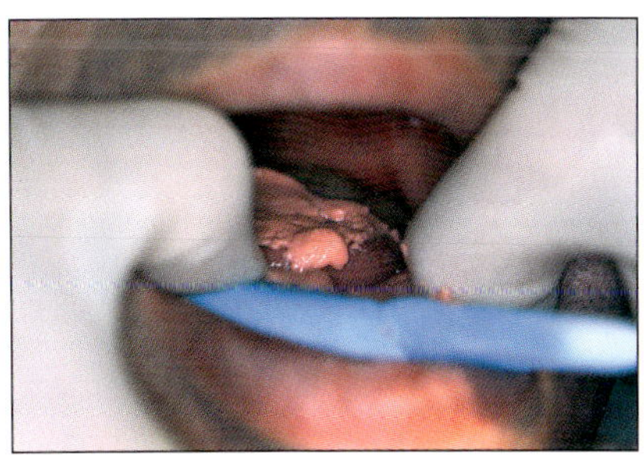

Fig. 10 Coating with adhesive agent (Technicol Bond®, GC Co.) for alginate impression material in advance.

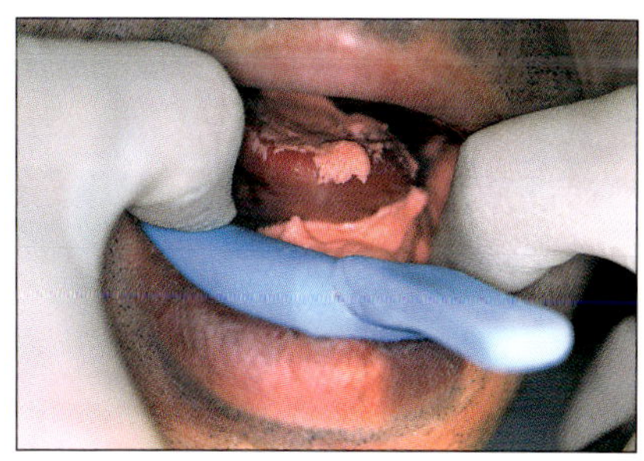

Fig. 11 Careful impression taking with border moulding.

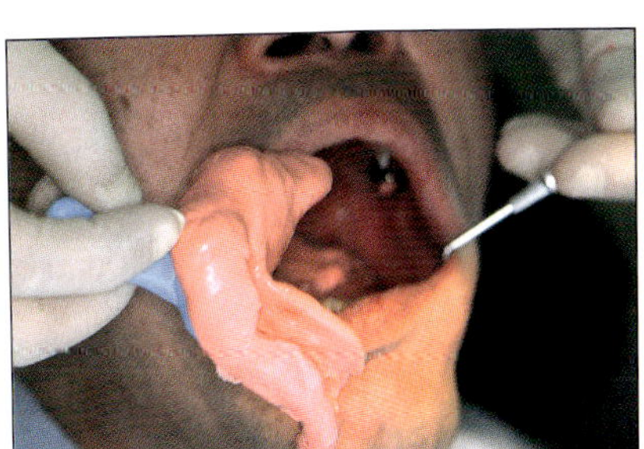

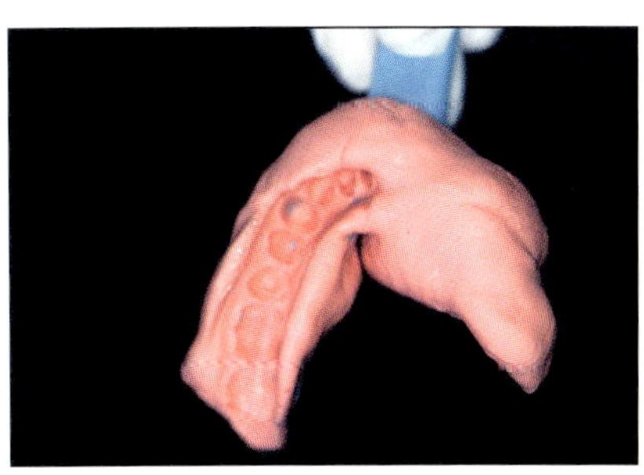

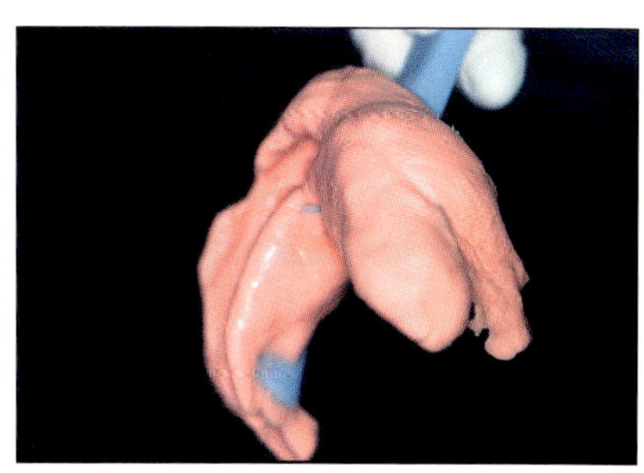

Figs. 12 to 14 The final impression is taken out.

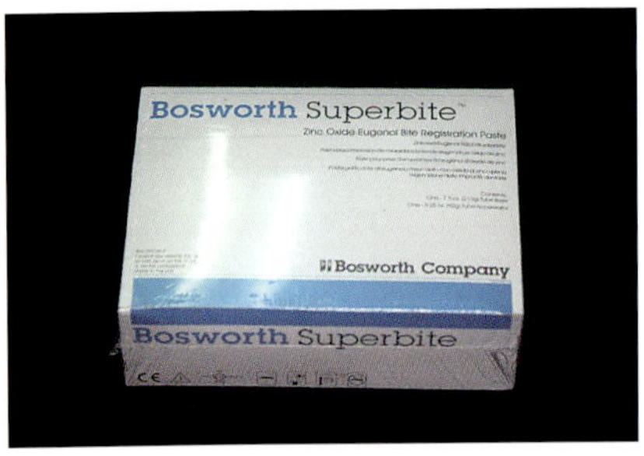

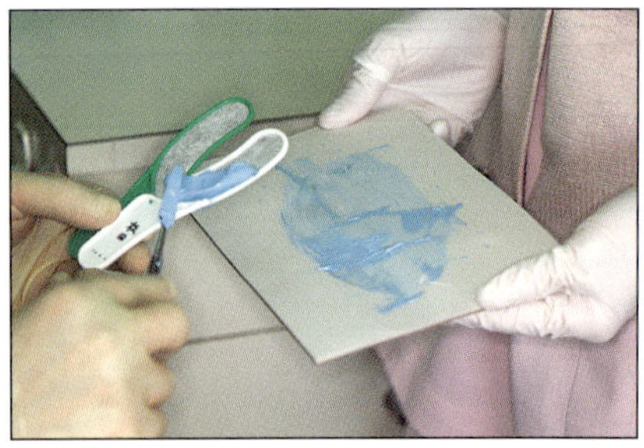

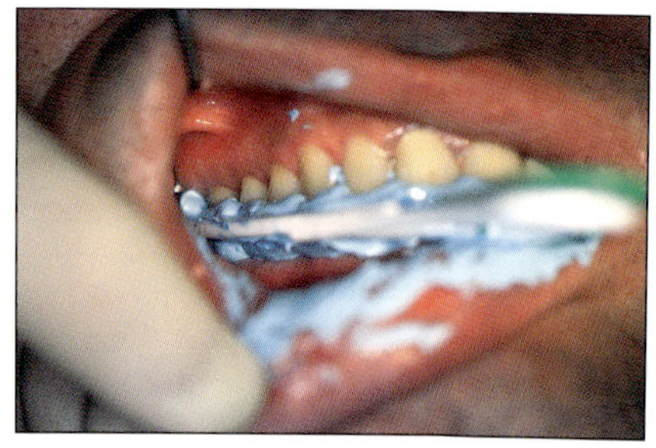

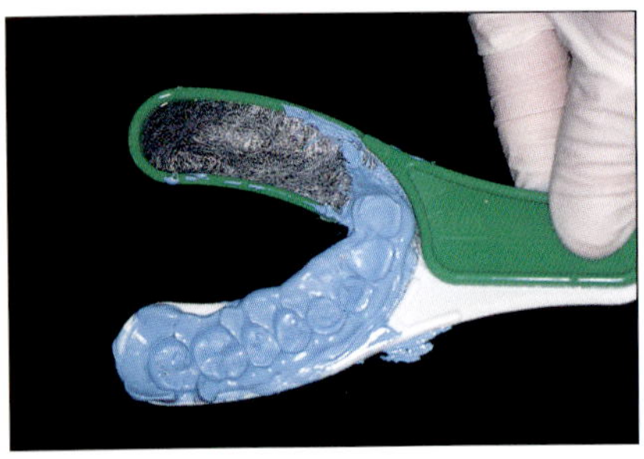

Figs. 15 to 18 Bite taking: When the intercuspal position is stabilized between the remaining teeth, registration of interocclusal relationship is done using bite paste. If possible, it is desirable to record not only the occlusal surfaces but also to record the counter-relations of teeth and gum(s). Bite paste used in this case: Bosworth Superbite®.

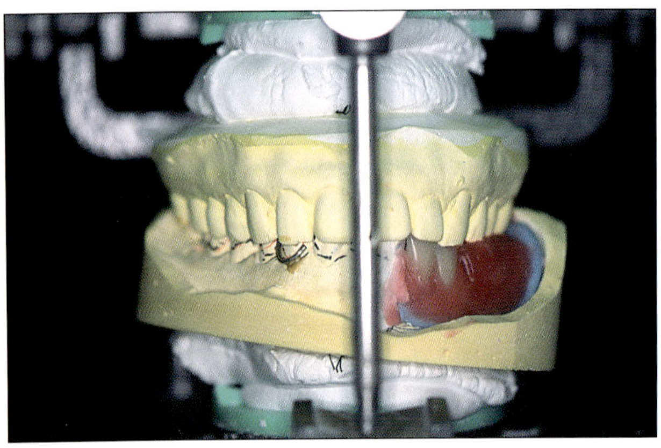

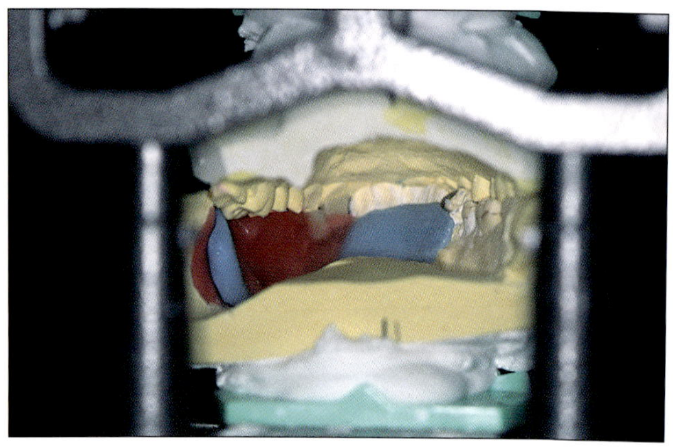

Figs. 19 and 20 The bite record taken is immediately placed on an articulator, and artificial teeth are arranged on the bite rim only in the front tooth region.

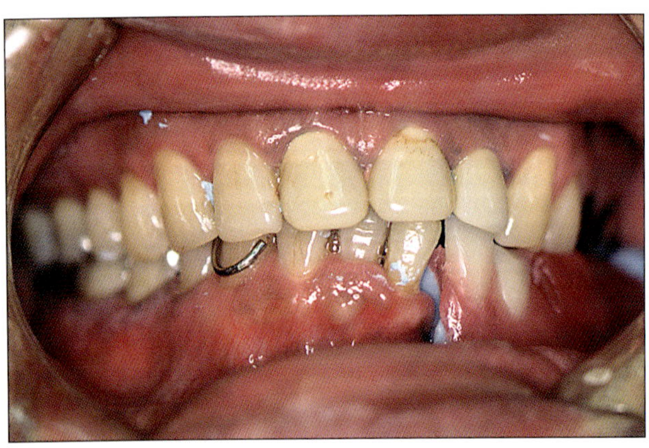

Fig. 21 Try-in: The compatibility of the prosthesis for the mandibular defect region is of far greater importance than the teeth; therefore doing a try-in for artificial teeth only in the region of the front teeth will suffice. In this case, a wire clasp was temporarily used for #43 for stabilization at the time of try-in. If the result of the try-in is good, the same process as for ordinary denture preparation is then carried out.

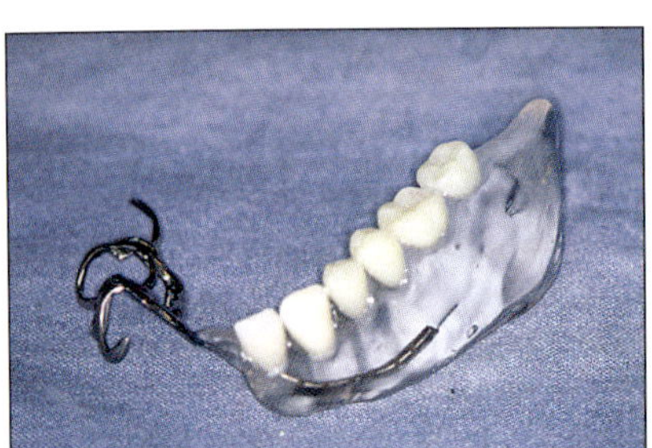

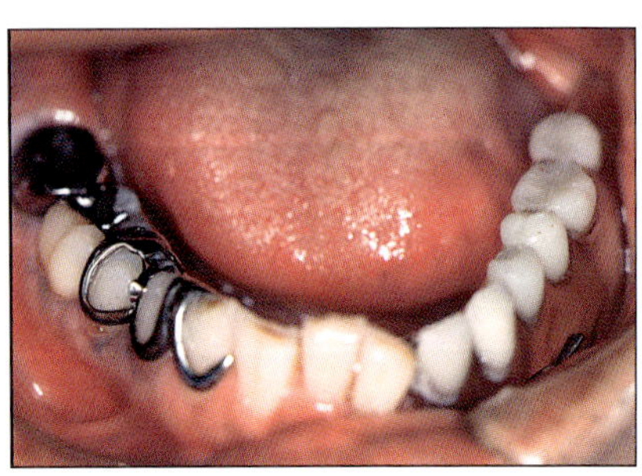

Figs. 22 and 23 A cast double clasp is used for #43, 44. The denture base was prepared using clear resin in order to provide easy control of the high pressure area from the prosthesis. The occlusal surfaces of artificial teeth are made smaller in consideration of the burden on the soft tissue; however, just how much the size of the occlusal surface affects the function of the whole maxillary defect prosthesis is unknown.

2. Mandibular defect prosthesis production method

Fabrication of insert-type mandibular prosthesis

Basic treatment policy for segmental mandibular defect is to reconstruct the mandibular arch whereby the mandibular shape and the ability to bear the masticating force can to be restored. In some specific cases, the following insert-type mandibular prosthesis may also be indicated by the formation of a pouch of split-thickness skin inlay graft as the prosthesis bed.

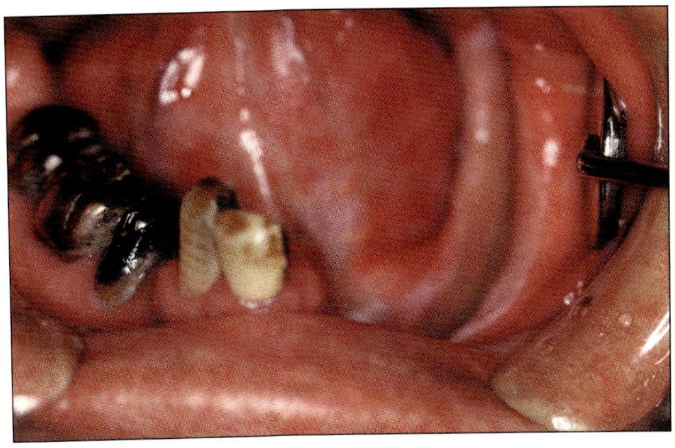

Fig. 24 A 61-year-old male patient had undergone left-side segmental resection (extirpation of mandible by intraoral method) due to left mandibular radiation osteonecrosis. A pouch from the mandibular angle toward mandibular condyle is formed by an inlay skin graft using split thickness skin. A resin bar was temporarily used as the core for the inlay skin graft. This bar supports the remaining-side mandible least deviated position. Remaining teeth were #17–27, and #43–47, with a gap between #44, 45.

Preliminary impression taking

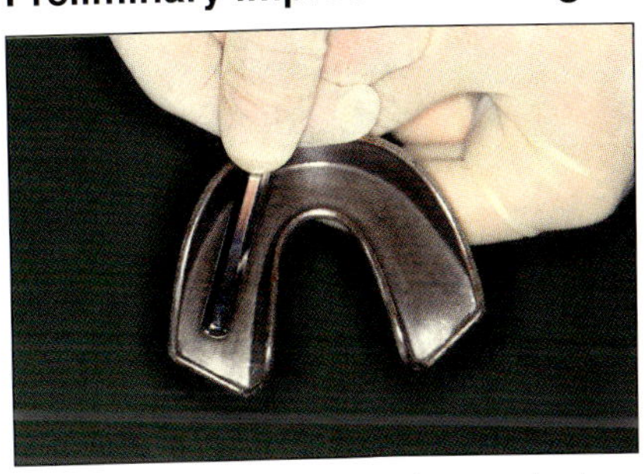

Fig. 25 Try-in of ready-made trays is done to select a suitable tray.

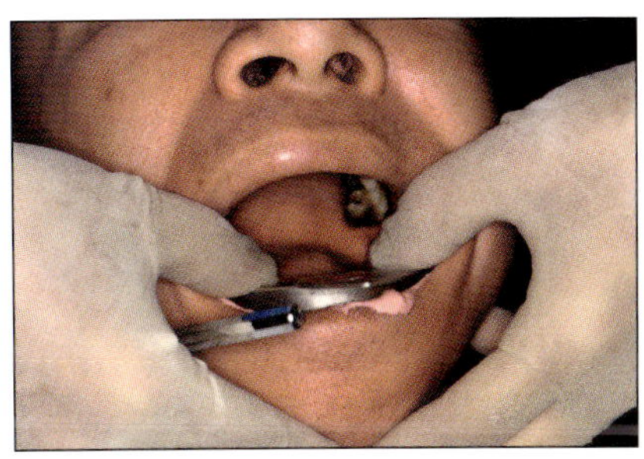

Fig. 26 As is done for ordinary impression taking, after the oral cavity is dried, using a spatula, the operator pushes the impression material into the pouch, then the impression tray is inserted to it. Have the patient to move tongue and cheek to make a rough impression of them.

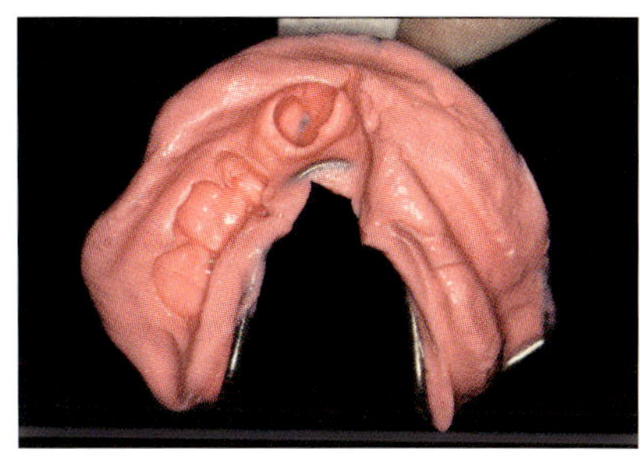

Fig. 27 Preliminary impression taken.

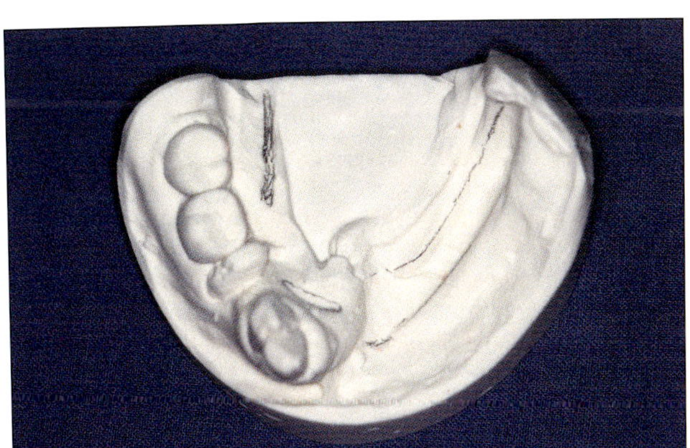

Fig. 28 A preliminary model for prosthetic examination is produced immediately, and a custom tray is made.

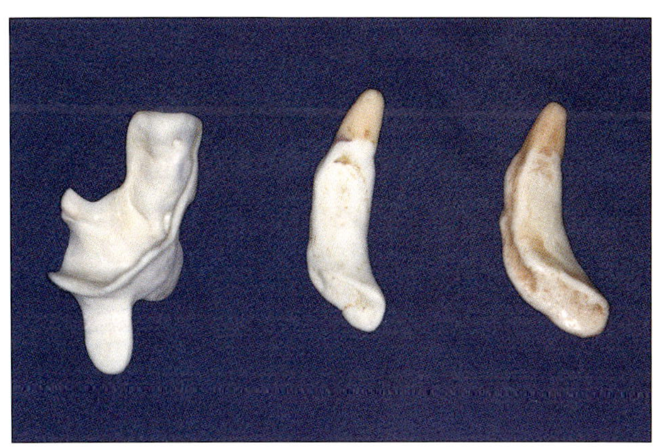

Fig. 29 The 2 pieces on the right side are duplicates of the spacer inserted into the space from where the mandible was extracted. One of these duplicates is used for the impression tray in combination with the left side piece in the photo. Using this set for the custom tray, combined impression taking for the entire mandible is executed. In addition, prepare another tray for taking the impression covering a wider scope than that shown in the left side of the photo, for precise reproduction of the transitional region from the remaining mandible to the defect part.

Taking working impressions

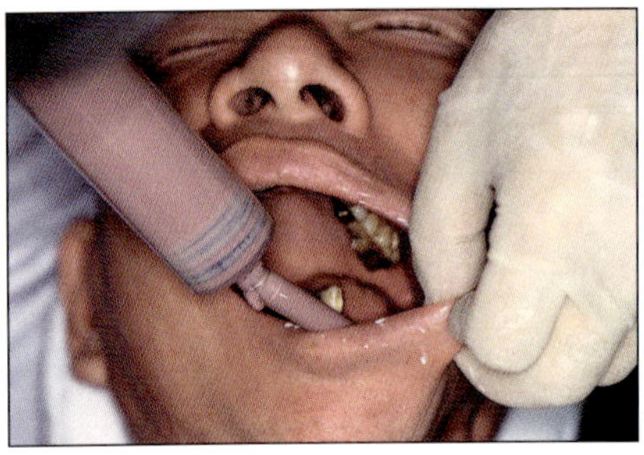
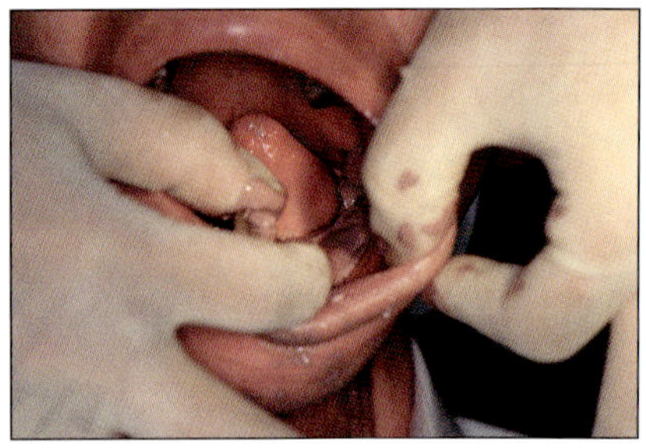

Fig. 30 *(left)* When taking the working impression, combined impression-taking is done using 2 kinds of impression materials. Use Thiokol rubber to take the impression of the defect-side insert part. Alginate-based impression material is used to take the impression of the entire region including the remaining mandible side.
Fig. 31 *(right)* First, using a syringe, inject Thiokol rubber into the pouch of the mandibular defect. Then, insert the tray coated with Thiokol rubber into the pouch.

Combined impression

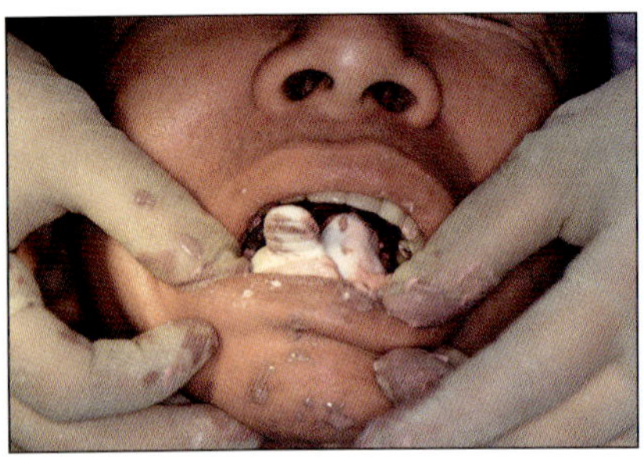
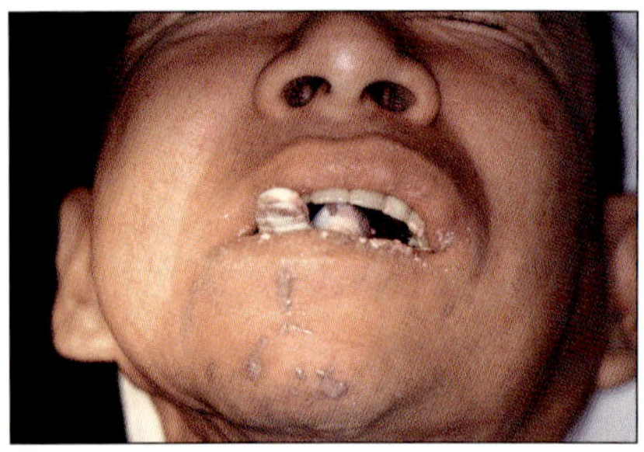

Fig. 32 *(left)* Immediately coat the remaining mandible side with alginate-base impression material, and insert the custom tray for the remaining mandible over the tray for the insert region.
Fig. 33 *(right)* Carry out muscle trimming while waiting for the impression material to cure. Note that there is a difference between the curing times of the impression materials used in the combined impression-taking.

Working impressions taken

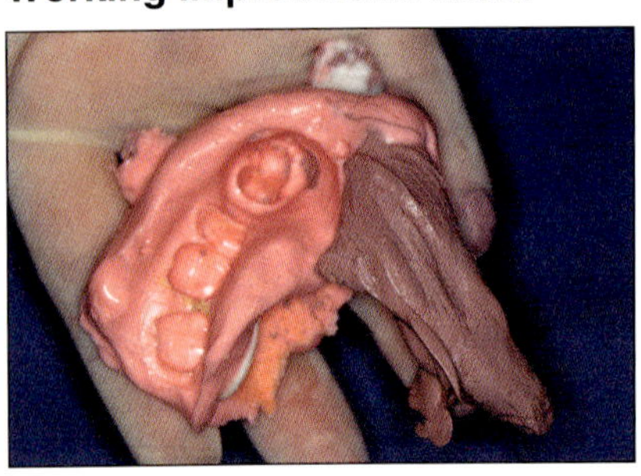
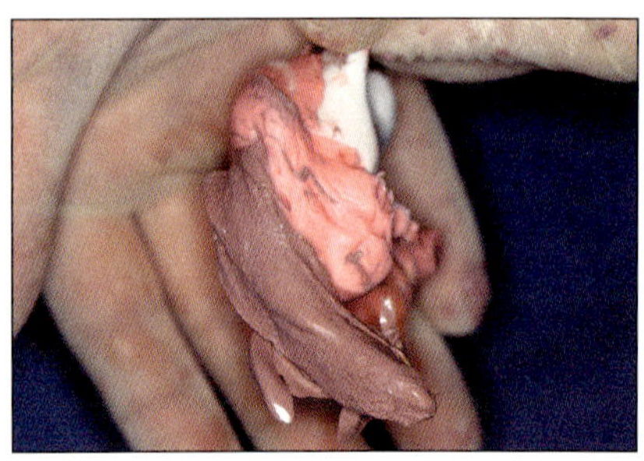

Figs. 34 and 35 These show the combined impressions.

Working model

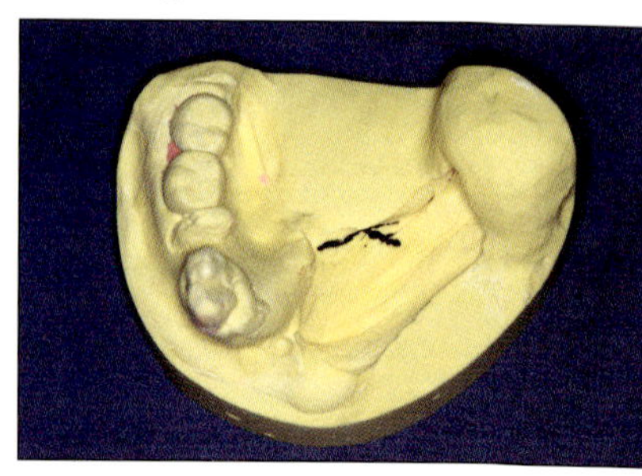

Fig. 36 Prepare 2 models from the defect-remaining side combined impressions; one for use as the working model and the other to be kept as a preserved model for study.

Bite-taking

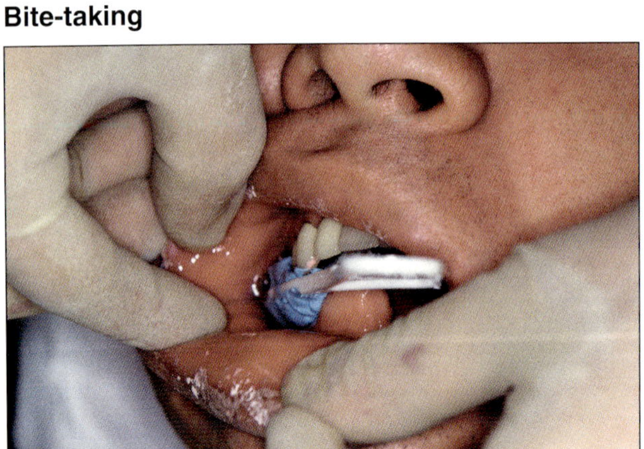
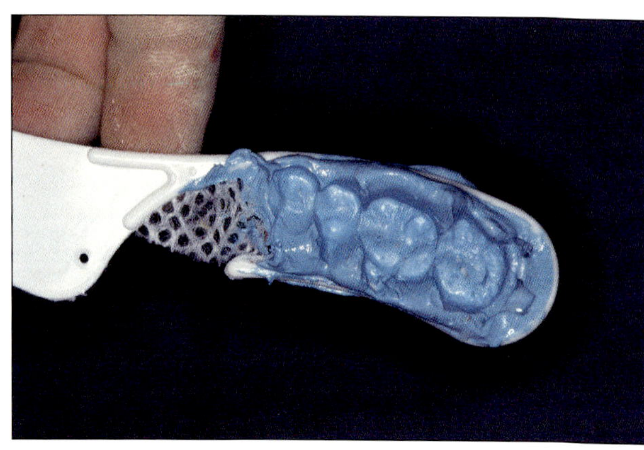

Figs. 37 and 38 If there are any remaining teeth, then, take the impression using eugenol paste. Using this bite impression, mount the entire mandibular working model on the articulator. Subsequent processes are similar with those for ordinary denture preparation; therefore only obviously different from ordinary denture preparation.

Retainer preparation

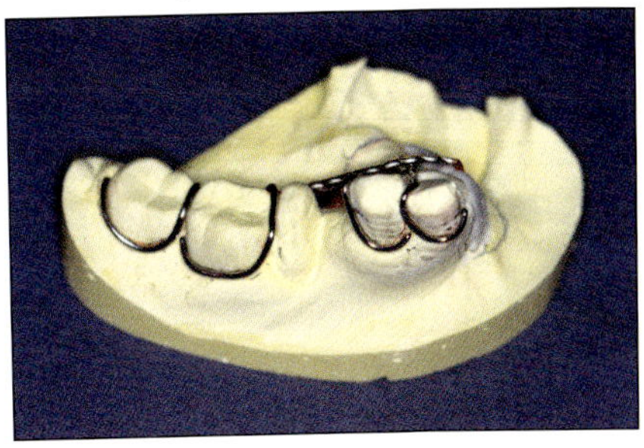

Fig. 39 On the model of the remaining mandible side alone the retainers (wire clasps in this case) are prepared. The gingival part of the remaining mandible side and wax rim are also prepared on this model.

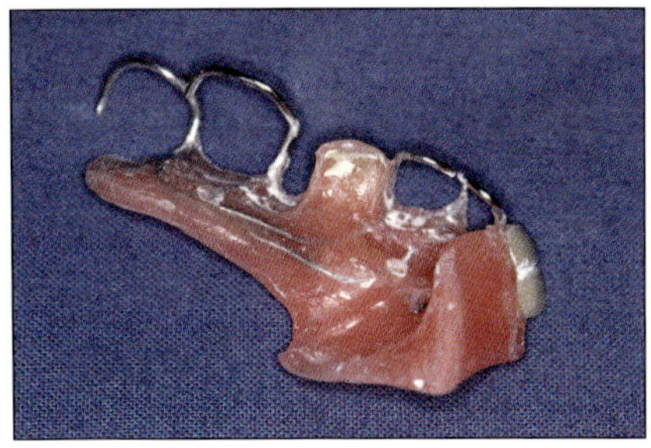

Fig. 40 For the remaining mandible side, displace the wax pattern with pour-type resin, then polish to finish. The whole of this part bears and disperses the pressure from the soft tissue of the insert part. The tentative name for this is the "anchor part".

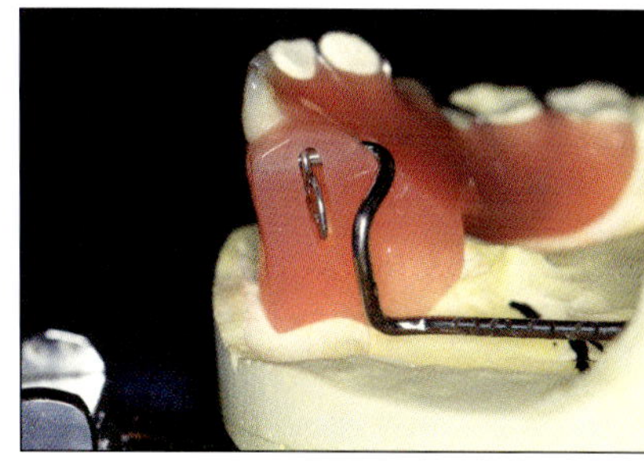

Fig. 41 Attach the prepared anchor part to the full-jaw working model mounted to the articulator, and wax up the defect side (insert part) on this working model. The "lock axis type" interlocking structure is shown here. As shown in the photo, a metal frame is prepared as the core of the insert part, which engages in the hole made in the anchor part. Prepare the insert part with wax. In this case, the artificial teeth for the defect part were prepared separately; therefore, only the insert part was prepared, and the upper surface was covered by Thiokol rubber as a negative mold for pour-type resin.

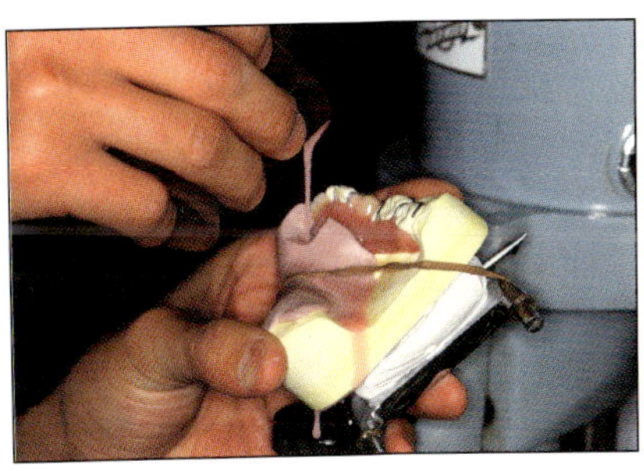

Fig. 42 After the junction part was made so that it could be separated easily, and after dewaxing, pour-type resin was infused.

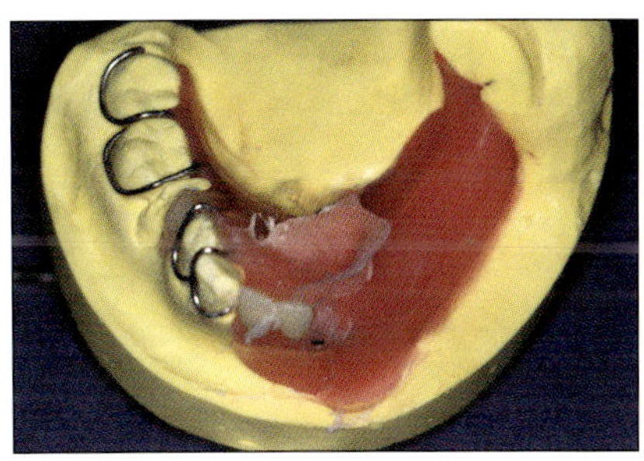

Fig. 43 Removing the negative mold after completion of polymerization, the condition of the junction part can be seen.

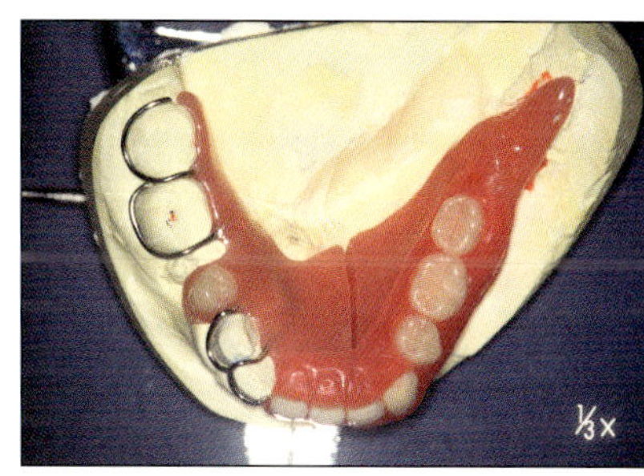

Fig. 44 Artificial tooth on the defect side were arranged and the displacement with resin and final polishing of each part is finished, the insert-type mandibular prosthesis is complete.

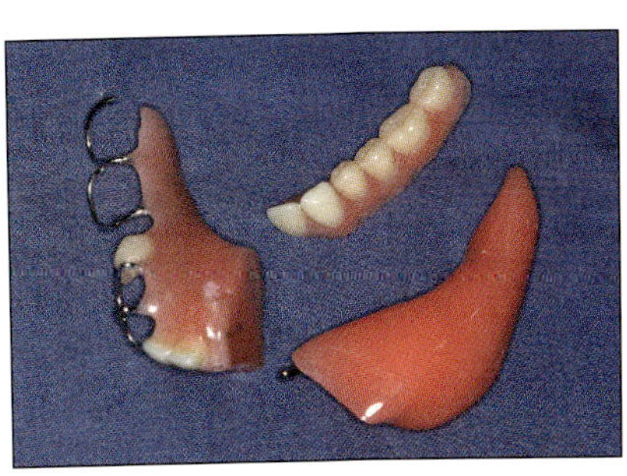

Fig. 45 A view of this insert-type mandibular prosthesis with the individual parts separated into anchor part, insert part, and artificial teeth part.

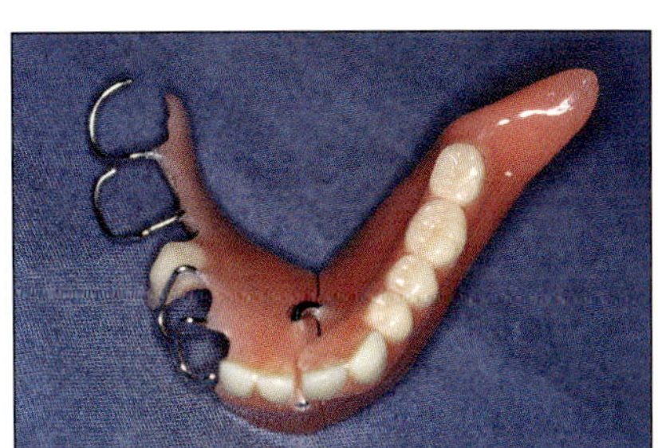

Fig. 46 All parts of this prosthesis joined together.

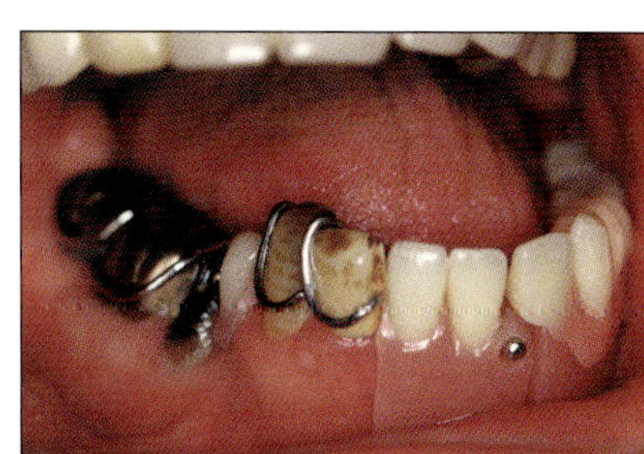

Fig. 47 The insert-type mandibular prosthesis is in place. There is some displacement of the prosthesis toward the remaining mandible side, but so far, the patient can chew.

CHAPTER 17

Retainer of mandibular prostheses

All conventional retaining methods used in ordinary prosthetics are to be checked for their applicability for maxillodental prosthetics, in our experience, however, some ordinary technology has been satisfactory in almost all cases. No particular method can be considered "the best" or "wrong" for maxillodental prosthetics.

This section shows examples of ordinary retainers such as wire clasp, cast clasp, continuous clasp, ball clasp, root attachment, swing lock attachment, spring denture, adhesive tape, and dental implant.

Wire clasp

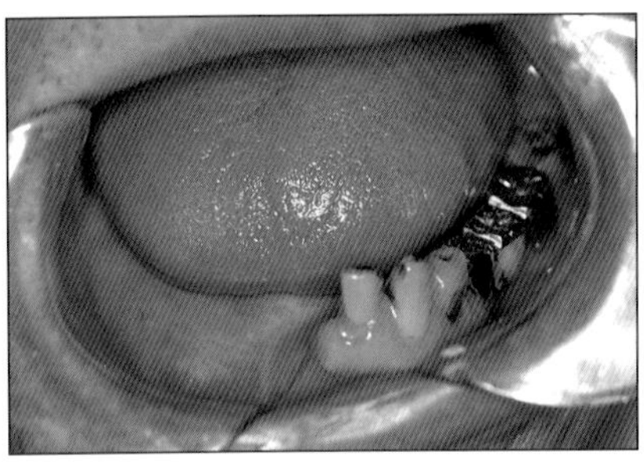

Fig. 1 Defect after excision of right mandibular margin in #43–47 region. #32–35, 37, 38 teeth remain and are firm, and there is a bridge supported by #35, 37 abutment teeth.

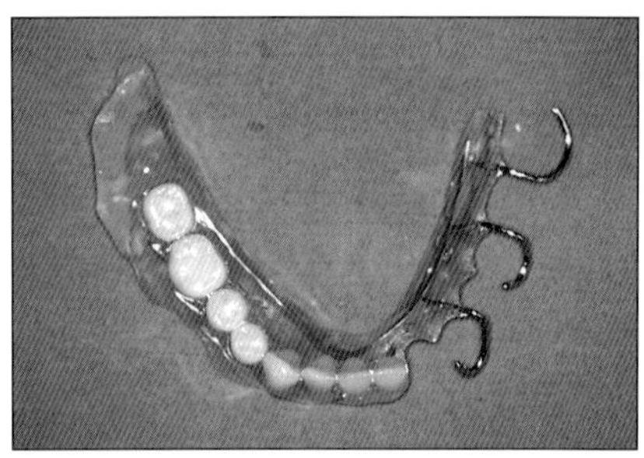

Fig. 2 Simple wire clasps were placed on #33, 35, 37 as retainers and clear resin was used as the denture base resin.

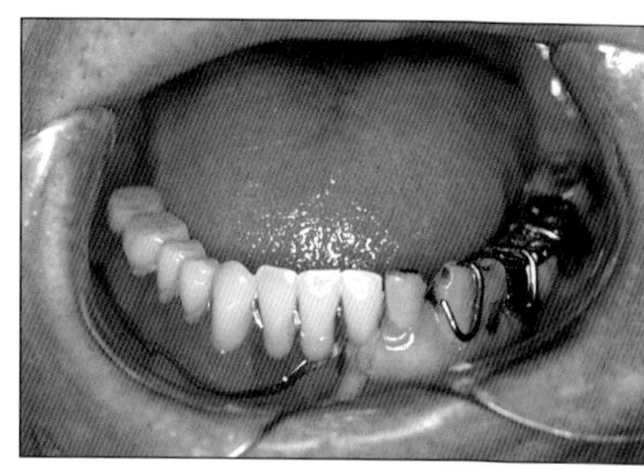

Fig. 3 View of the mandibular prosthesis in place. The stability of this prosthesis is good both with wire clasps and with cast clasps which were lateral replaced.

Continuous clasp

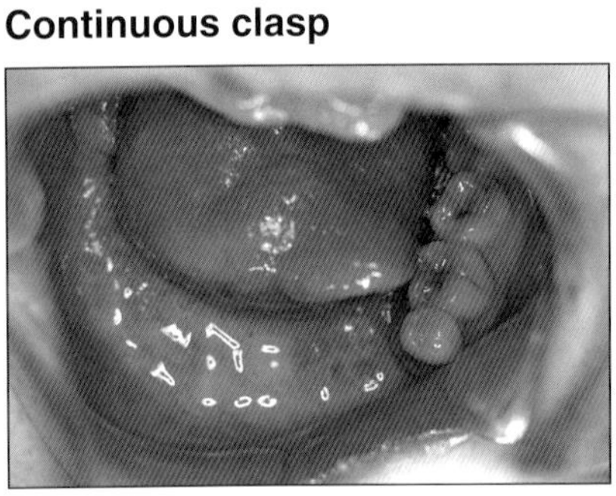

Fig. 4 After segmental resection of mandible with oral floor, free fibulae for mandible and pectoralis major myocutaneous flap for soft part are used. Remaining teeth of #48, #36–38 have 1 degree of mobility, and #35 has 2 degrees.

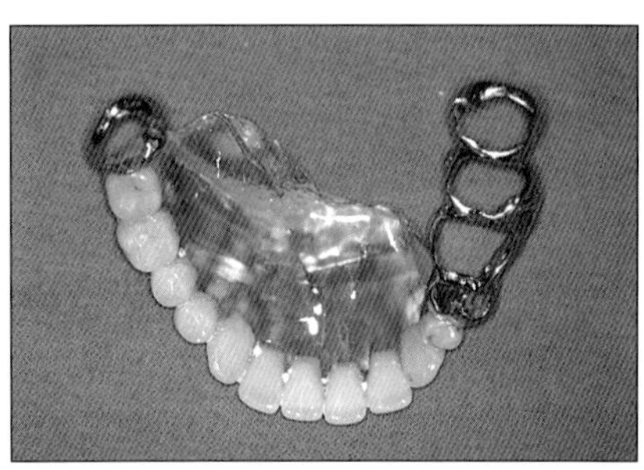

Fig. 5 Mandibular prosthesis using cast clasp for #48 and cast continuous clasps for #35–38 as the retainers is shown. Clear resin is used for the prosthesis base.

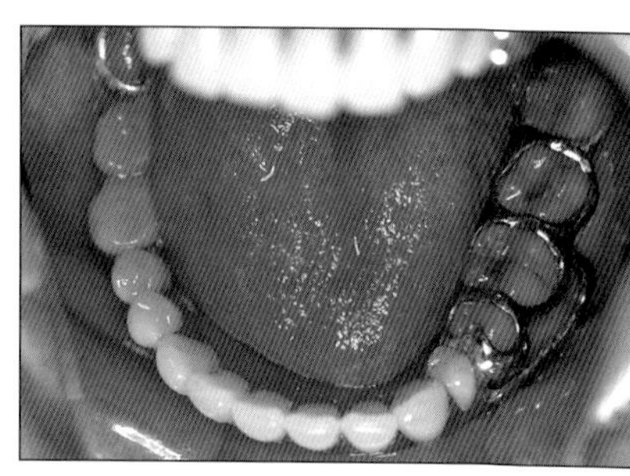

Fig. 6 Stability of mandibular prosthesis is not always good. Any improvement in ingestion disorders using this prosthesis is not clear.

Ball clasp

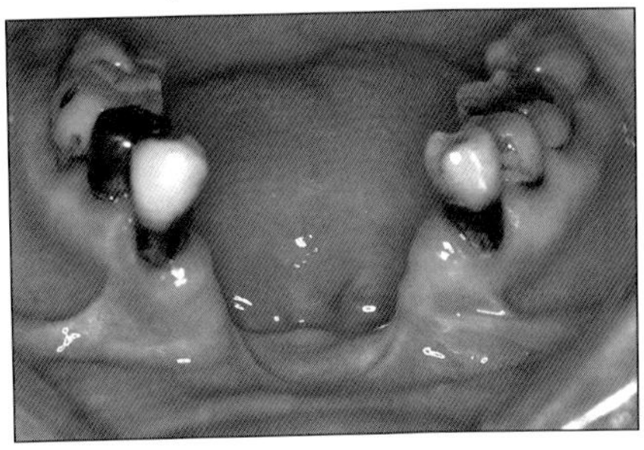

Fig. 7 Defect after marginal mandiblectomy in the median region. The height of the remaining mandible is about 1cm and is quite poor. The remaining teeth, #34–37, 44–47, are securely rooted into bone.

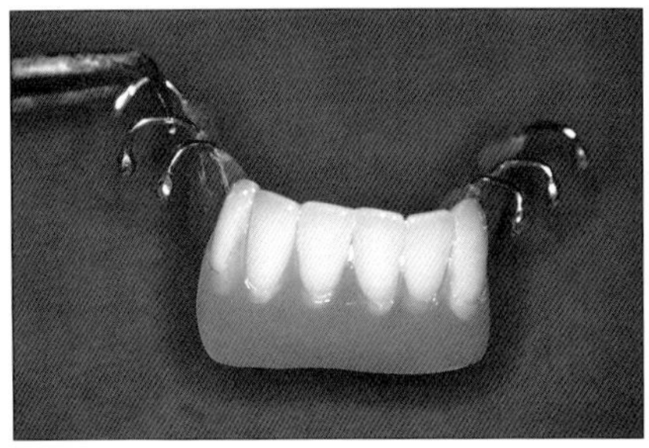

Fig. 8 Two ball clasp units using the embrasures of #34–36, 44–46 were applied.

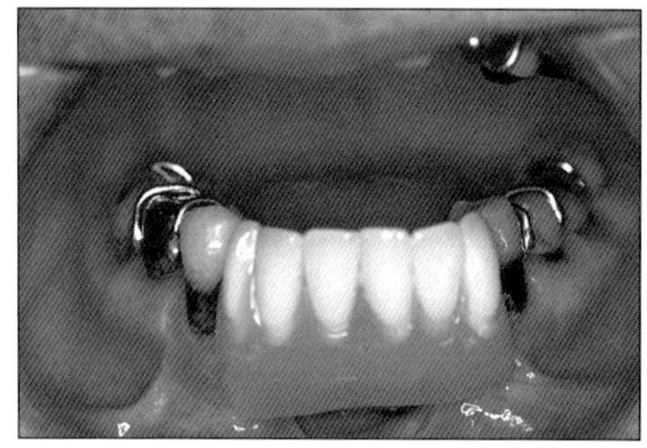

Fig. 9 Stability of mandibular prosthesis is good.

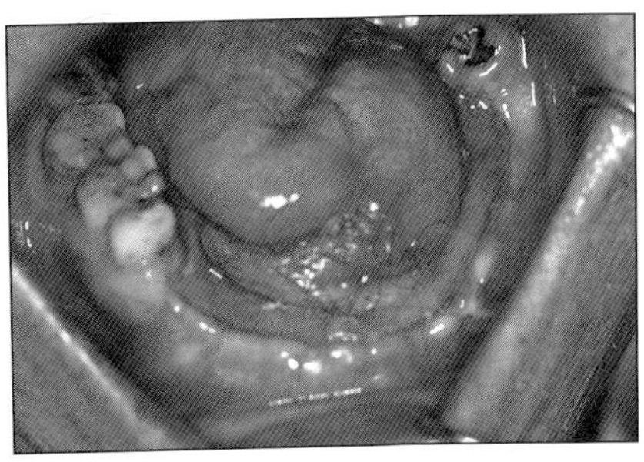

Fig. 10 Case of marginal mandiblectomy and resection of the anterior floor of the mouth. A soft tissue defect in anterior oral floor is reconstructed by a forearm free flap. #38, 45–48 teeth remained. #45–47 teeth are inclined inward, and there is no available undercut on the cheek side. #38 is mobile.

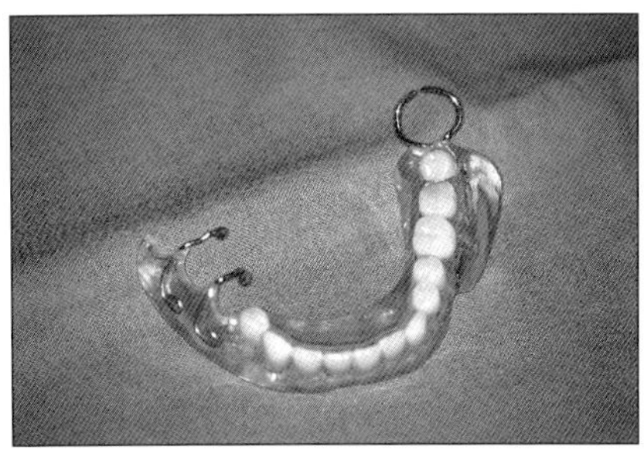

Fig. 11 In addition, as the skin flap was too near the lingual cervical area of the #45, 46 teeth, ball clasps are used in reverse toward the lingual side. A double-armed wire clasp is used for #38.

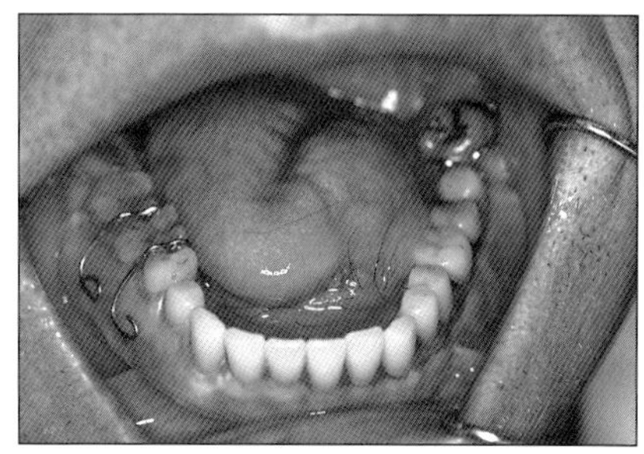

Fig. 12 Mandibular prosthesis stability is poor due to mobility of the flap, although the ingestion disorder has improved.

Root surface attachment

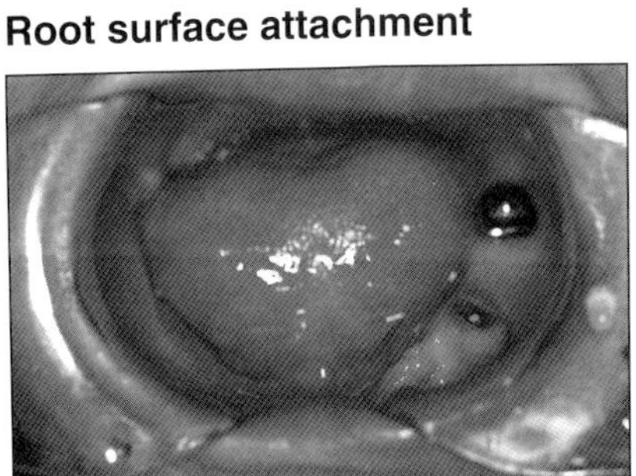

Fig. 13 After segmental resection of right mandible, the mandibular arch was restored using reconstruction plate and hydroxyapatite block. Only the roots of #35, 38 teeth remained. After endodontic treatment for #35, 38, a root cap and the female part of an attachment were fixed to the #38 tooth root. (GPC stud type attachment, Hader Co.)

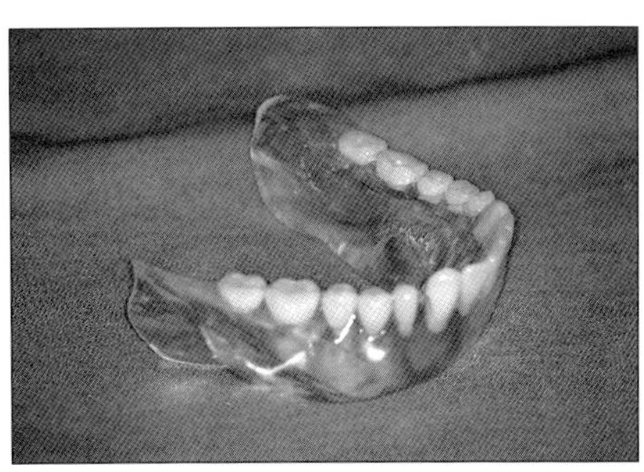

Fig. 14 The male part of the attachment was placed to the mucosal side of the full denture type mandibular prosthesis.

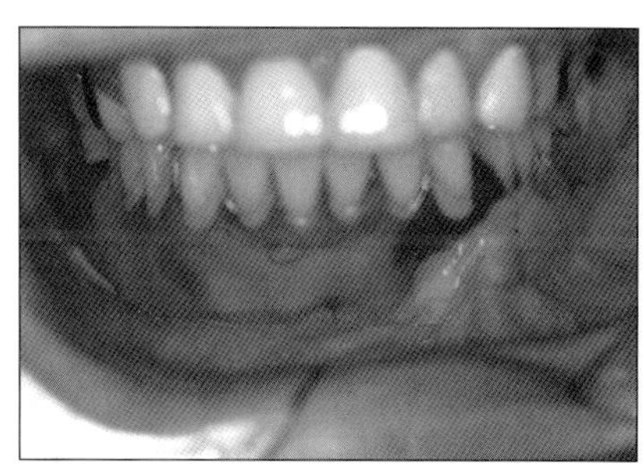

Fig. 15 As the retention of mandibular prosthesis by some structure on the right, or defective, side could not be expected, so we planned to retain it by using this attachment and the alveolar ridge remaining on the left side. Stability of the mandibular prosthesis is good and ingestion disorder has somewhat improved.

Swing lock attachment

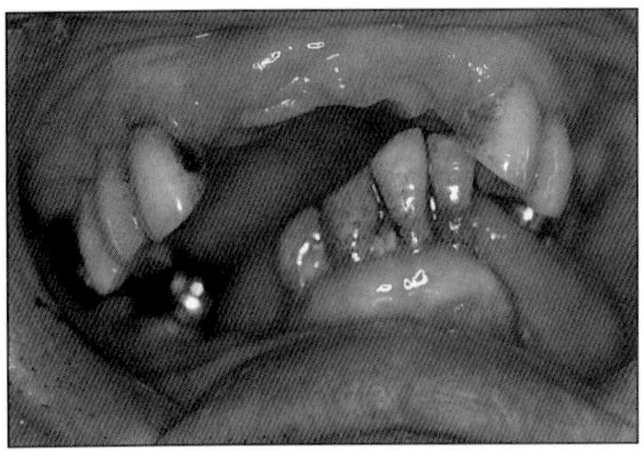

Fig. 16 Segmental mandibular defect of #31–37 area after excision. The reconstruction by PMMC and bridging plate was removed due to infection. Remaining teeth are #13–16, 23–27 and #41, 44–46. The mandible has severely deviated to the left side.

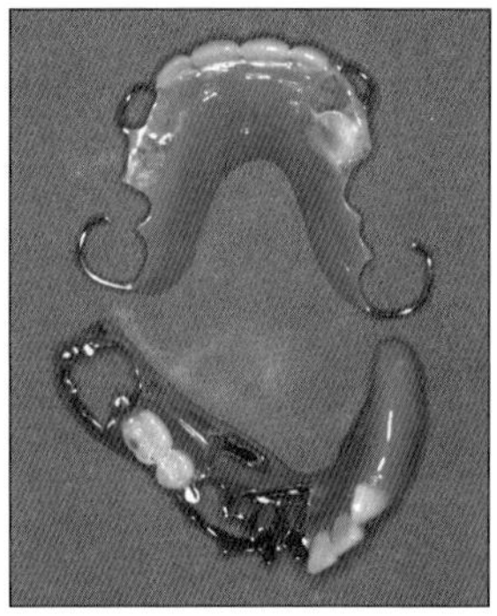

Fig. 17 Swing Lock attachment with I-bar for #41–44, 46 teeth was used in order to secure a firm retentive force. #33 artificial tooth was placed in a slightly extruded manner to accept occlusive guidance on the palatal surface of the #23 artificial tooth.

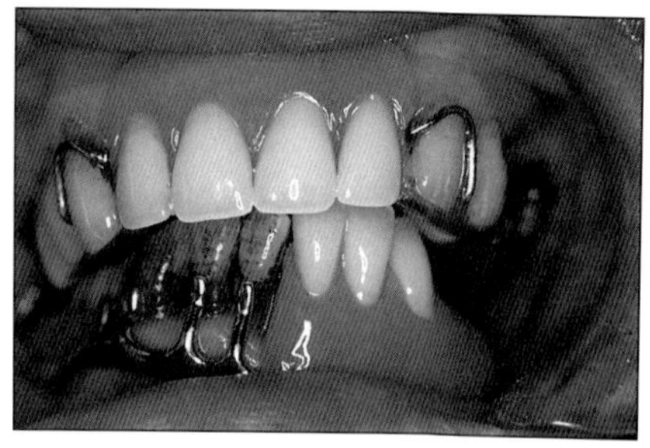

Fig. 18 The lower jaw is well guided to bite with remaining teeth on the healthy side. The mandibular prosthesis has stabilized, and improvement of ingestion disorder has been achieved.

Spring denture

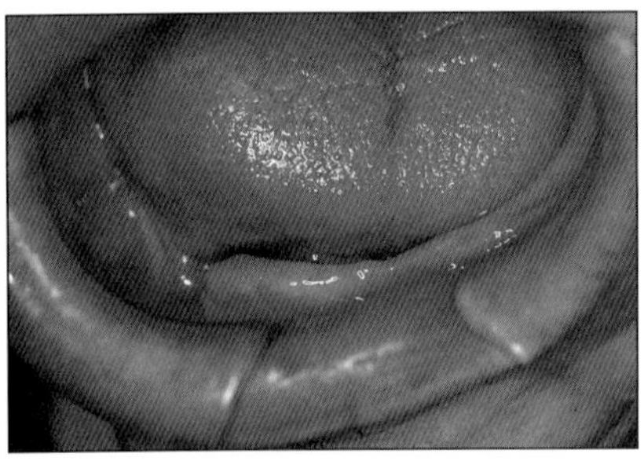

Fig. 19 This edentulous patient has had a right segmental resection of the mandible (#43–47 area). The remaining alveolar ridge has atrophied.

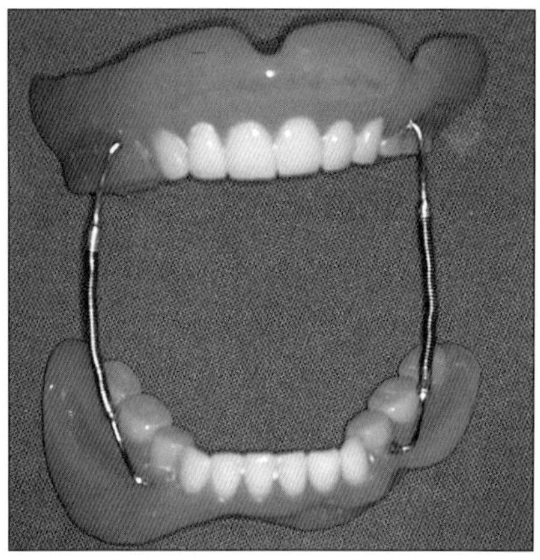

Fig. 20 Springs were attached to the maxillary denture bilaterally used as the anchorage unit, to retain and stabilize the mandibular prosthesis.

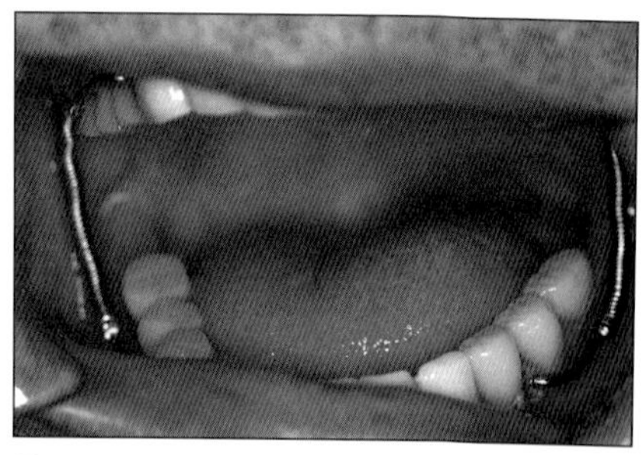

Fig. 21 The mandibular prosthesis is almost stable during the movement of opening the mouth for eating, but the prosthesis is unstable at his maximum mouth opening.

Adhesive tape

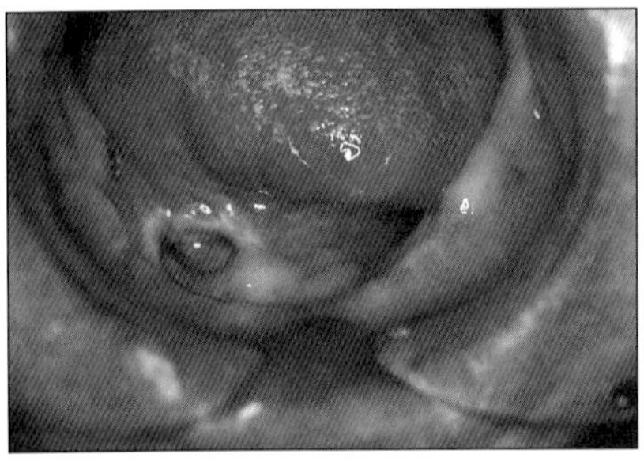

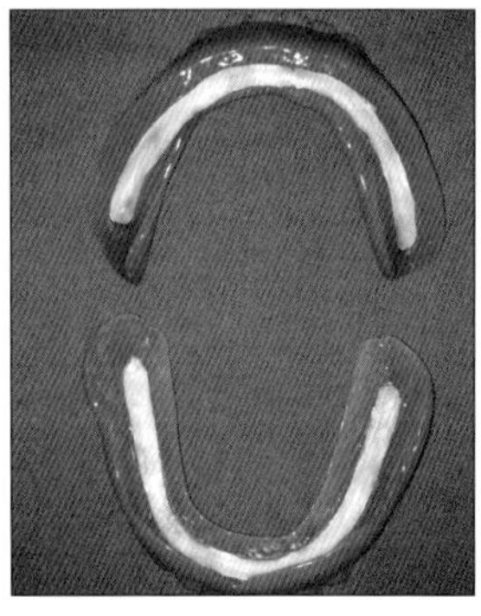

Fig. 22 *(left)* Free skin graft was performed after resection of tongue and anterior oral floor with marginal mandiblectomy of #35–46 area. There are no remaining teeth.
Fig. 23 *(right)* Full-denture type prosthesis was made using ordinary denture stabilizing material.

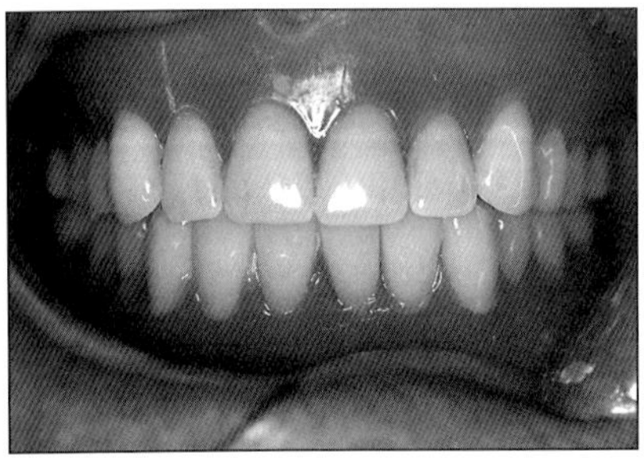

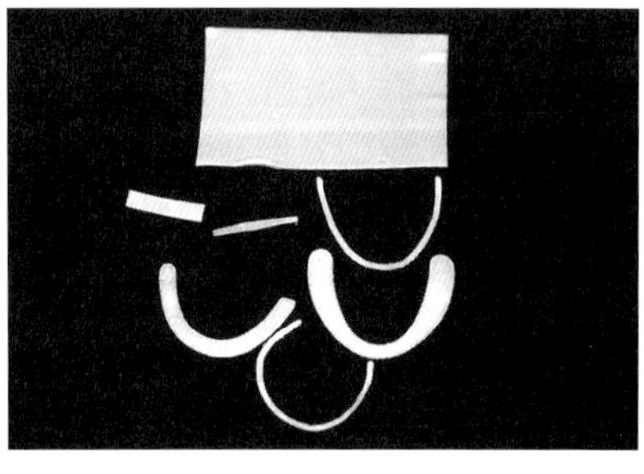

Fig. 24 *(left)* View of full-denture type lower maxillary prosthesis in place.
Fig. 25 *(right)* Ordinary denture stabilizing material (TOUCH CORRECT 2®, Shionogi & Co., Ltd.). This material is dissolved by saliva.

Cast clasp and sacciform region

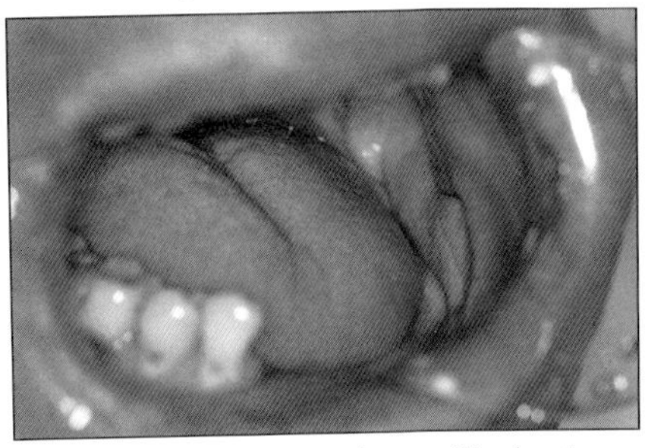

Fig. 26 After left hemimandibulectomy extended to the contralateral canine area, mandibular, reconstruction using fibula osteocutaneous flap and reconstruction plate with condyle was done. (Leibinger Co.). Remaining teeth are #17, 15–27 and #44–48.

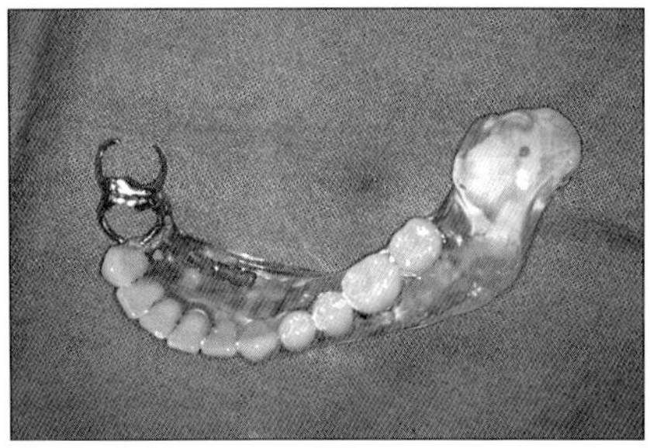

Fig. 27 Placing the mandibular prosthesis on the reconstructed skin flap is not very likely to improve the ingestion disorder, but the sacciform part, with a depth of about 20mm in the skin flap section near the retromolar trigon area on the defect side, and a double clasp for #44, 45, were used for retention in this case.

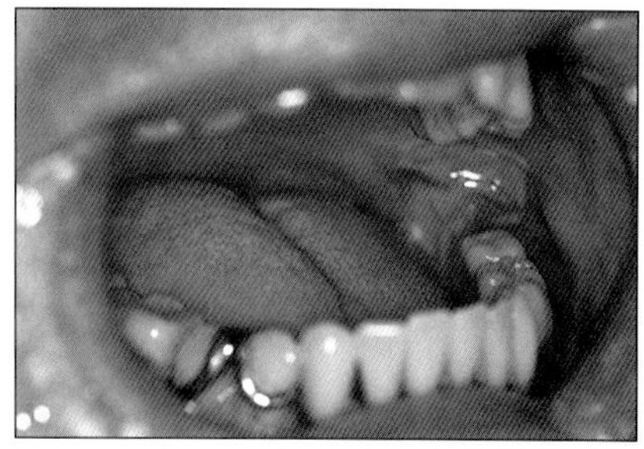

Fig. 28 In this case, the mandibular prosthesis on the skin flap did not result in improvement of the ingestion disorder, but did achieve improvement of esthetics.

Retention by dental implants

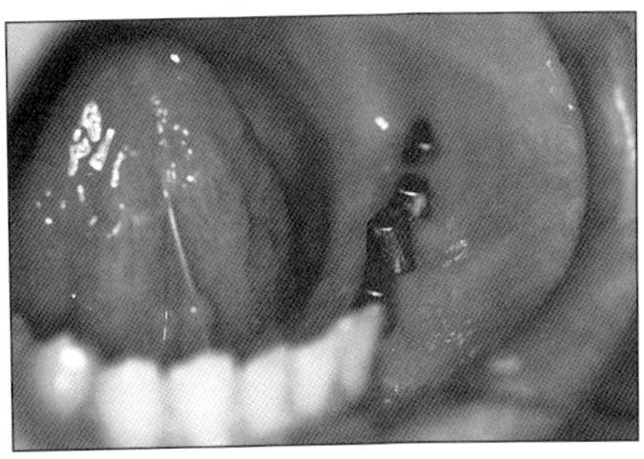

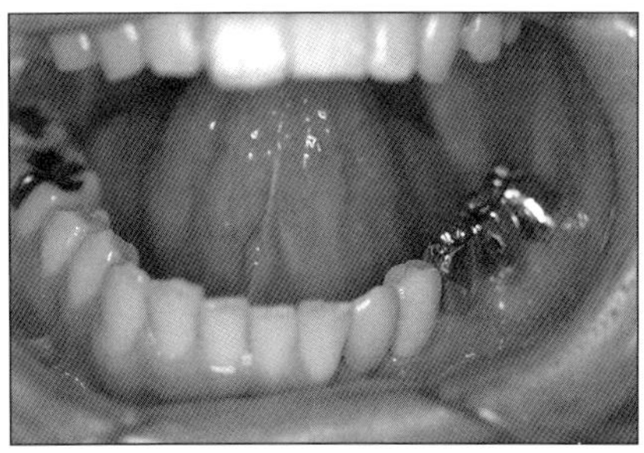

Fig. 29 *(left)* After segmental resection of left mandible, secondary bony reconstruction of mandible is carried out by free iliac graft Four dental implants were installed in the area of #33–37 of the grafted bone.
Fig. 30 *(right)* A superstructure prosthesis has been placed on the implants.

Full denture type

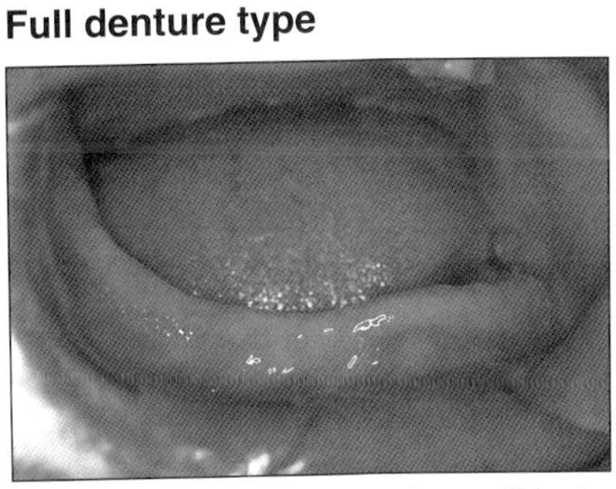

Fig. 31 View after segmental mandiblectomy from #35 area to left condylar neck. The mandible has deviated to the defect side, in this edentulous case.

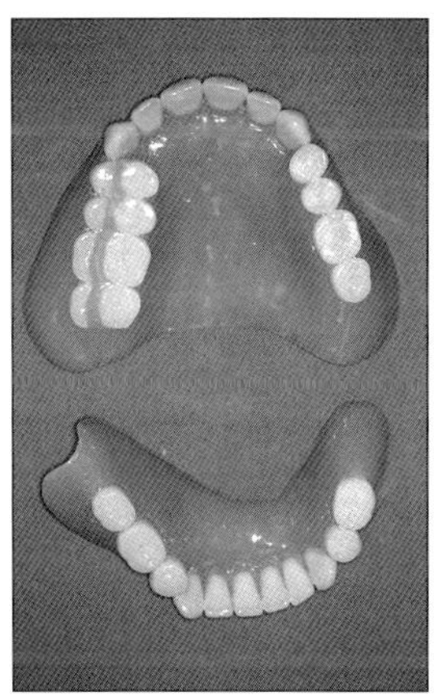

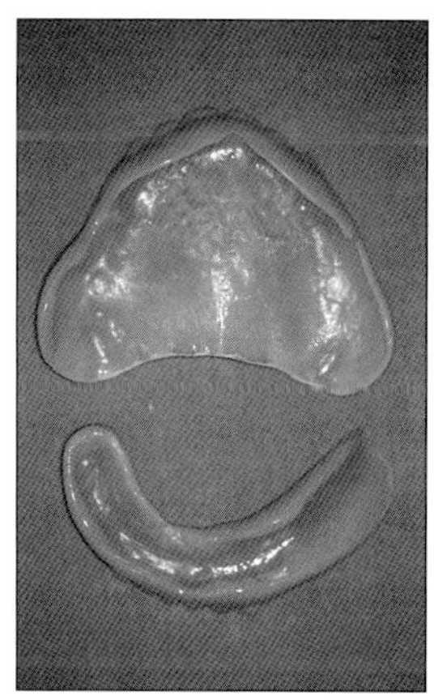

Figs. 32 and 33 A denture base was prepared up to #34 region, and the artificial teeth are arranged from #46 to #35 on to the remaining mandible. Its form resembles an ordinary denture with part cut off. Mandibular prosthesis stability was maintained by giving a second row of artificial teeth palately to the molar region of the right non-affected side of the upper jaw, corresponding to the displacement of the mandible to the defect side (occlusal hump).

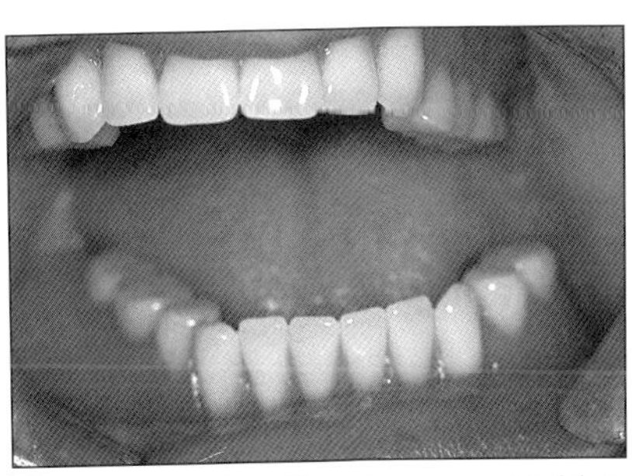

Fig. 34 Ingestion disorder was considerably improved.

Full denture type

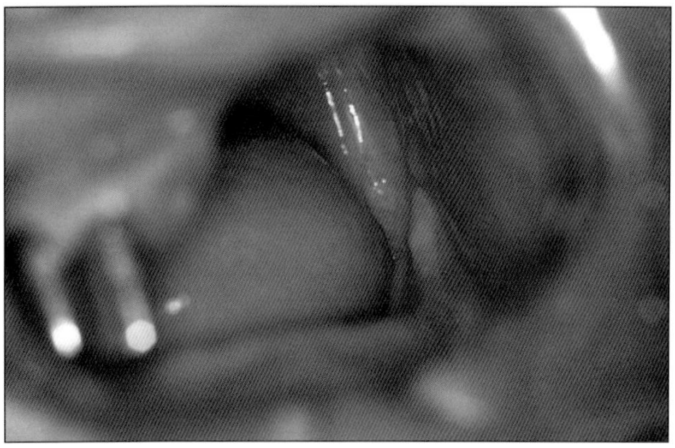

Fig. 35 View after segmental resection of left mandibular ramus from #38. The only remaining teeth are #12, 13, and the mandible has deviated to the defect side.

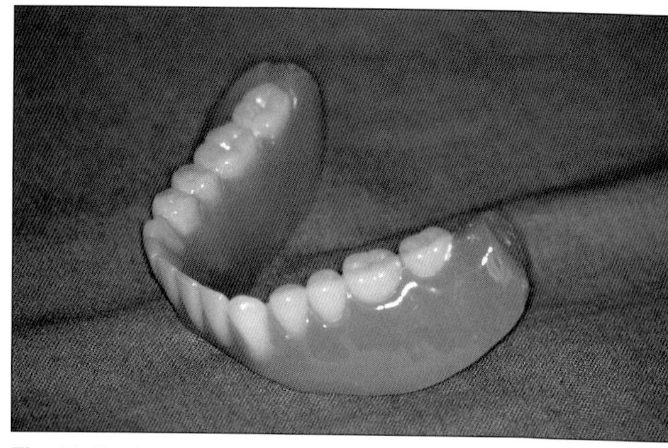

Fig. 36 The lower maxillary prosthesis was prepared in the same form as an ordinary denture, but a crossbite arrangement of the artificial teeth on the defective side.

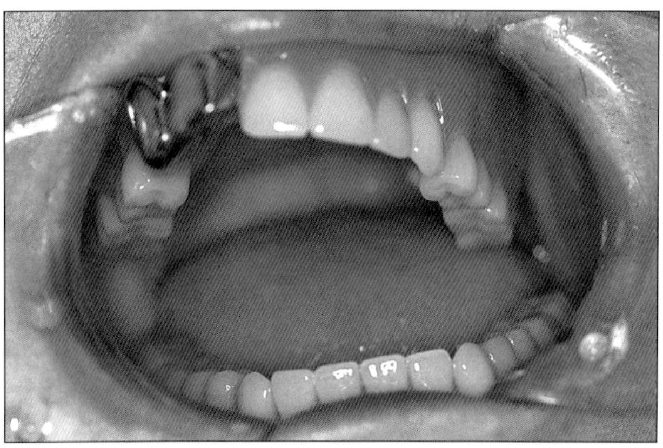

Fig. 37 Ingestion disorder improved without any problems.

CHAPTER 18

From placement of implants to fabrication of prostheses

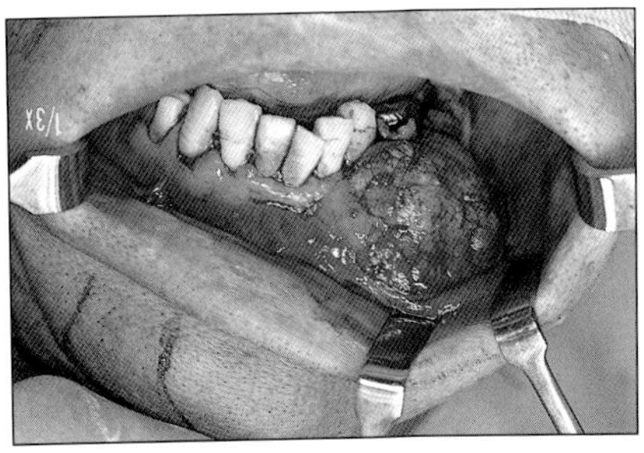

Fig. 1 This case of ameloblastoma developed in the left side of the mandible of a 48-year-old male.

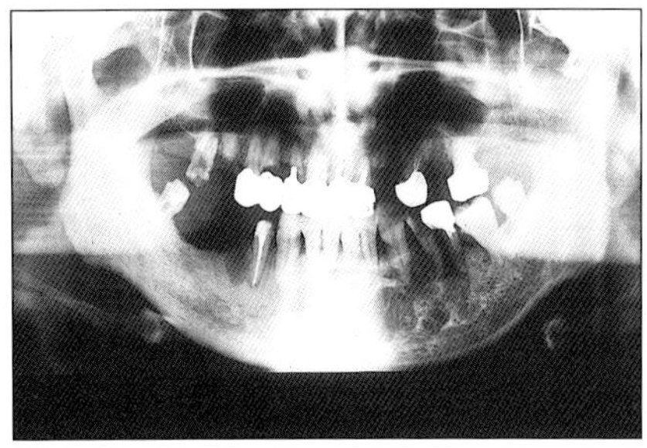

Fig. 2 Radiography showed multilocular radiolucency in the left mandible.

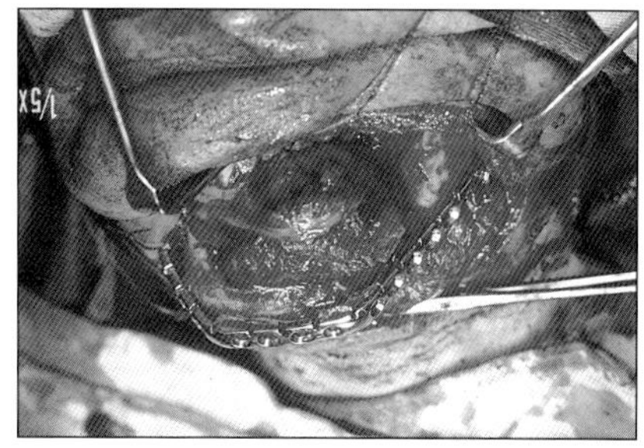

Fig. 3 Segmental mandibulectomy was conducted to resect the ameloblastoma, followed by reconstruction of the mandible with a mandibular reconstructive plate.

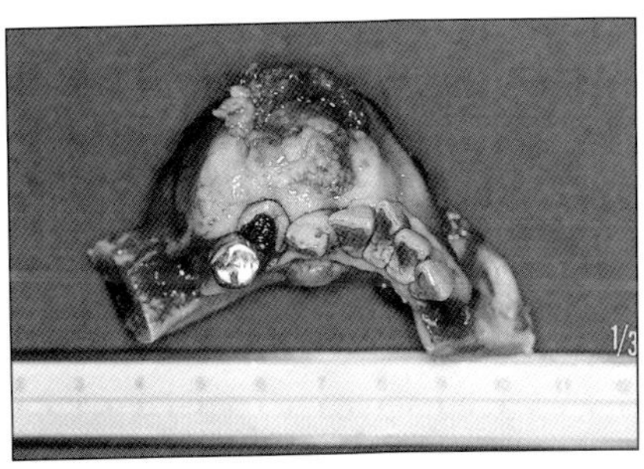

Fig. 4 Segmental mandibulectomy was performed, with a safety range of 10mm from the tumor.

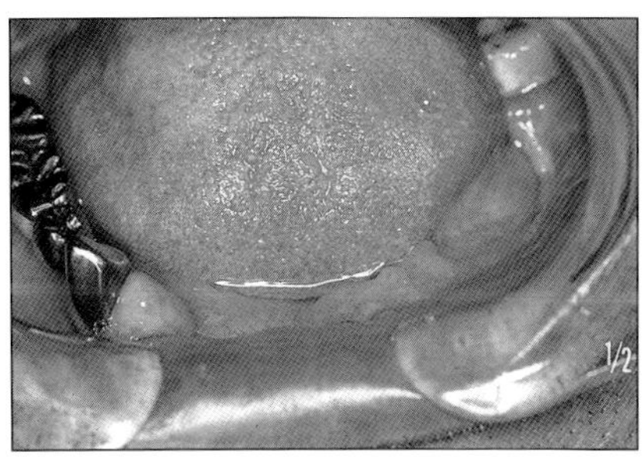

Fig. 5 The defect of the residual ridge due to tumor resection made placement of a denture difficult, so that functional restoration of mastication was difficult to achieve.

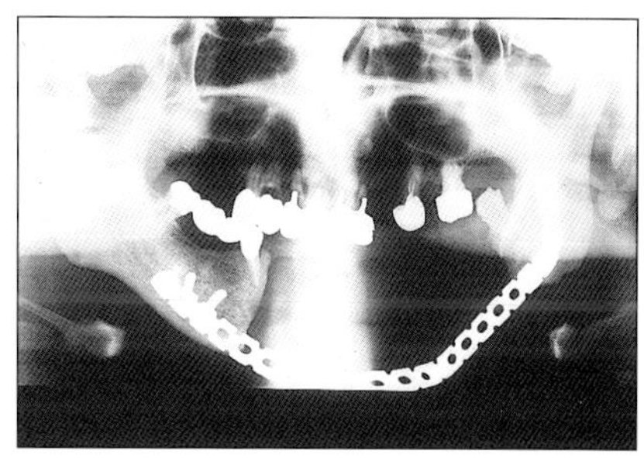

Fig. 6 Panoramic radiograph after segmental mandibulectomy.

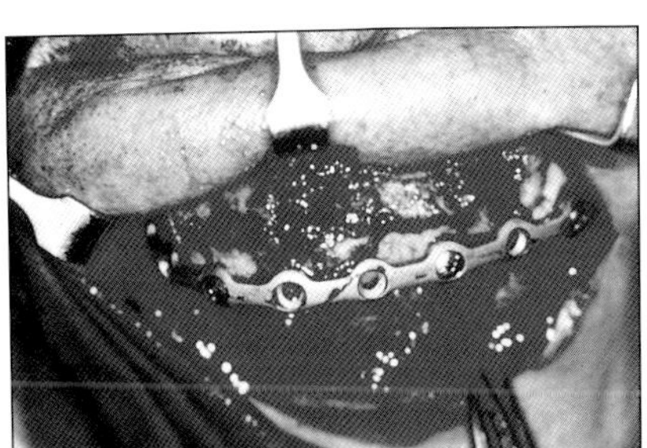

Fig. 7 Placement of prosthesis supported with osseointegrated implants was planned. Transplanting an iliac bone graft into the bone defect after segmental mandibulectomy for improvement of masticatory function had been carried out.

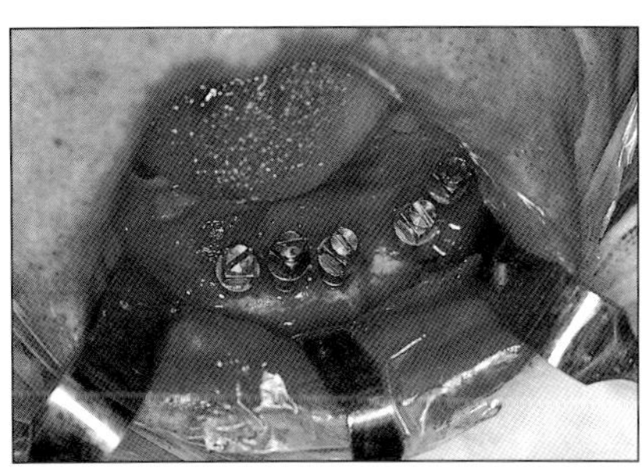

Fig. 8 Five implants were placed in the bone 6 months after the iliac transplant was done.

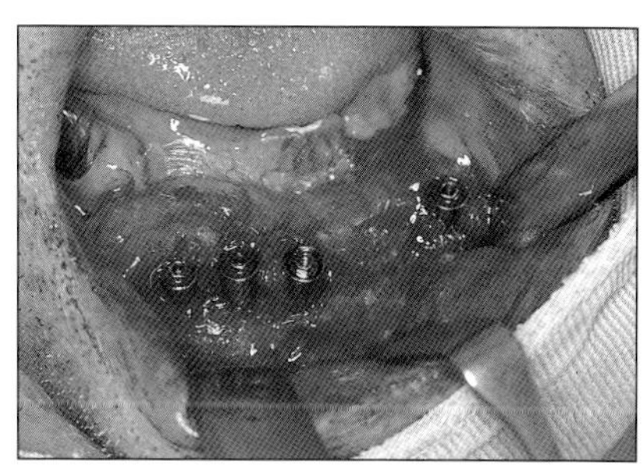

Fig. 9 A secondary operation to connect abutments was conducted 6 months later. Since it was impossible to place an abutment into the second distal implant owing to its inadequate positioning. Four abutments were connected into the other implants.

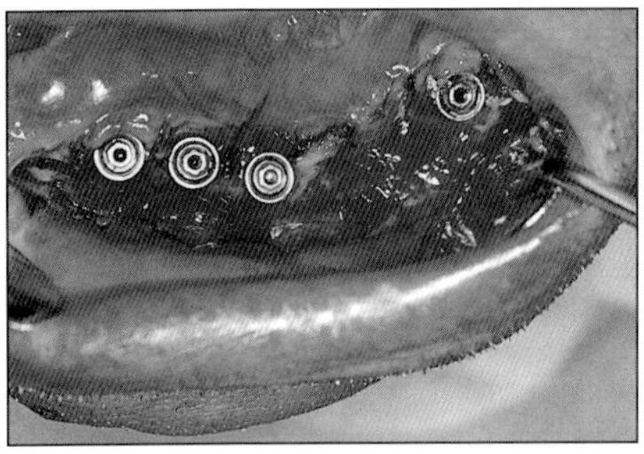

Fig. 10 The mucosa around the abutments was movable tissue, and the oral vestibule was lost. Therefore vestibuloplasty was performed by a free mucosal graft.

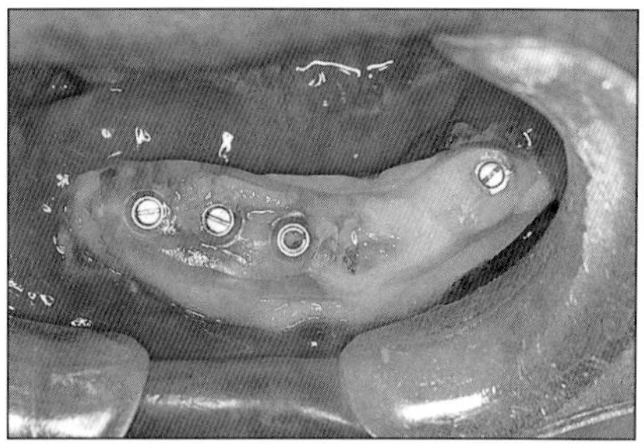

Fig. 11 A plate to fix the grafted mucosa under compression was secured to the abutments with screws.

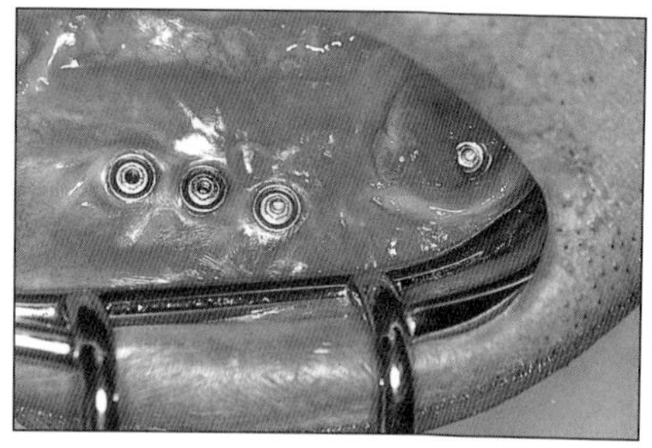

Fig. 12 The periphery of the implants became immovable mucosa due to the free mucosal graft with formation of an oral vestibule.

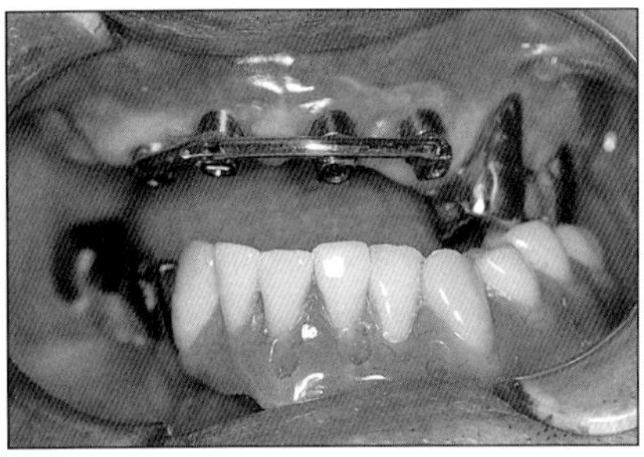

Fig. 13 A fixed bridge supported by 4 implants was connected to the lower implants. Four implants were placed, then a bar attachment was placed to the maxilla.

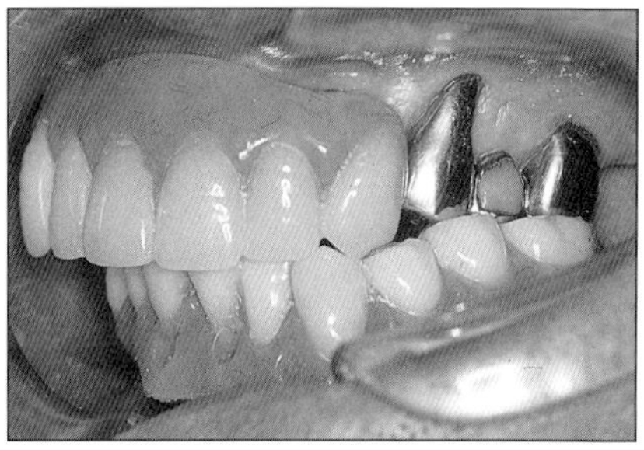

Fig. 14 This intraoral photograph shows the prostheses placed to the maxilla and mandible. Masticatory function after placement of prosthesis was improved as compared with previously.

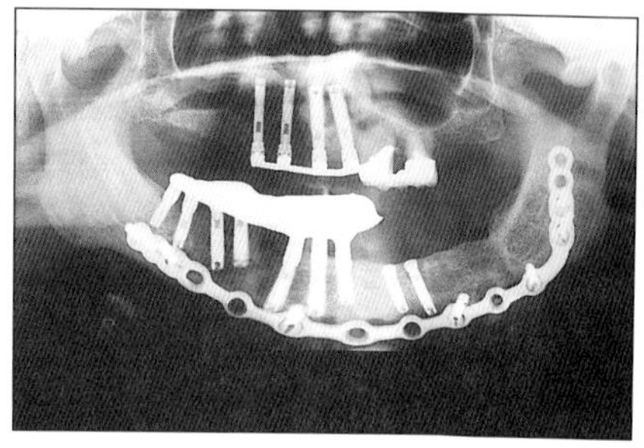

Fig. 15 Since the mandibular right posterior teeth were lost after 3 years, 4 implants were placed on the right posterior region of the mandible. Three old implants in the grafted bone were connected with the new implants to fabricate a new fixed implant bridge. Two lower implants on the left side were slipped under the mucosa.

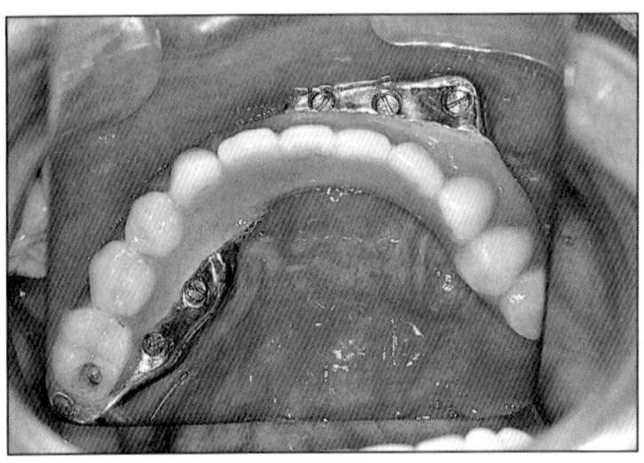

Fig. 16 Occlusal view of renewal implant prosthesis of the mandible.

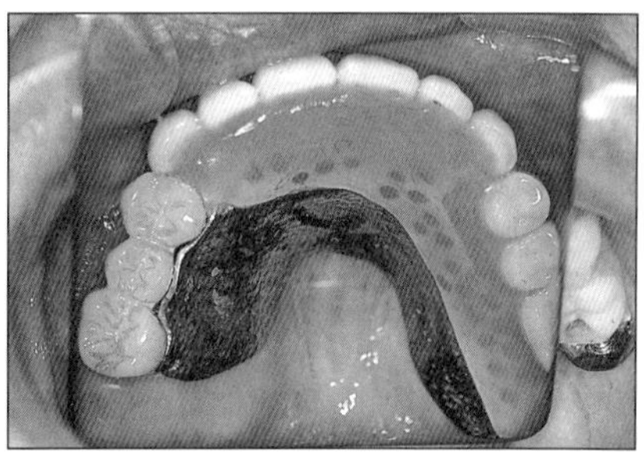

Fig. 17 With the maxillary residual bridge renewed, an upper implant prosthesis was also fabricated.

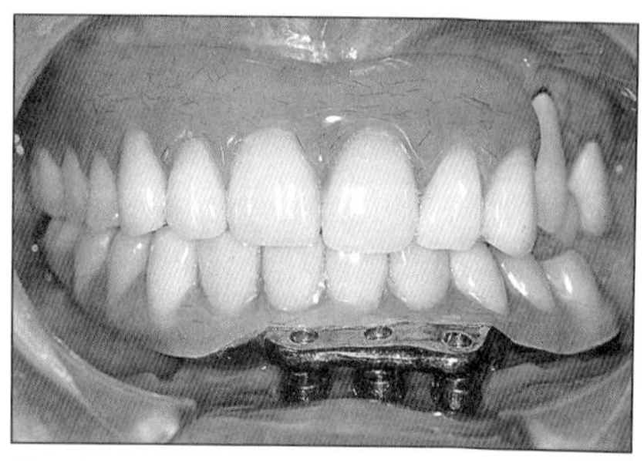

Fig. 18 Improvement in mastication was found after reconstruction of the maxillary and mandibular prostheses.

Fabrication procedures for implant prosthesis

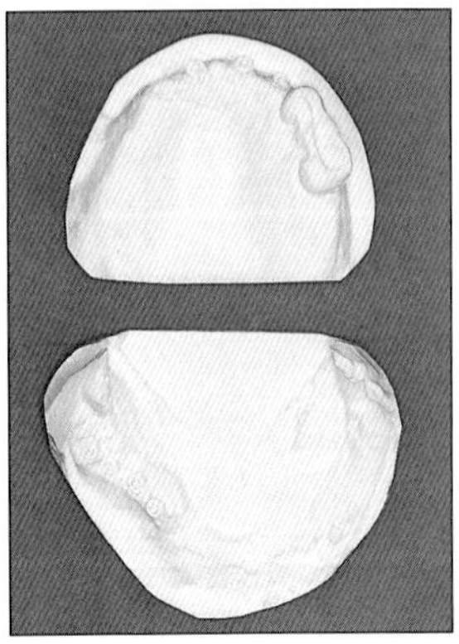

Fig. 19 After connecting the abutments and while waiting for the intraoral mucosa to heal, snap impressions were taken with an alginate impression material in order to fabricate study casts.

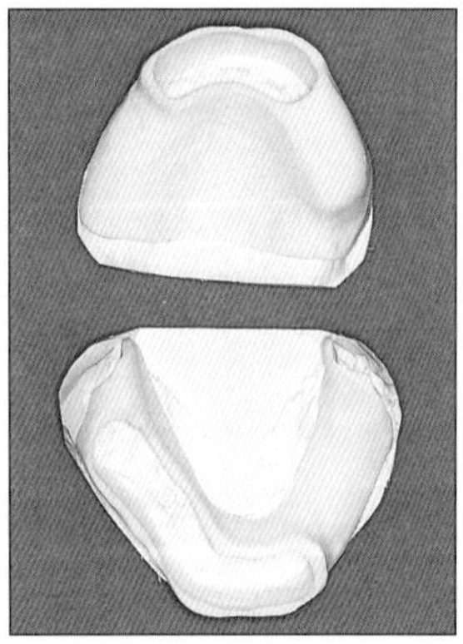

Fig. 20 Individual trays were fabricated on the study casts for precise impression.

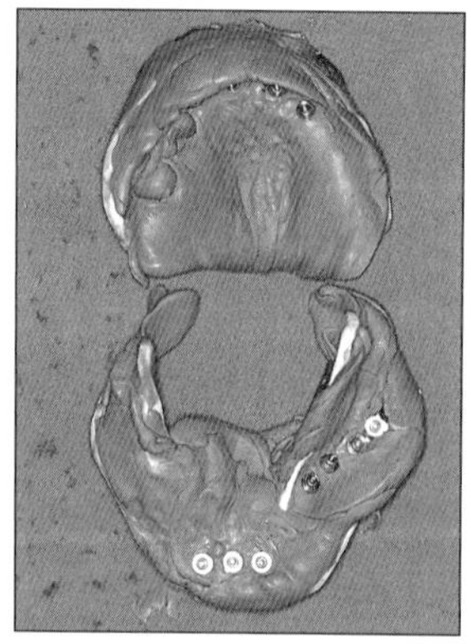

Fig. 21 Exclusive copings for impression were inserted on the abutments, then the copings were connected and reinforced using an acrylic resin. The individual trays were filled with a silicon impression material to take precise impressions.

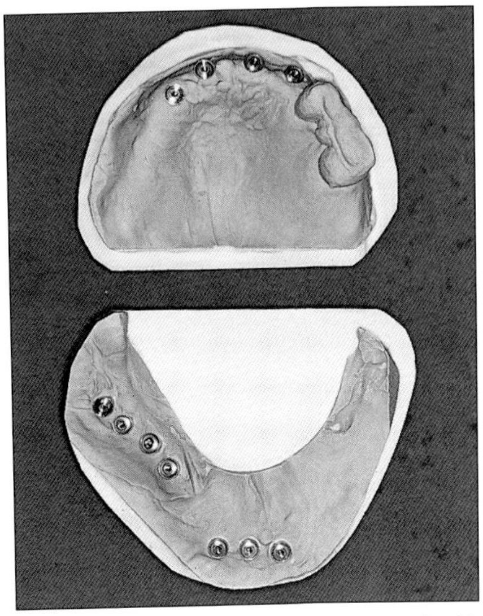

Fig. 22 Working casts were fabricated with super-hard plaster poured into the precise impressions.

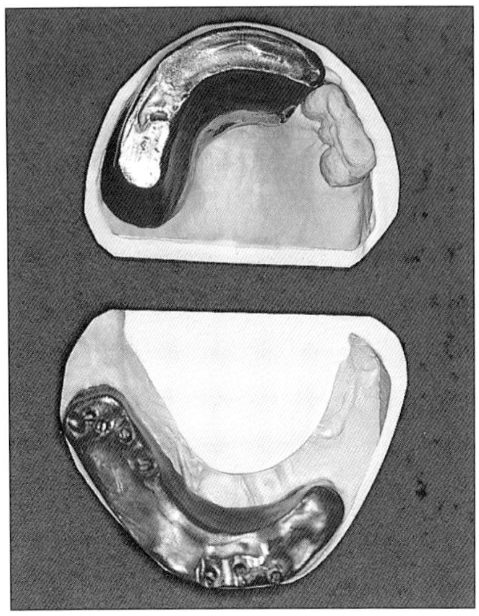

Fig. 23 Wax occlusion plates were fabricated for bite taking, then the working casts were mounted on an articulator.

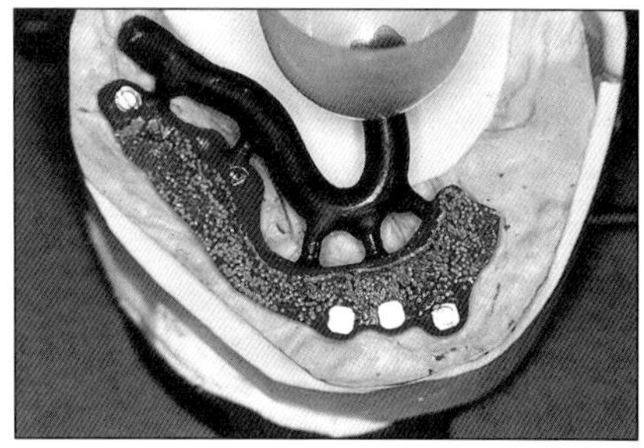

Fig. 24 For the mandible, a metal frame was "waxed-up" for the fixed implant prosthesis.

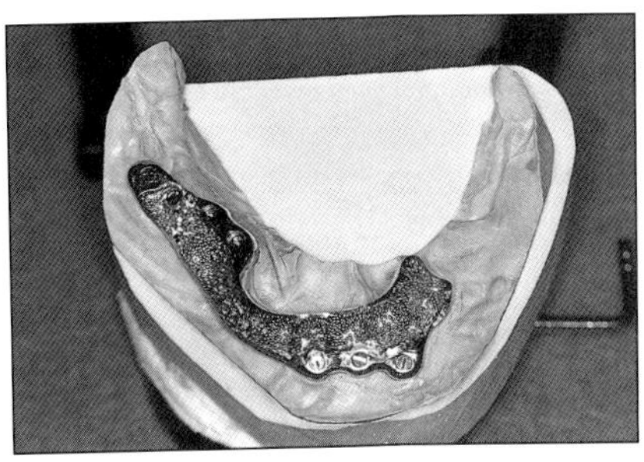

Fig. 25 The frame was cast using gold-platinum alloy.

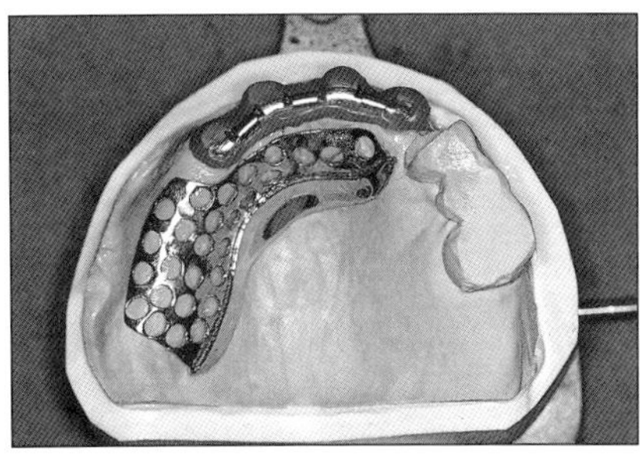

Fig. 26 For the maxilla, it was decided to fabricate a removable prosthesis retained by a CM rider attachment. Gold cylinders were soldered to a bar. The metal base of the removable prosthesis was made using a cobalt-chromium alloy.

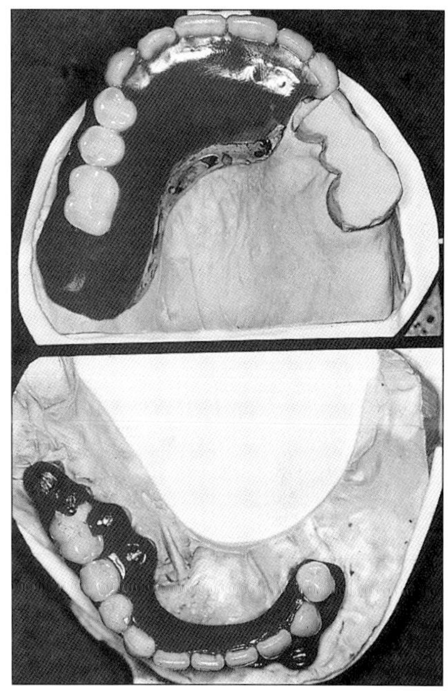

Fig. 27 Arrangement of artificial teeth on the waxed-up denture.

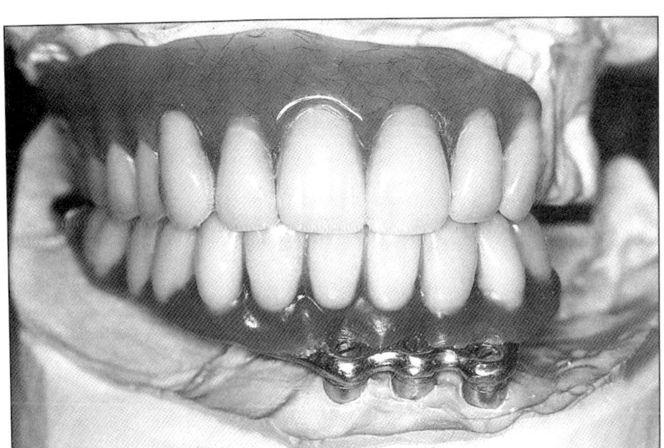

Fig. 28 The implant prostheses were completed using a pour-type resin.

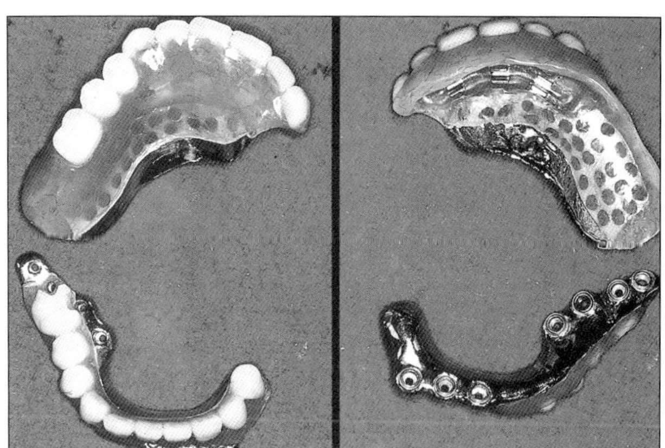

Fig. 29 Occlusal surface and mucosal surface views of the implant dentures.

CHAPTER 19

Alveolar reconstruction

1. Case with distraction osteogenesis of alveolar ridge

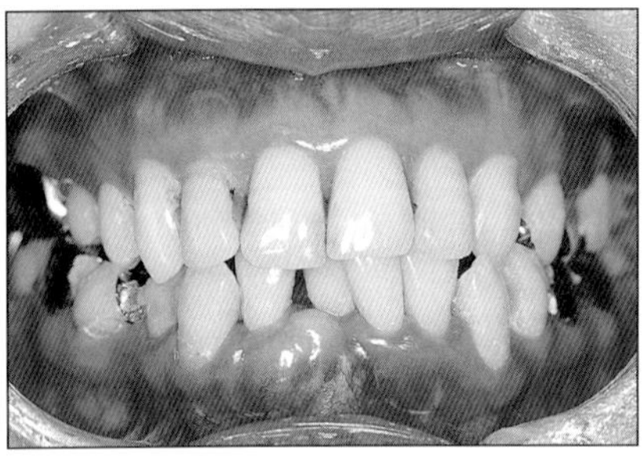

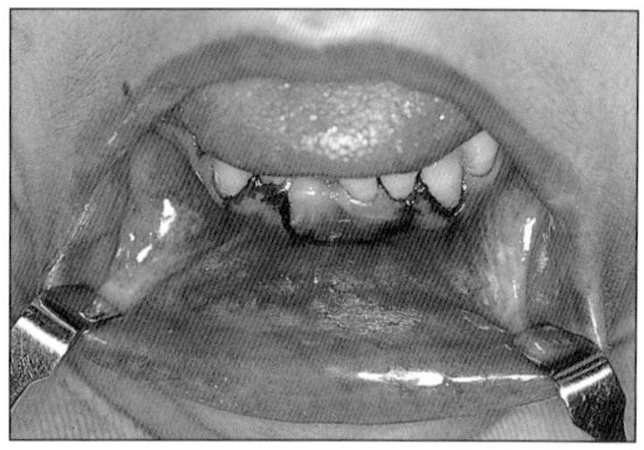

Fig. 1 *(left)* In this case a nerve sheath myxoma developed in the roots between the bilateral mandibular lateral incisors of a 38-year-old woman.
Fig. 2 *(right)* For resection of the tumor, incision lines were established at the level of the margin of the mandibular canines on both sides including an anterior part of the lower gingiva.

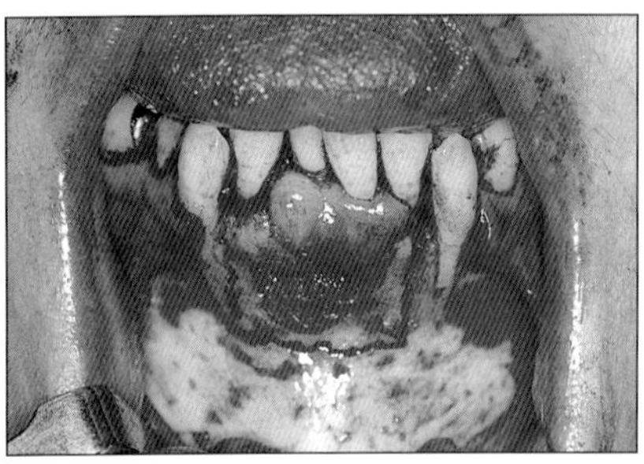

Fig. 3 Longitudinal ostectomy was performed between the mandibular lateral incisor and canine, and horizontal ostectomy was performed below the tumor.

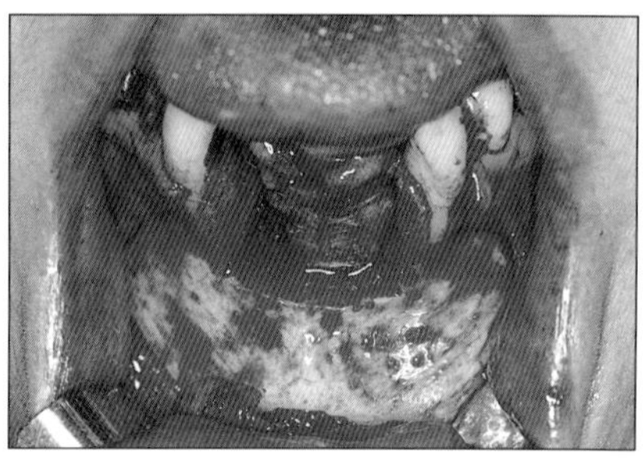

Fig. 4 The alveolar bone including the tumor was resected, and the wound was closed.

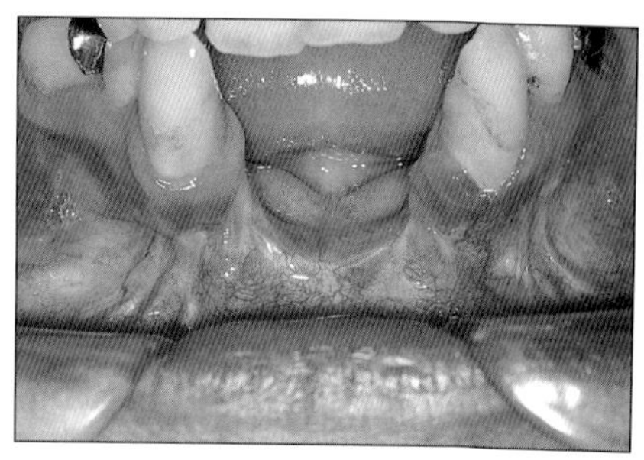

Fig. 5 The loss of residual ridge after removal of the tumor made the placement of implants difficult.

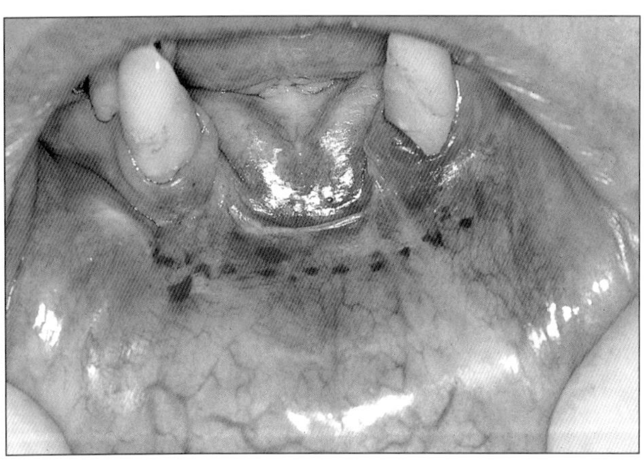

Fig. 6 It was decided to restore the alveolar bone with distraction osteogenesis at 9 months after the removal of the tumor. The vestibule was incised horizontally between the bilateral mandibular-canines, then only the labial mucoperiosteal flap was reflected.

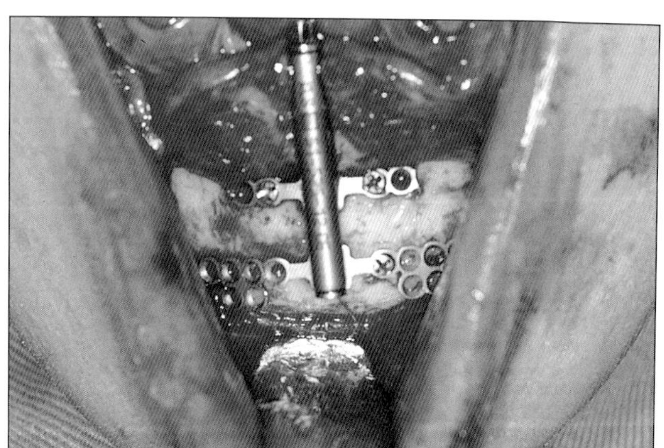

Fig. 7 According to preoperative measurement, a 9mm elongation of the alveolar ridge would be required. The distractor used was a TRACK 1.5mm Distractor, made by Martin Co (distraction length 10mm). With this distractor, a longitudinal cylinder was aligned in the direction of bone distraction, and a microplate 0.6mm in thickness, bent to fit the ostectomy site, was fixed with screws 1.5mm in diameter and 4 – 5mm in length.

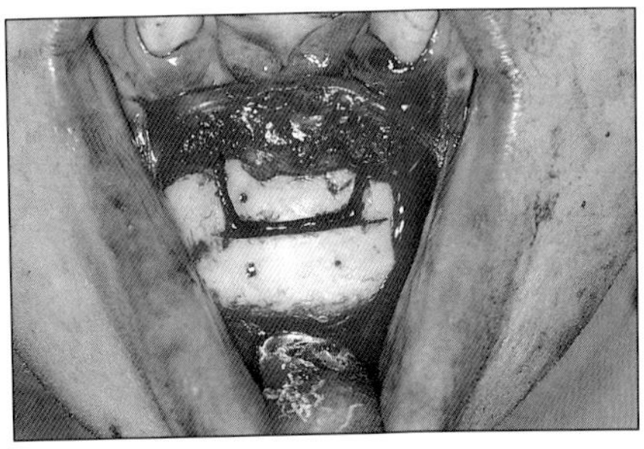

Fig. 8 The temporarily fixed distractor was removed for osteotomy of the transport segment.

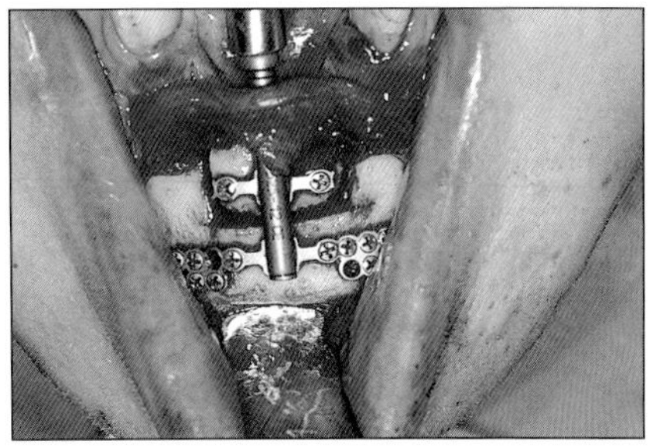

Fig. 9 Following replacement of the distractor, the transport segment was confirmed to be movable, by using a screwdriver to turn the screw of the cylinder in the center.

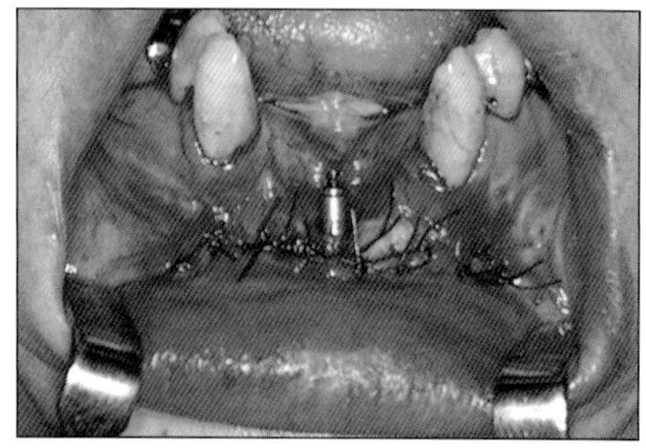

Fig. 10 The wound was closed by replacing the mucoperiosteal flap. Starting 8 days postoperatively, distraction of 0.9mm a day (3 times a day by 0.3mm each time) was performed for 10 days.

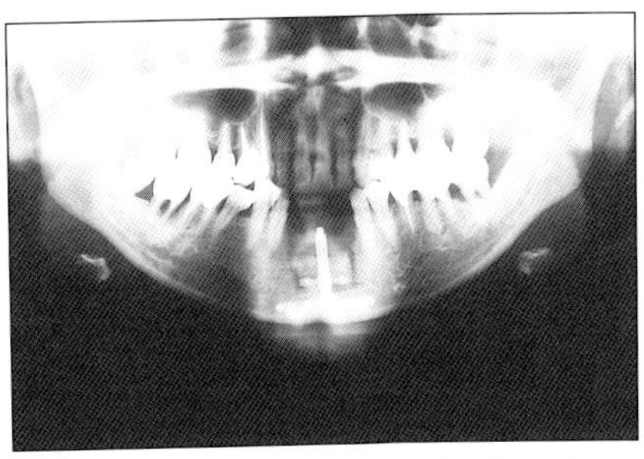

Fig. 11 Panoramic radiograph after placement of distractor.

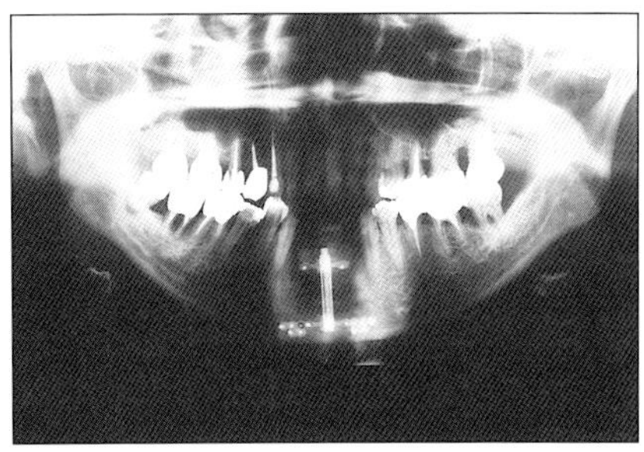

Fig. 12 Panoramic radiograph at completion of distraction osteogenesis.

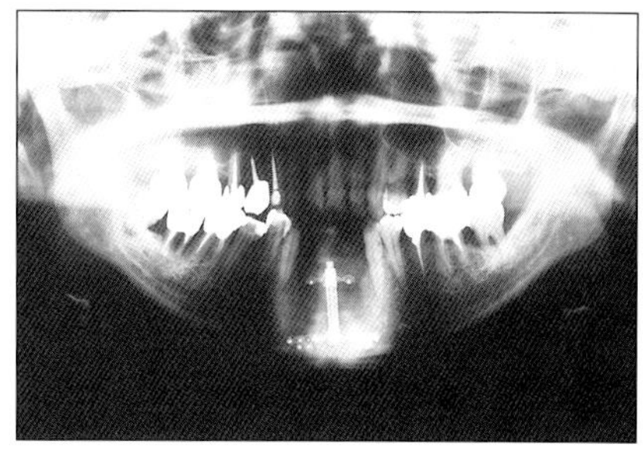

Fig. 13 Panoramic radiograph just before placement of dental implants. The removal of the distractor and placement of implants were planned to follow a retention period of about 5 months after distraction osteogenesis.

Fig. 14 *(left)* The distractor was removed following incision of the alveolar crest and reflection of the mucosa. Bone was augmented in the distracted region.
Fig. 15 *(right)* Two osseointegrated-implants, each 18mm in length, were placed in the bone-augmented region.

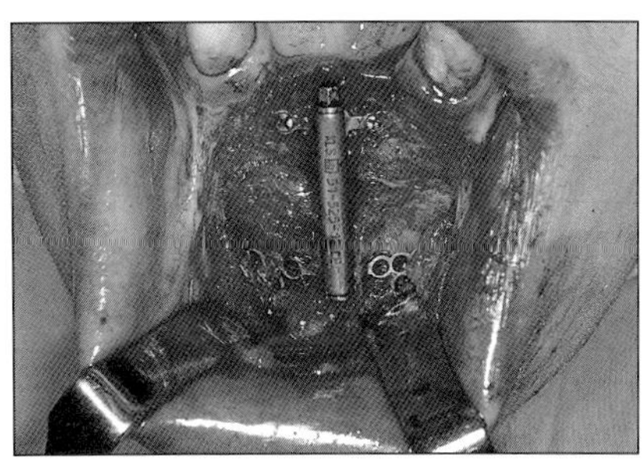

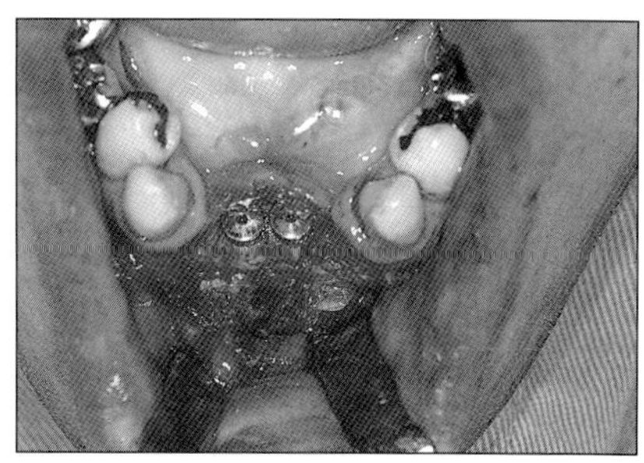

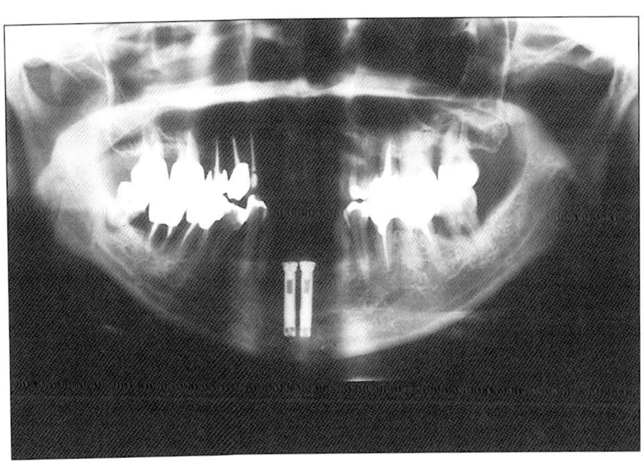

Fig. 16 Panoramic radiograph after placement of implants.

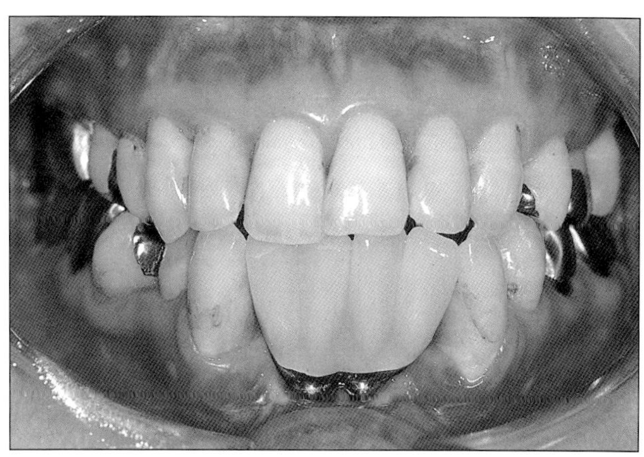

Fig. 17 A fixed implant-denture was inserted at 5 months after placement of implants.

2. Alveolar reconstruction with vascularized bone graft

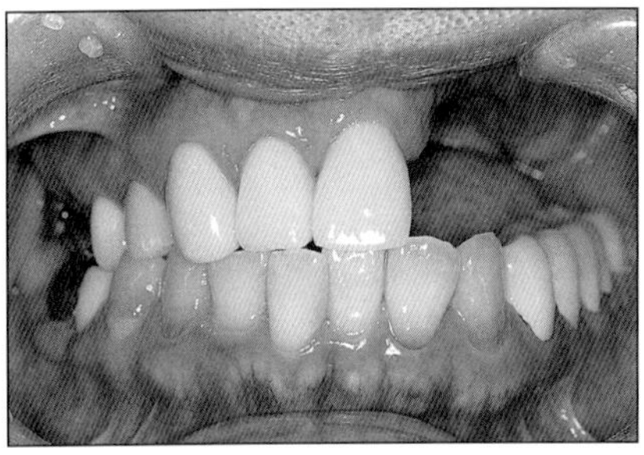

Fig. 18 In this case, a 36-year-old woman had undergone partial resection of the maxilla following a diagnosis of dentigerous cyst at 5 years of age. The alveolar bone below the anterior nasal aperture was lost with the left maxilla.

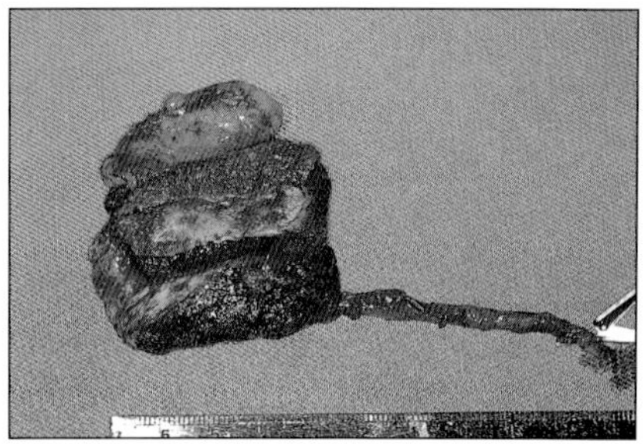

Fig. 19 A free iliac bone flap with a deep iliac circumflex artery to provide nutritional blood vessels and an accompanying vein was obtained.

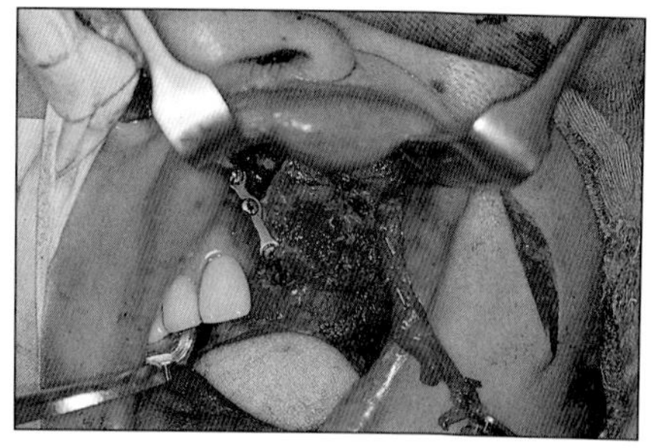

Fig. 20 The free iliac bone obtained was fixed to the residual maxilla with a mini plate and screws, and the deep iliac circumflex artery and vein accompanying it were sutured to a facial artery and vein. The flap covering the bone transplanted into the alveolar crest was sutured to the circumferential mucosa.

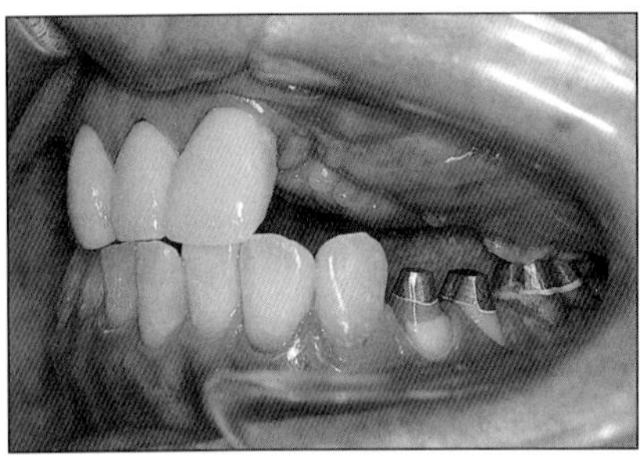

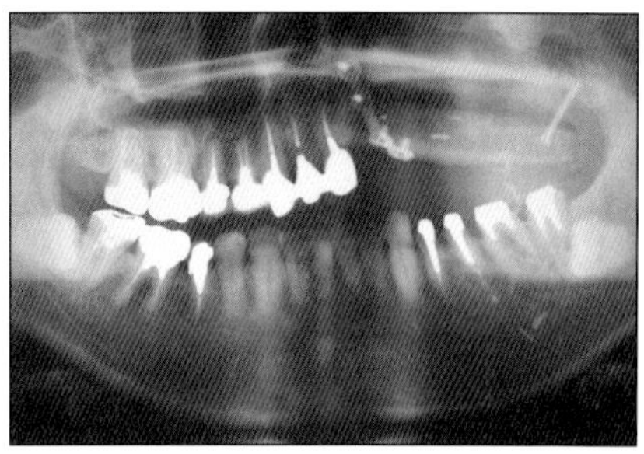

Fig. 21 *(left)* Sufficient alveolar ridge was reconstructed by the transplantation of the vascularized free iliac bone flap.
Fig. 22 *(right)* With the smooth osseous joint between the transplanted iliac bone and the residual maxilla confirmed radiographically, the placement of implants was planned after 5 months.

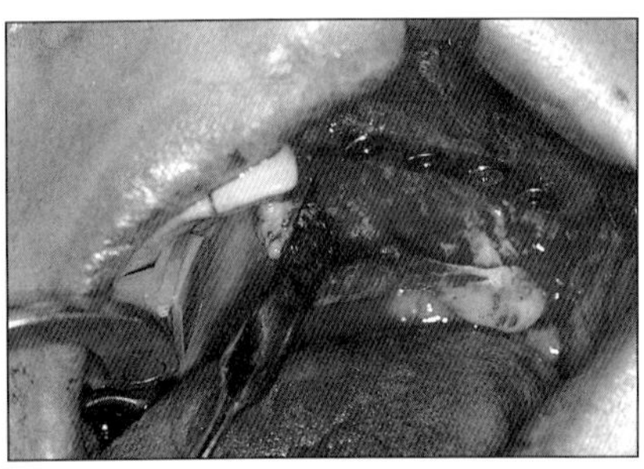

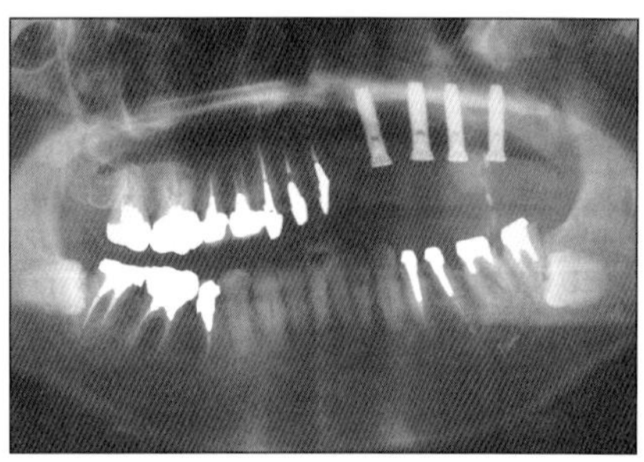

Fig. 23 *(left)* Four osseointegrated-implants were placed following removal of the mini plate and screws with which the free iliac bone had been secured.
Fig. 24 *(right)* Panoramic radiograph after placement of implants.

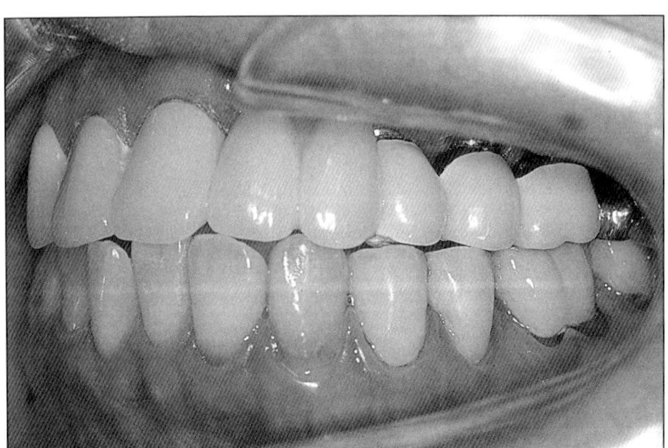

Fig. 25 Fixed implant-denture (lateral view).

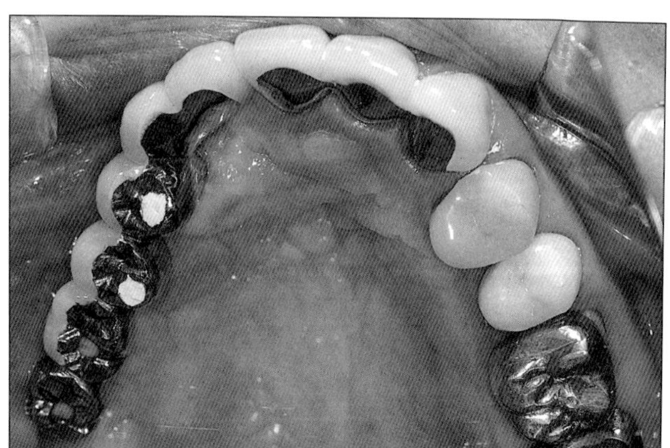

Fig. 26 Fixed implant-denture (occlusal view).

SECTION 5

Facial Defects

CHAPTER 20

Patterns and classification of facial defects

Facial defects can be caused by the treatment of intraorbital or maxillary malignant tumors, maxillofacial injuries, and congenital malformations. In Japan, most such cases follow the resection of malignant tumors, and there are various defect states. It is difficult to imagine the defective state even when a detailed description of the facial defect pathosis is given; this can be shown most clearly by photographs and drawings. However, universal scientific data should be provided when discussing treatments and effects. It is essential to use some sort of symbols to classify defective pathoses according to their severity and degree of difficulty of treatment. So, in 1981, the authors prepared an FC classification of the mid-face defects with highest frequency among patients subject to facial prosthetic treatment.

In this classification, the mid-face was divided into 4 regions on the grounds that the smaller the facial defect to be covered, the easier facial prosthetic treatment becomes, and that achieving a marginal seal is impossible on highly mobile sites, although it is possible on sites where the form is unaffected by facial movements. With limited orbital defects, the facial prosthesis remains within the eyeglass frame area, providing easy camouflage. However, with defects extending to the infraorbital region, the margin extending beyond the eyeglass frame causes esthetic problems. When the zygomatic region has been removed, the facial prosthesis becomes quite large, resulting in serious problems with retention and esthetics. A defect extending to the upper lip and buccal region may result in functional disorder as the form changes with movement, making a marginal seal difficult to achieve. Ugly shapes resulting from defects can involve not only facial skin defects but also concavity of the remaining skin; therefore the range covered by the prosthesis must extend over both such areas. FC classification represents each type of pathosis by indicating the regions where there are skin defects and concavities of the remaining skin.

FC classification of facial defects

To assess facial skin defects (F) and concavities of the mid-face (C), the mid-face as subject to facial prosthetic treatment is divided into 4 regions: 1. orbit; 2. infraorbital region; 3. zygomatic region; 4. buccal region and upper lip (Fig. 1). When the facial skin defect extends to Region 2 from Region 1 and the concavity of the mid-face extends to Region 3 from Region 2, the defect is represented as $F_{12}C_{23}$. Defects limited to F_1 are represented as F_1C_0, and this F_1C_0 is subdivided into three types, depending on the condition of the defect : F_1 (deep orbital defect), F_{1a} (shallow orbital defect), and F_{1b} (defect caused by insufficient reconstruction).

1. Facial skin defect (F)

F_0 : no facial skin defect
F_1 : skin defect to within the orbit
Cases of skin defect limited to the orbital region (F_1C_0) are divided into 3 subdivisions
F_1 : deep orbital defect
F_{1a}: shallow orbital defect
F_{1b}: defect caused by insufficient reconstruction
F_2 : skin defect in the infraorbital region
F_3 : skin defect over the zygomatic region
F_4 : skin defect on the upper lip and in the buccal region

2. Concavity of the mid-face (C)

C_0 : no concavity of the mid-face
C_1 : concavity of the orbital region
C_2 : concavity of the infraorbital region
C_3 : concavity of the zygomatic region
C_4 : concavity extending to the upper lip from the buccal region

External nasal defects (N) and auricular defects (E) are represented as N(+) or E(+) respectively.

Notational examples are shown in Figs. 2 – 5.

Representation of facial defect

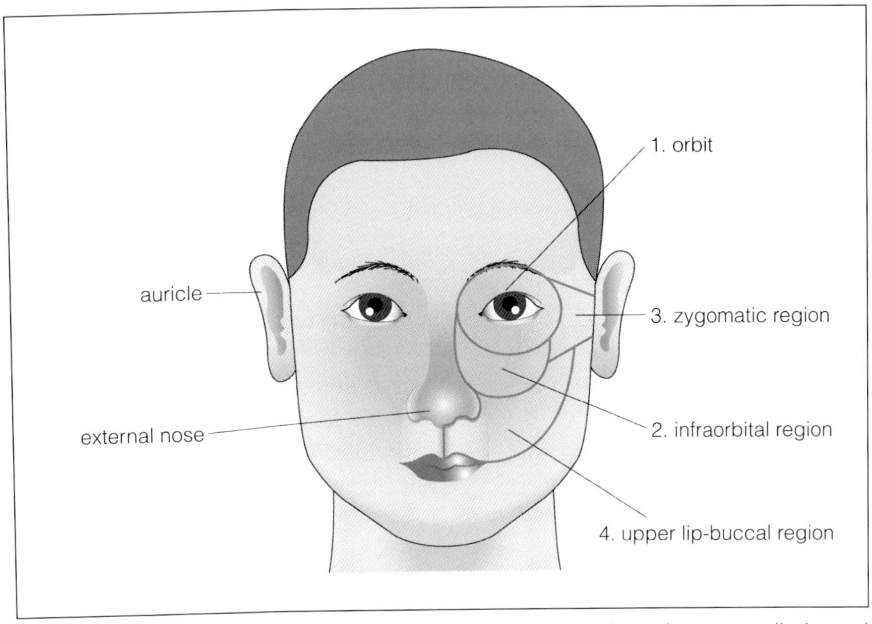

Fig. 1 Mid-facial regions: orbit; infraorbital region; zygomatic region; upper lip-buccal region. The external nose and auricle are also subject to facial prosthetic treatment.

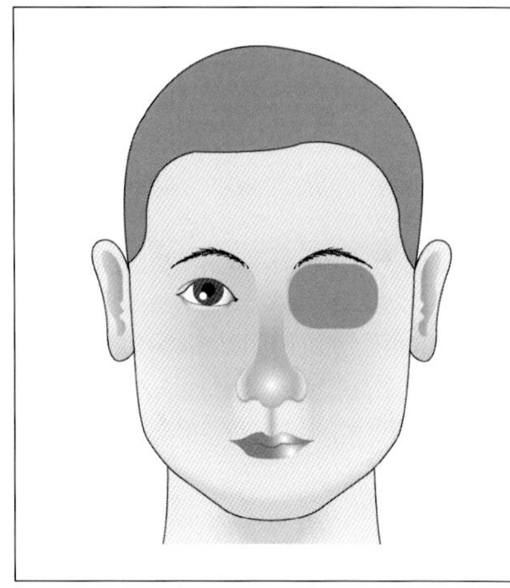

Fig. 2 This deep orbital defect is represented as F_1C_0 because there is no skin defect or concavity of the mid-face on other sites.

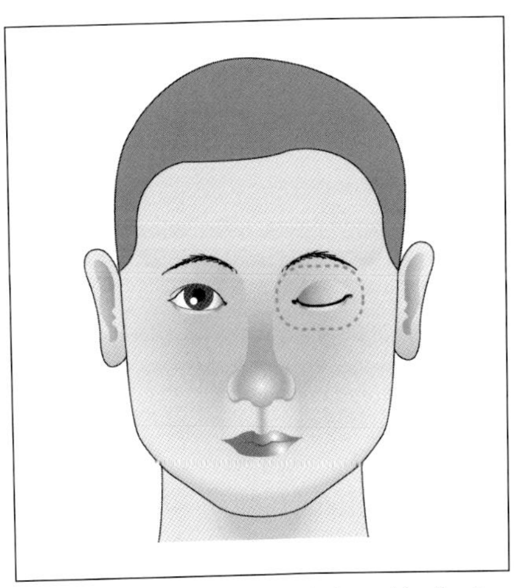

Fig. 3 The eyelids and the skin in the orbital region have been preserved, but the orbital content has been removed, resulting in remarkable concavity in the orbital region. This defect is represented as F_0C_1.

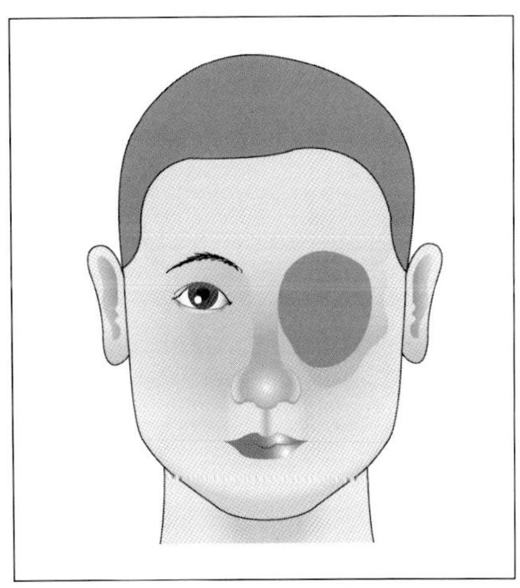

Fig. 4 This skin defect involves the orbital and infraorbital regions, and the skin on the zygomatic region and upper lip-buccal region is concave. This defect is represented as $F_{12}C_{34}$.

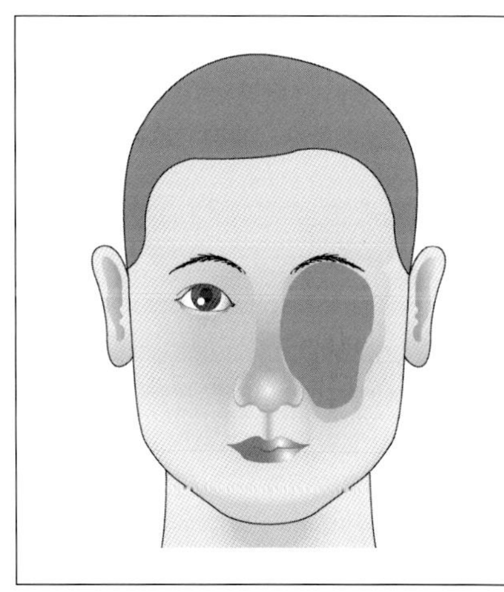

Fig. 5 This skin defect involves the orbital, infraorbital, and upper lip-buccal regions, and the skin on the zygomatic region and upper lip-buccal region is concave. This defect is represented as $F_{124}C_{34}$.

CHAPTER 21

Fabrication methods of facial prostheses

Restorations of facial defects arising from operations for tumors are classified broadly by method into those done by means of reconstructive operations and those made using artificial materials. In either method there is extreme difficulty in achieving a natural harmonization of the restored site with the original face as a part of the face, regardless of the various scales of defect sites and defect ranges. Particularly for an extensive defect including the orbit, restoration by means of reconstructive surgery cannot satisfy the patient because the defect site is situated in the center of the face. In such cases there are many problems, although facial prostheses using artificial materials provide more excellent esthetics than do reconstructive operations. Therefore, whether patients accept and attach facial prostheses for constant use depends on freedom from a sense of disharmony with each patient's face and on secure retentive force so that the prosthesis will never suddenly fall off in public. The former problem has been resolved by excellent materials and the skilled techniques of makers; the latter problem has been solved by implants, adhesives and mechanical retention, or combinations of these. Different facilities use various methods for the fabrication of facial prostheses. We also describe measures taken in different facilities for the resolution of problems, including techniques for obscuring retainers and the margins of facial prostheses, and for resolving problem such as the feeling that appearance is unnatural due to immovable ocular prostheses and eyelids and the degeneration of colors and materials occurring in short periods of 1 to 2 years.

Fabrication of facial prosthesis to be retained by adhesive

For the contour of a facial prostheses using adhesive, the largest possible portion of the prosthesis should be applied to less-mobile facial soft tissue around the defect in order to provide better retention, with the smallest possible portion of the prosthesis covering more mobile areas, thus avoiding the danger of detachment. Therefore, when using adhesives for retention, the contours of facial prostheses must be larger than those of prostheses using other retentive measures.

Facial snap impression

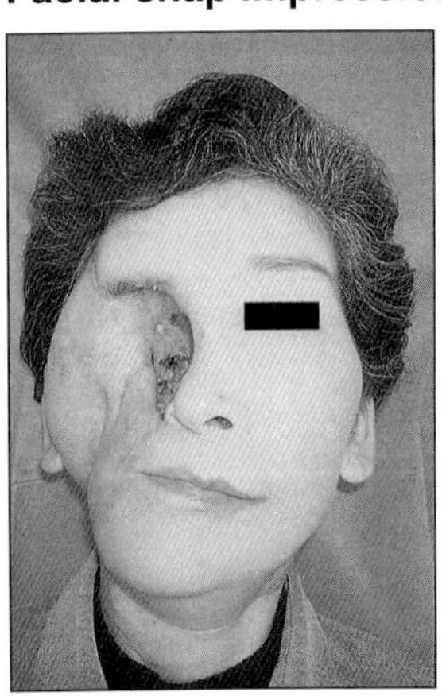

Fig. 1 Case 1 (extensive defect including orbit, from right side of the midface): In this case, a 60-year-old woman suffered a primary malignant neoplasm of the right maxillary sinus, with extensively evolved squamous cell carcinoma from the cranial base to the skin. Following right maxillary resection, orbital exenteration, and radical neck dissection, the facial defect was reconstructed using a rectus flap and forearm flap. The defect status was an extensive defect from the right orbit to the buccal region.

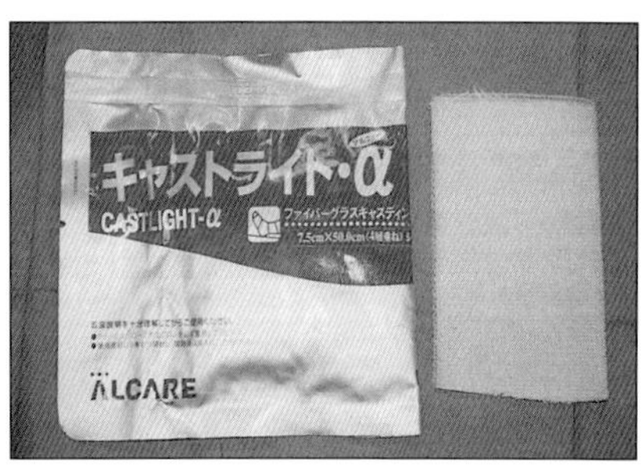

Fig. 2 The materials prepared for facial snap impression are materials for fabricating a barrier to keep impression material from flowing out off the face, gauze, and an alginate impression material. To prevent the outflow of impression material, we use silicon putty impression material, clay, and cardboard: our department also uses CASTLIGHT®, a water-settable plastic gypsum bandage commonly used in the orthopaedic field.

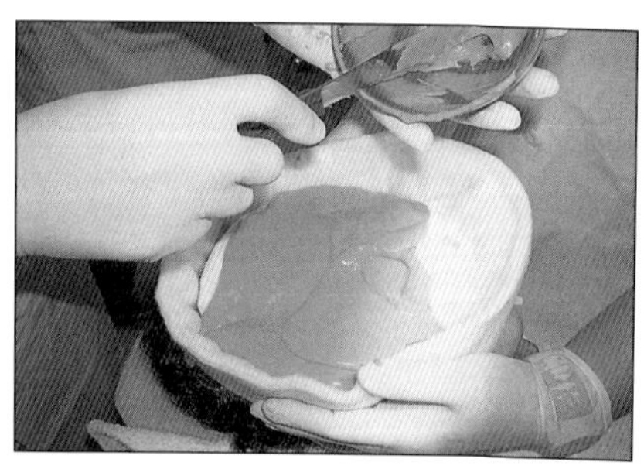

Fig. 3 CASTLIGHT® is cut with scissors to fit around the circumference of the face then wetted with water so it will start to harden. Gauze is applied around the patient's hair and elsewhere to prevent leakage of the impression material. First, the opening through the defective facial region and oral cavity is protected with gauze, then the facial impression region is surrounded with protective walls to prevent the outflow of impression material, and rubber tubes for respiration are inserted in the mouth and external naris to ensure respiration paths. Then an impression of the whole face is taken with alginate impression material.

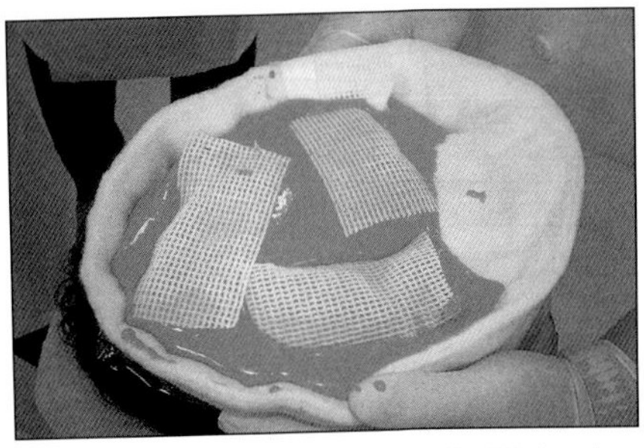

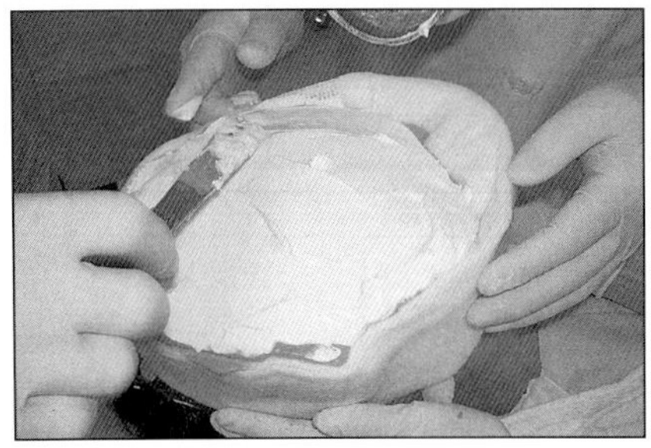

Figs. 4 and 5 Some CASTLIGHT® is placed in the impression material as a mechanical bonding material for reinforcement, and tapped down to allow bonding with the cast.

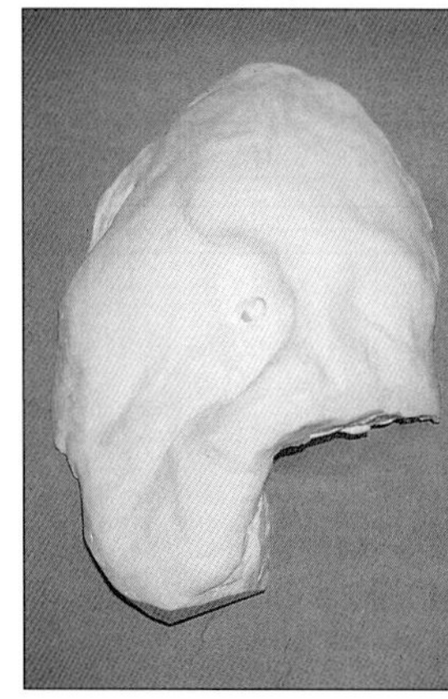

Fig. 6 A study cast is fabricated from the facial snap impression.

Facial impression, and fabrication of facial cast and frame for reinforcing silicon

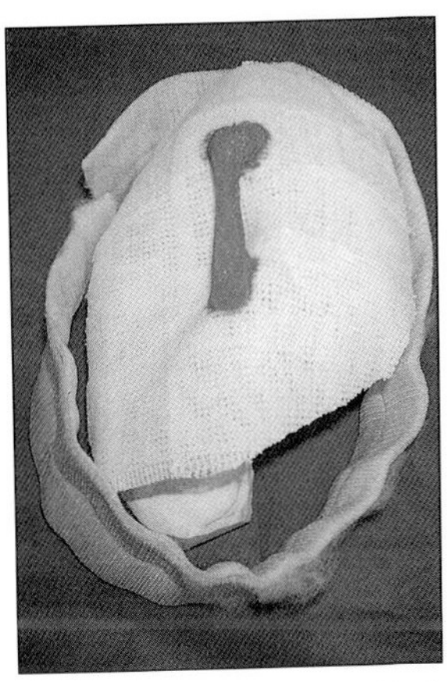

Fig. 7 A protective wall of CASTLIGHT® to prevent the outflow of impression material used for impression, and a tray for reinforcing the alginate impression material, are fabricated on the cast.

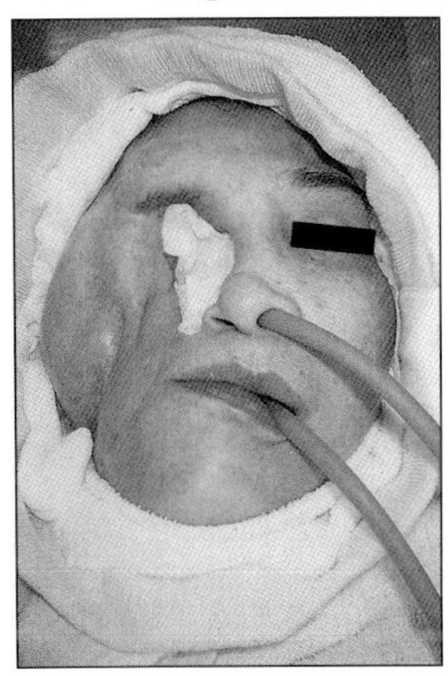

Fig. 8 As was done for the snap impression, a breathing path is ensured by rubber tubes for respiration, and the defective region and oral cavity are isolated using gauze.

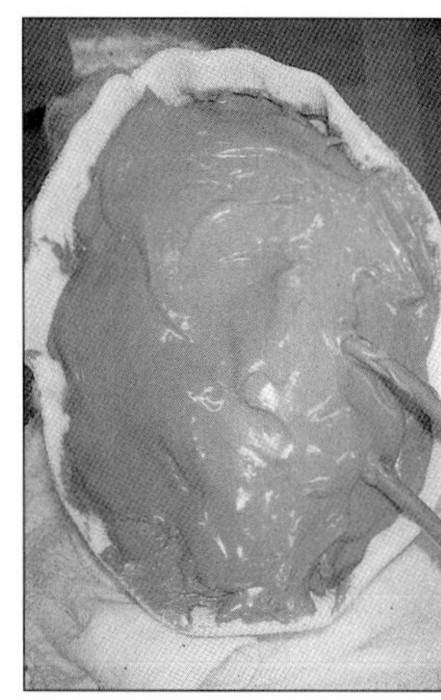

Fig. 9 Alginate impression material is fully applied to the entire face to take the impression.

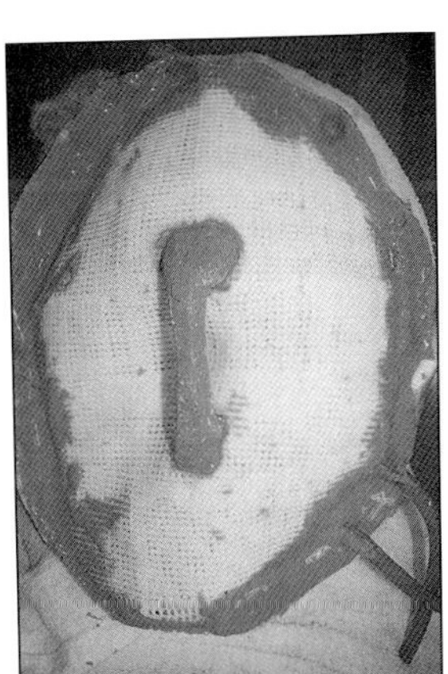

Fig. 10 The whole cast is covered by a tray to reinforce the impression material to prevent deformation of the alginate impression.

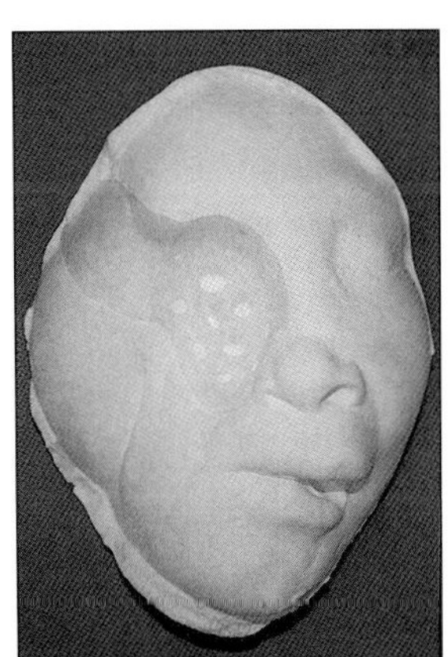

Fig. 11 A working cast is fabricated of modified hard plaster.

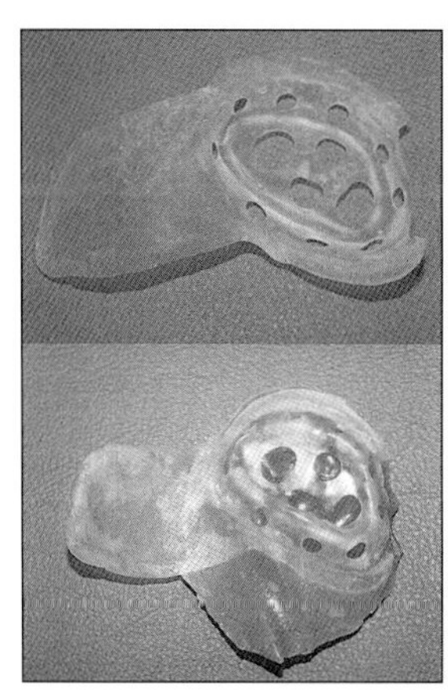

Fig. 12 A frame for reinforcing silicon is fabricated using self-curing resin to reinforce the center of the facial prosthesis. The upper photo in Figure 12 shows the inside of the resin frame for reinforcement centering on the orbital region, and the lower photo shows wax for facial formation retained through the resin for reinforcement.

Facial formation with wax

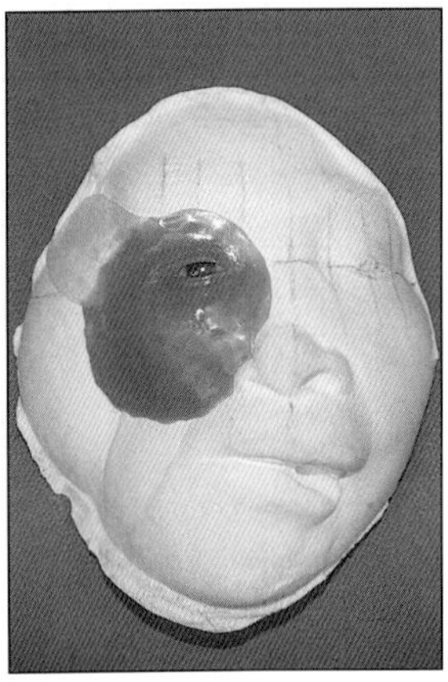

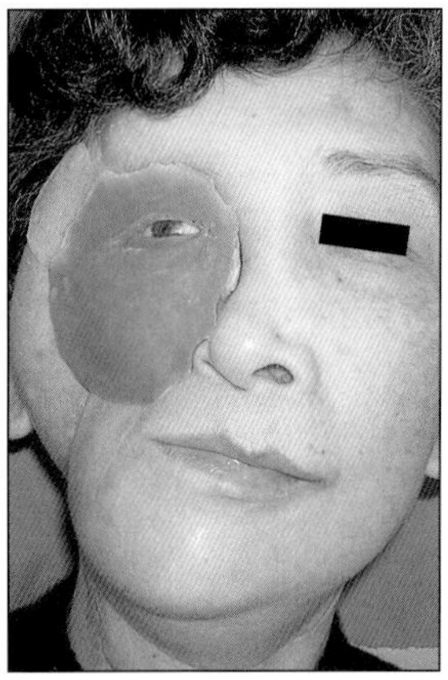

Fig. 13 *(left)* The central region of the defect is waxed up first to precisely determine the position of the eyeball.
Fig. 14 *(right)* The position of the eyeball is adjusted by trial fitting on the patient.

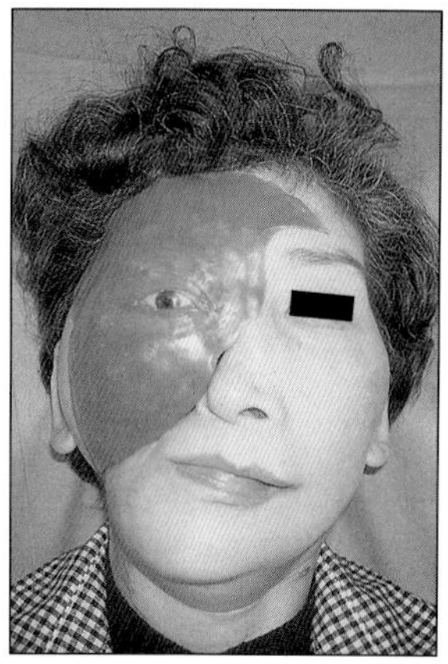

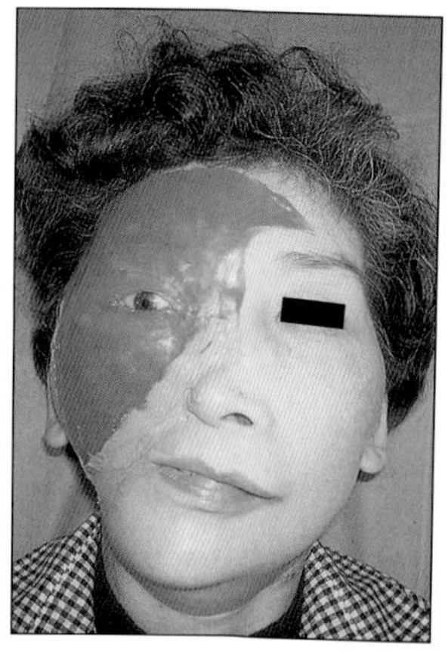

Fig. 15 *(left)* With this method, the contour should be extended as much as possible to facial regions where there is less movement, to secure a larger area for bonding. Therefore, with the forehead as the main retention source in this case, the reconstructed flap of the anterior earlobe and the median nose should be used for additional retention.
Fig. 16 *(right)* Following checking of eyeball and eyebrow positions, misadaptations between the right nasal wing and upper lip are corrected with silicon impression material.

Silicon vulcanization for facial prosthesis

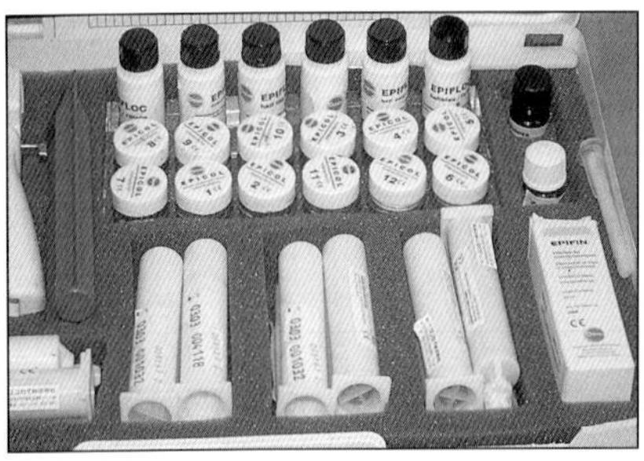

Fig. 17 Silskin® (Trackray, England) is used as the silicon material for the facial prosthesis, and to match the facial skin color, the facial prosthesis fabricated is modified with silicon colors manufactured by GMBH.

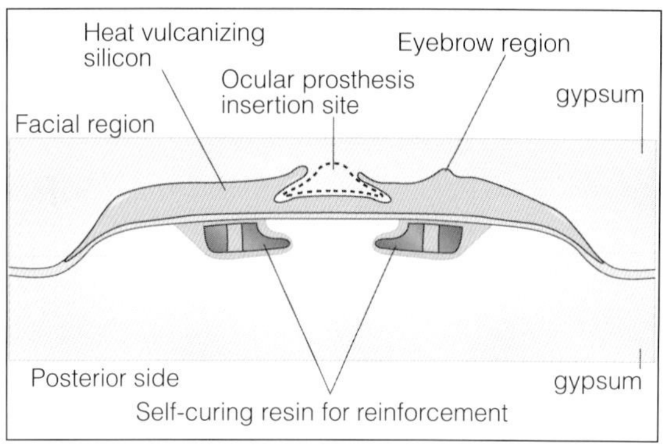

Fig. 18 The wax facial prosthesis with self-curing resin frame to reinforce the silicon is invested in the plaster for flasking, the flask is boiled out, the wax is then melted by boiling water, and finally, the silicon is poured into the cavity of the wax facial prosthesis via the retainer holes in the resin provided for mechanical retention.

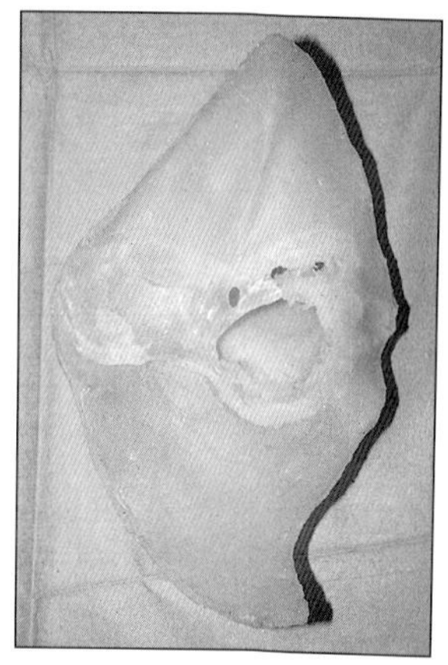

Fig. 19 Vulcanization for 2 hours at 150°C allows the silicon to cure.

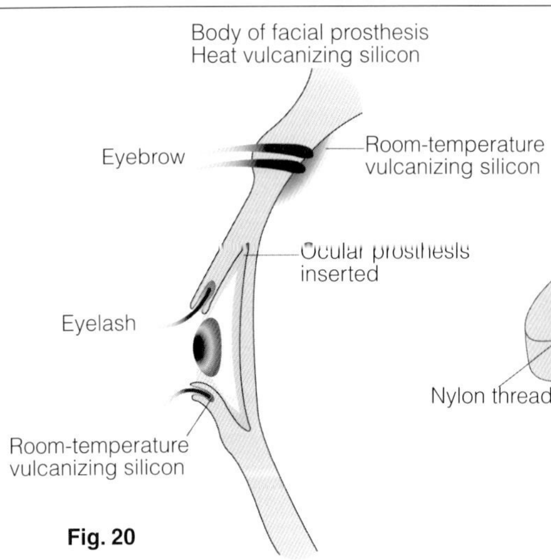

Fig. 20

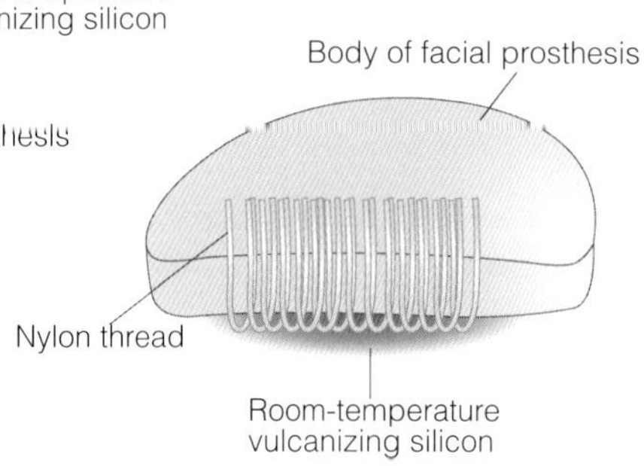

Fig. 21

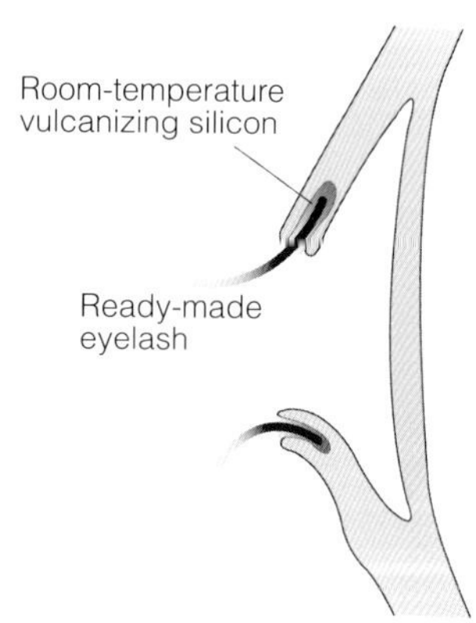

Fig. 22

Fig. 20 An ocular prosthesis eye is inserted into the silicon after vulcanization followed by fine-tuning of the position of the eyeball.
Fig. 21 An eyebrow is fabricated by carefully sewing fine nylon thread into the silicon.
Fig. 22 Modified ready-made sets of women's eyelashes are placed in the edges of the eyelids and fixed with room-temperature vulcanizing silicon.

Insertion of facial prosthesis

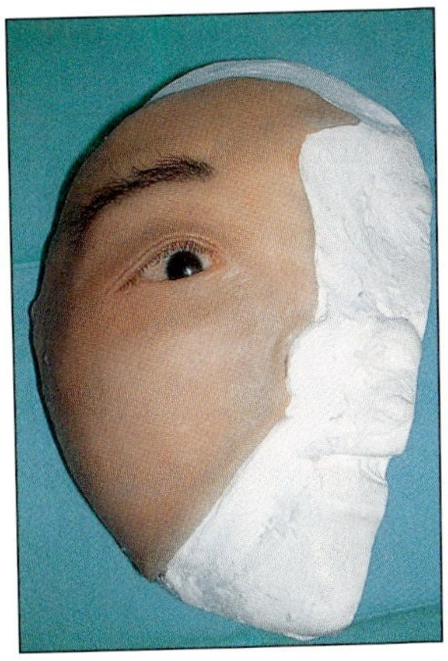

Fig. 23 The facial prosthesis is complete after overall adjustments.

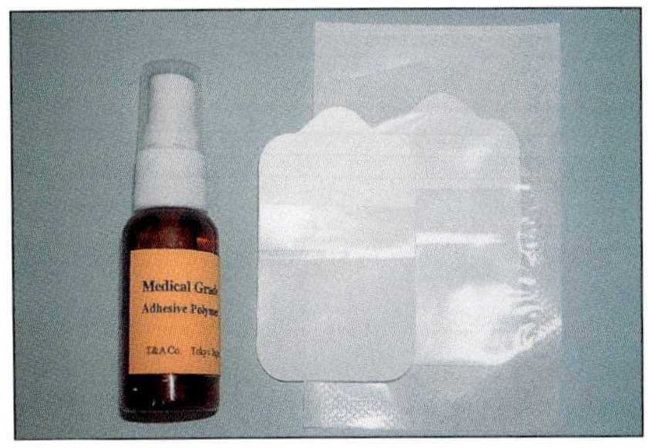

Fig. 24-1 Prosthesis adhesion method. Medical bandage material made of polyurethane sheet coated with acrylic-based adhesive agent, a medical silicon bioadhesive agent containing poly-dimethyl siloxane, and remover, are needed for adhesion of prostheses made of silicon.

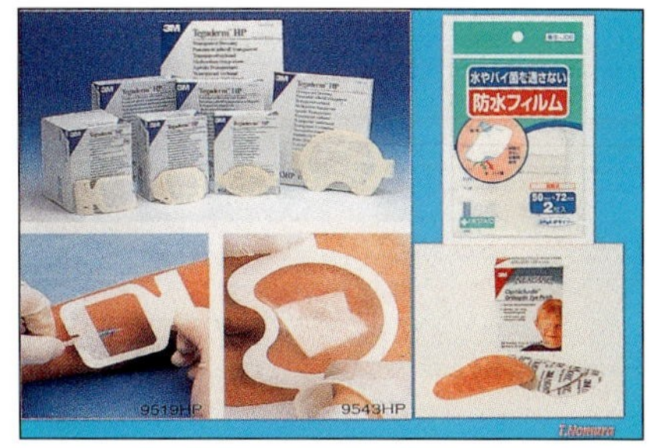

Fig. 24-2 Medical bandage material made of polyurethane sheet coated with acrylic-based adhesive agent. (The material shown at left is made by 3M; the material shown at upper right is bandage material made of polyurethane and marketed through drugstores, etc.)

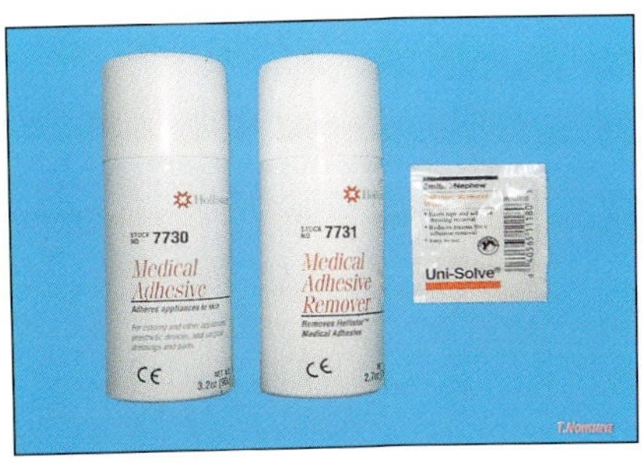

Fig. 24-3 Medical silicon bioadhesive agent containing poly-dimethyl siloxane (left), and remover (2 items at right). Prosthesis adhesion is done in the following 2 stages. First, the polyurethane sheet, divided into small pieces, is adhered to the entire marginal area of the rear surface of the prosthesis. Next, the surface of the acrylic-based adhesive agent on the polyurethane sheet is adhered to the patient's skin. Adhesion is done in the order shown in a~h in Fig. 24-4-7.

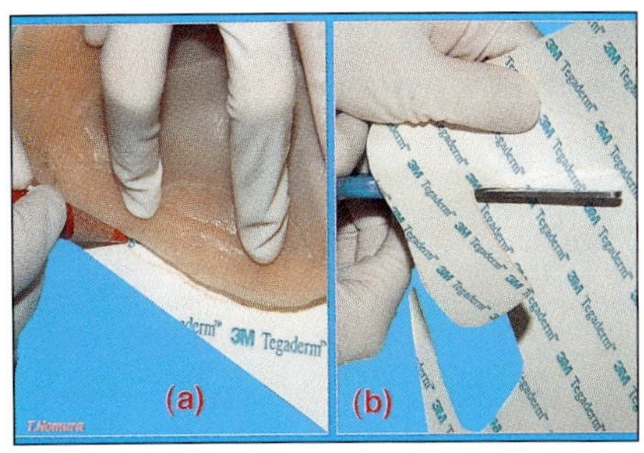

Fig. 24-4 a: Keep the acrylic adhesive agent coated side of the medical polyurethane sheet upward, place the rear surface of the prosthesis on top of the adhesive agent surface, and use a red pencil to mark the shape of the prosthesis. **b:** Keeping the acrylic adhesive agent coated side of the medical polyurethane sheet upward, cut the sheet to roughly fit the shape of the prosthesis.

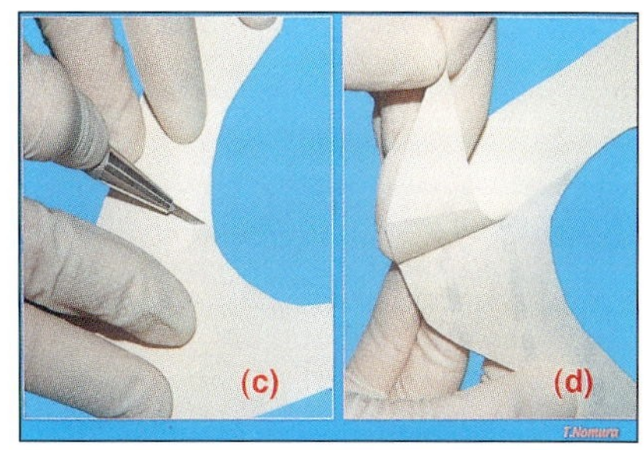

Fig. 24-5 c,d: After the urethane sheet has been cut, turn it over, lightly cut notches on the protective sheet on the non-adhesive surface, then remove the protective sheet.

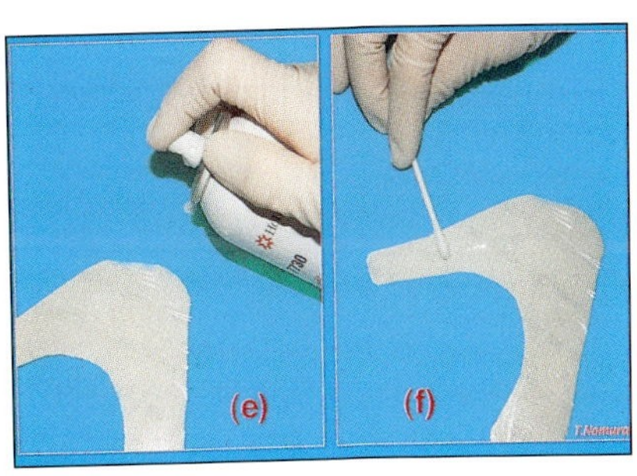

Fig. 24-6 e,f: After the protective sheet has been removed, spray the non-adhesive surface with medical silicon bioadhesive agent containing poly-dimethyl siloxane, and use a swab to evenly distribute the coating of the sprayed-on adhesive agent.

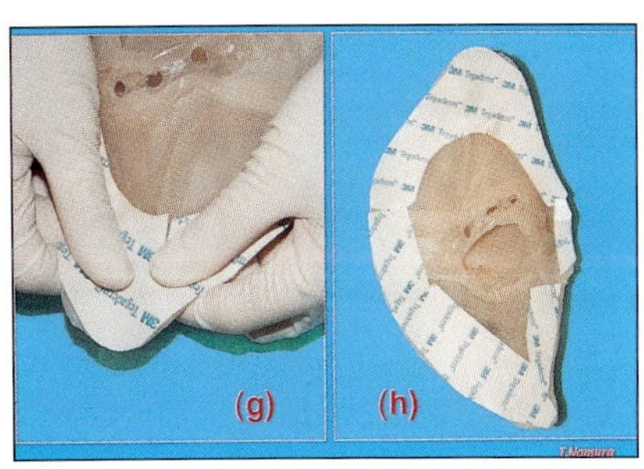

Fig. 24-7 g: After the adhesive agent has dried for several minutes, press-weld this surface coated with adhesive agent to the rear surface of the prosthesis to adhere the urethane sheet to the prosthesis. Repeat this operation for the number of sheets needed. **h:** Photo shows the medical bandage material divided into several parts and adhered to the marginal area of the rear of the prosthesis.

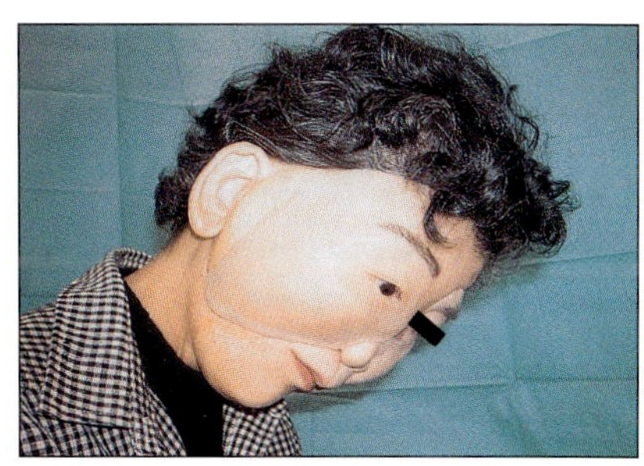

Fig. 25 In order to adhere the prosthesis to the living body, peel off the printed surface sheet which is protecting the acrylic-based adhesive agent shown in the previous photo, and press-weld the prosthesis to the living body. Confirm that the prosthesis does not fall off even when the patient faces downward.

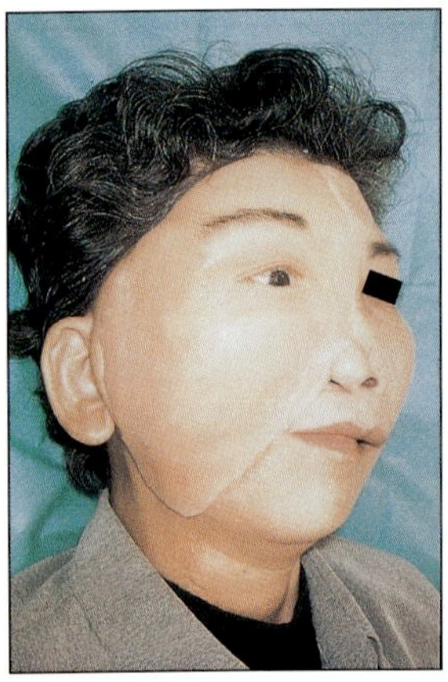

Fig. 26 Further fine-tuning of position is done after attaching the facial prosthesis to the face.

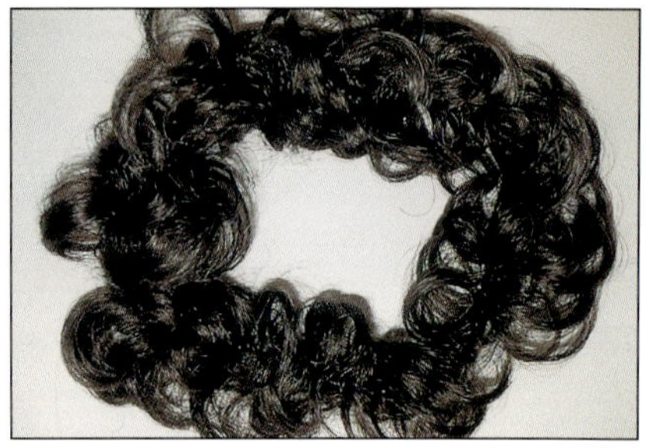

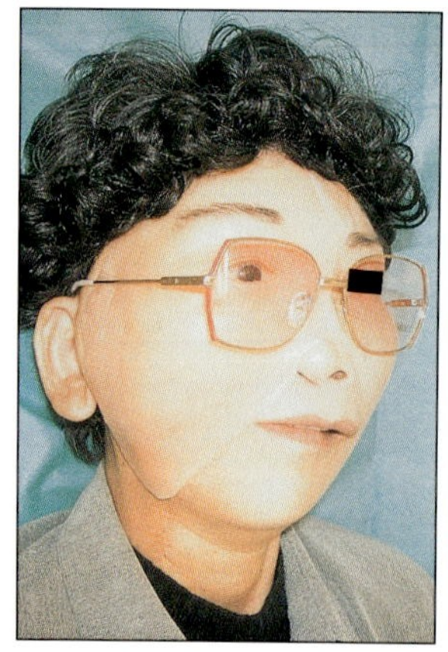

Figs. 27 and 28 A hairpiece and eyeglasses are worn to camouflage the facial prosthesis.

Small-size defect case

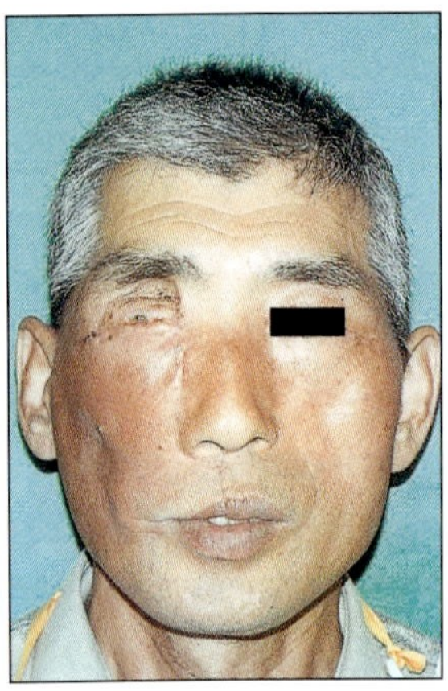

Fig. 29 Case 2 Case of small shallow defect in right orbit: in this case a 65-year-old man had undergone right maxillary resection and right orbital exenteration due to right maxillary squamous cell carcinoma 3 years earlier. The upper and lower eyelids had been preserved and the orbit had been closed.

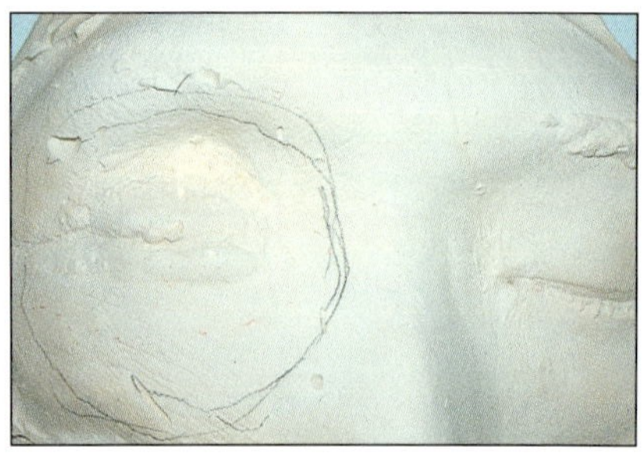

Fig. 30 Impression only in and around the orbit was taken with an alginate impression material to fabricate a working cast.

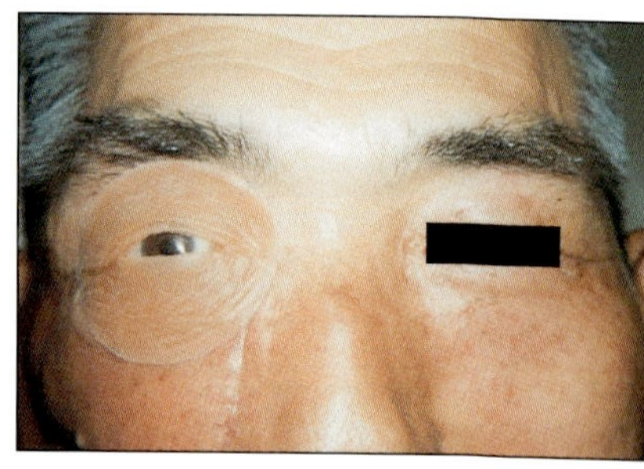

Fig. 31 A facial prosthesis was fabricated with Silskin.

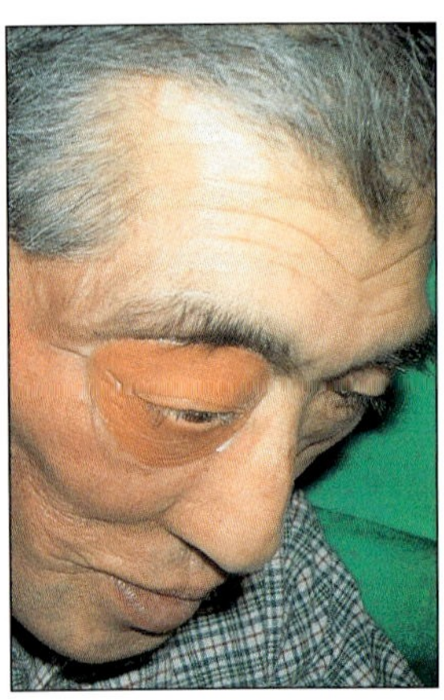

Fig. 32 It was ensured that the facial prosthesis would not fall off even when the patient was facing downward.

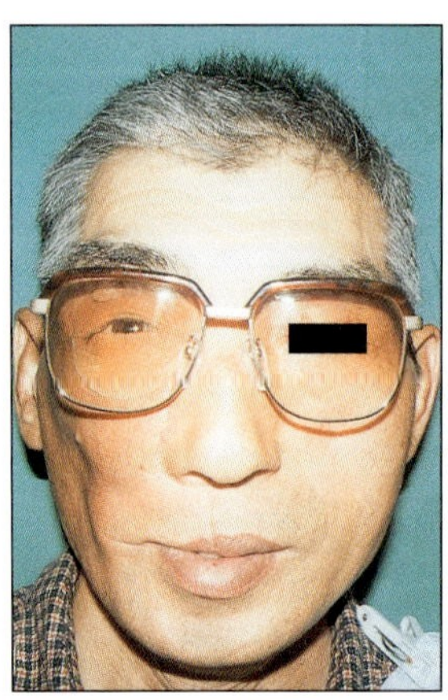

Fig. 33 Completion after camouflaging with eyeglasses.

CHAPTER 22

Retention methods for facial prostheses

To keep a facial prosthesis in place, some methods of retaining the prosthesis are needed. Since olden times, facial prostheses have been retained by the wearing of eyeglasses or wigs, or the facial prosthesis has been made as a continuation of a maxillodental prosthesis, or the facial prosthesis has been adhered to facial skin. Magnets, undercuts, adhesive agents, adhesive tape, etc., have been used as retaining methods.

In addition, various types of facial implants have been introduced in recent years.

This section shows methods which are relatively less invasive, such as the customary methods using adhesive agents, double-sided adhesive tape, eyeglasses or wigs to hold facial prosthesis in place.

An adhesive agent has been often applied using a brush, etc., to the part of the prosthesis that contacts the skin. Adhesive agent use has the disadvantages that the diluent for the adhesive agent is difficult to apply due to its quick-drying property, and that also, once applied, the adhesive agent is difficult to peel off. On the other hand, its advantages are that its adhesion to the defective part is good and that closure is also good. The advantages of improved double-sided adhesive tape for facial prosthesis use are that the tape can be quite easily adhered to the prosthesis, the seal between the prosthesis and skin is good, secondary surgery is not needed, and tape can be used from the beginning, immediately after surgery in so far as the surrounding skin is sound.

The application of facial implants has recently advanced. Facial implants have the advantage of being able to attach the prosthesis firmly to the patient's face, but secondary surgery is needed to install the implants; the disadvantages are that the cost for implant surgery is expensive.

Retention of facial prosthesis by eyeglasses and magnet

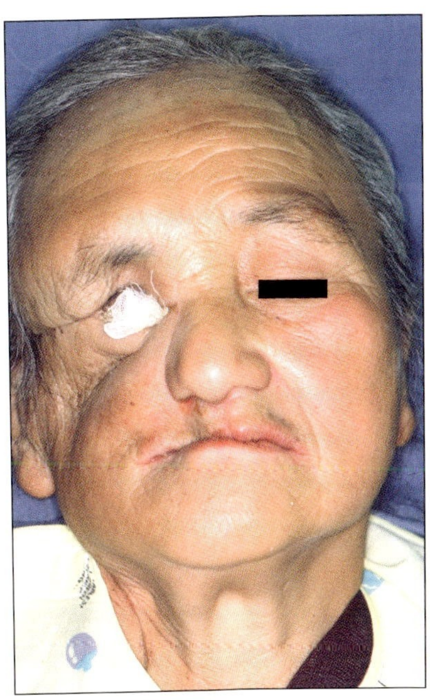

Fig. 1 66-year-old female with skin defect 29 × 11mm in size around the right lower eyelid. The orbit, infraorbital and zygomatic area are concave. FC classification is F_1C_{123}.

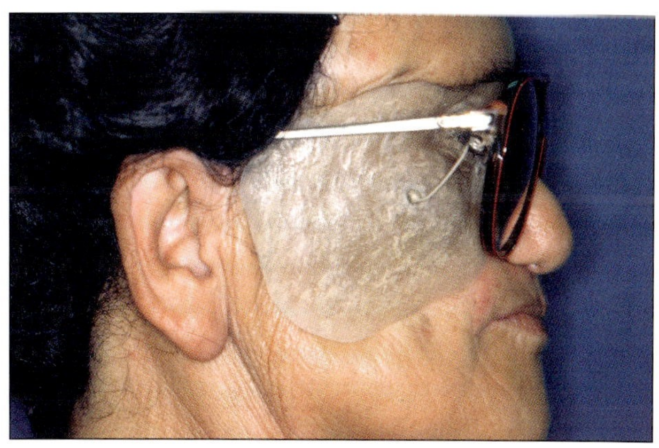

Fig. 2 Eyeglasses are connected to the facial prosthesis using magnets as the retainers. The patient uses 3 kinds of eyeglasses: for going out, for at-home use and for presbyopia.

Retention of facial prosthesis by joining with maxillodental prosthesis using a magnet (Case 1)

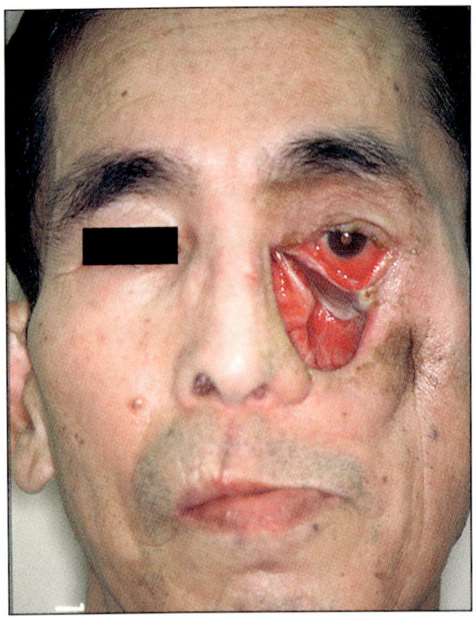

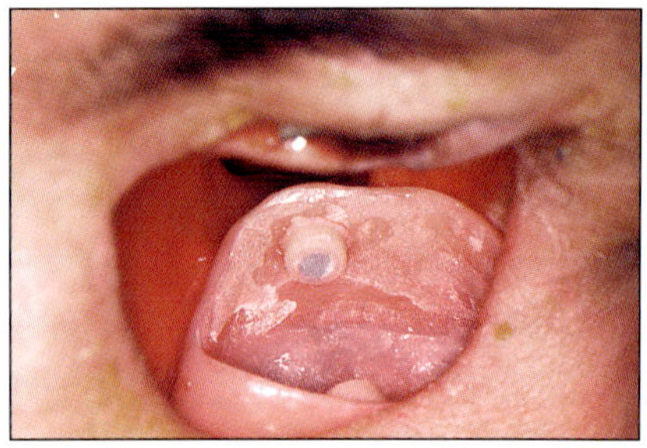

Fig. 3 *(left)* 60-year-old male with skin defect 36 × 32 mm in size on the lower part of the left orbit, which reaches the mobile portion of the upper part of the upper labiobuccal region. There is a concavity on the front of the malar bone area. FC classification: F_2C_{34}.
Fig. 4 *(right)* The magnet attached to the extended part of the obturator of the maxillodental prosthesis is used as the retainer for the facial prosthesis.

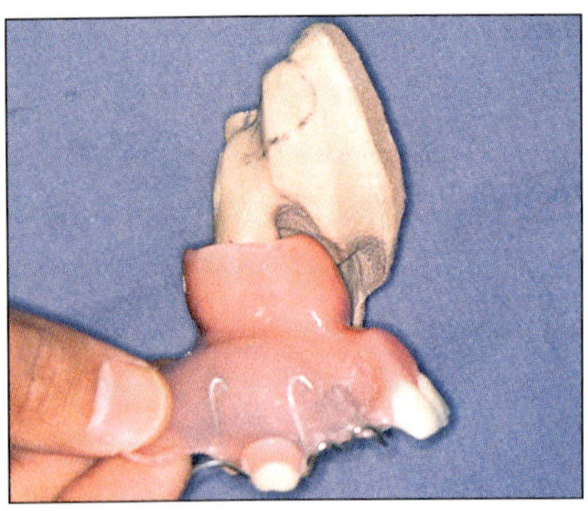

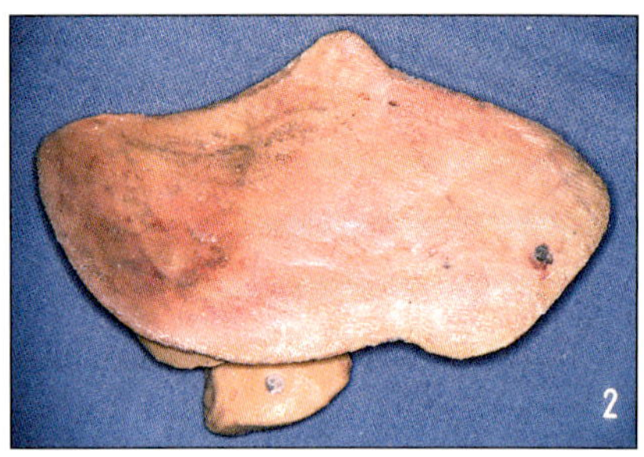

Figs. 5 and 6 View of maxillodental prosthesis joined to facial prosthesis. Closure by facial prostheses is not always good in this, defect cases that include the mobile portion of the upper labiobuccal region. The photo at right shows the surface of the facial prosthesis.

Retention of facial prosthesis by joining with maxillodental prosthesis using a magnet (Case 2)

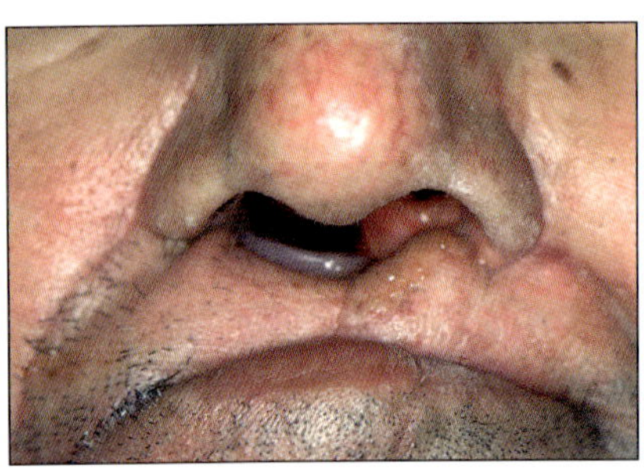

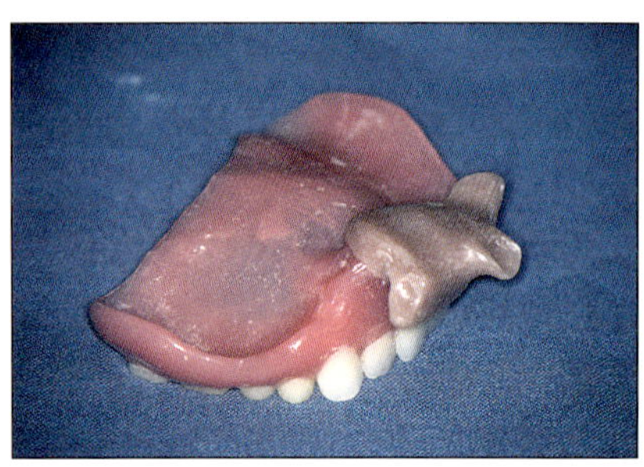

Fig. 7 *(left)* 60-year-old male with defect of columella and upper half of upper lip, size 7 × 15mm.
Fig. 8 *(right)* A magnet is used for retention of the facial prosthesis to the maxillodental prosthesis.

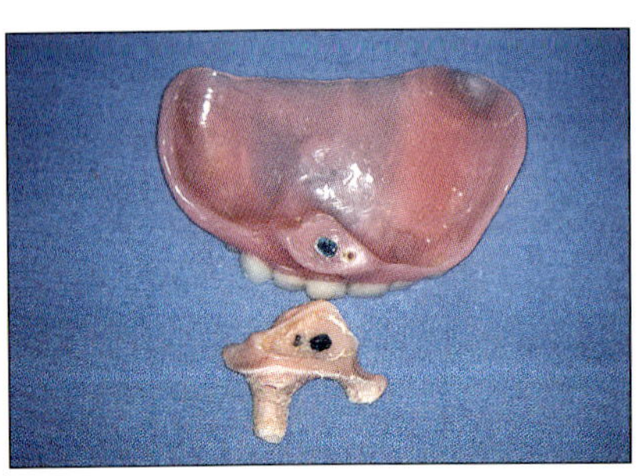

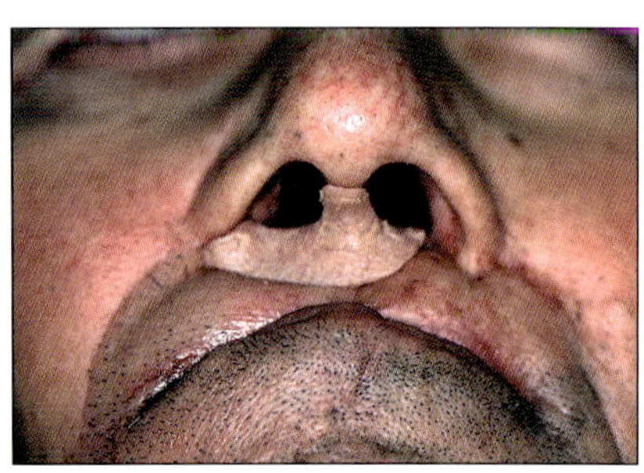

Fig. 9 *(left)* The magnet has been buried in the upper edge of the obturator of the maxillodental prosthesis. Hole to prevent rotation of the prosthesis is provided.
Fig. 10 *(right)* View of facial prosthesis in place. Rhinorrhea could not be stopped.

Retention by assembly

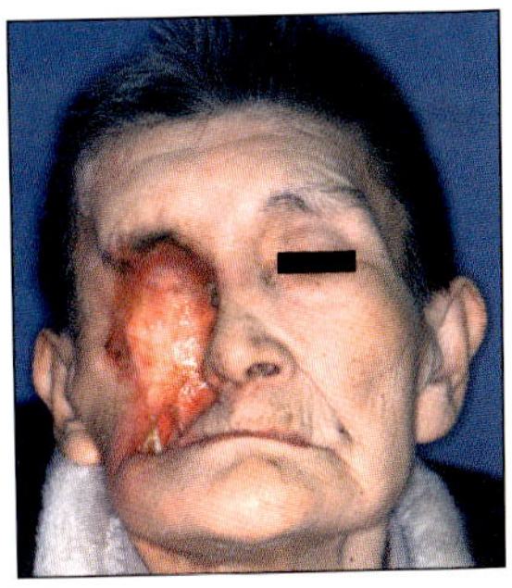

Fig. 11 74-year-old female, wide-ranging facial defect covering 76 × 75mm including right orbit infraorbital region, cheek, zygomatic, and upper lip region. Opening size is 40mm. This patient suffers from senile dementia and is now in a nursing home facility. FC classification is $F_{12345}C_3$. Facial prosthetics was started while the patient was still in hospital after surgery, to prevent the outflow of food during eating.

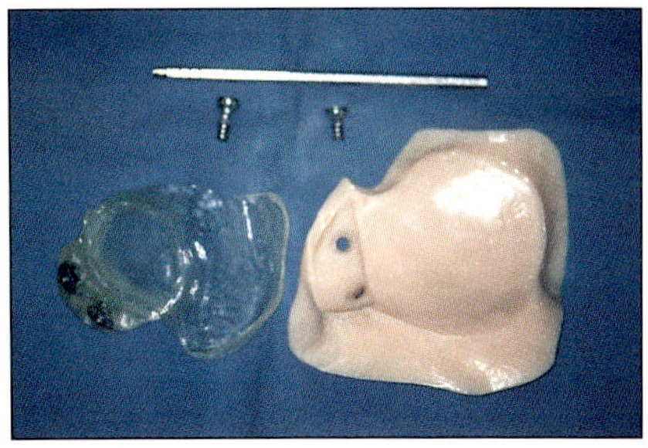

Fig. 12 Because of her dementia, she cannot detach the prosthesis by herself, so we decided to fix the facial prosthesis to the maxillodental prosthesis using screws. In the photo, the item on the left is the maxillodental prosthesis, the item on the right is the facial prosthesis, and the screws and exclusive screwdriver are shown above them.

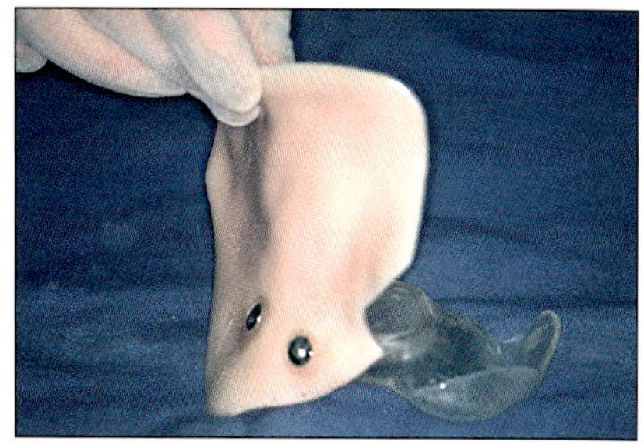

Fig. 13 The photo shows the combined assembly of prostheses.

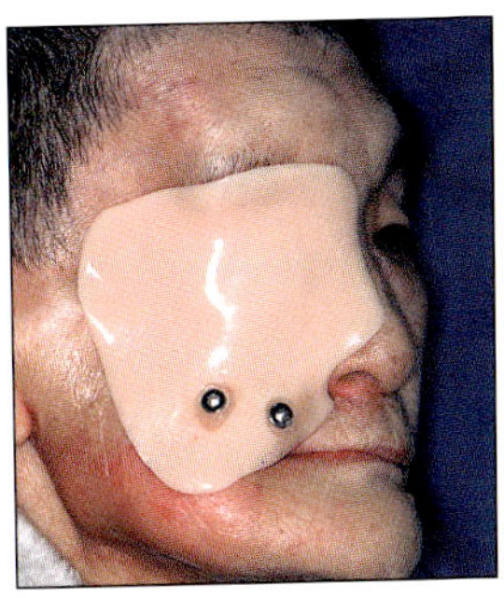

Fig. 14 The photo shows the facial prosthesis in place.

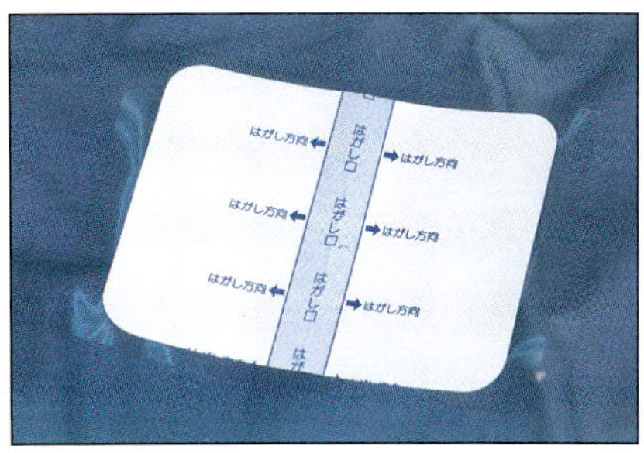

Fig. 15 For dressing was attached to the part where the prosthesis contacts the skin of the mandibular angle, to prevent the leakage of liquids.

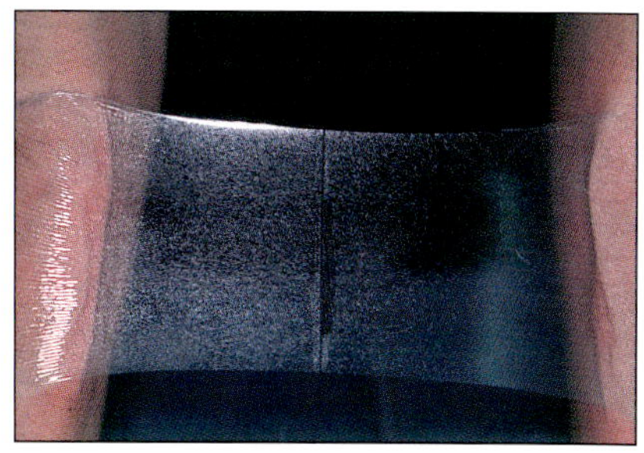

Fig. 16 The 2 sheets of tape shown are elastic; they have adhesive property on only one side (Cateri Tape®, Nichiban K.K.).

Retention using double-sided adhesive tape (Case 1)

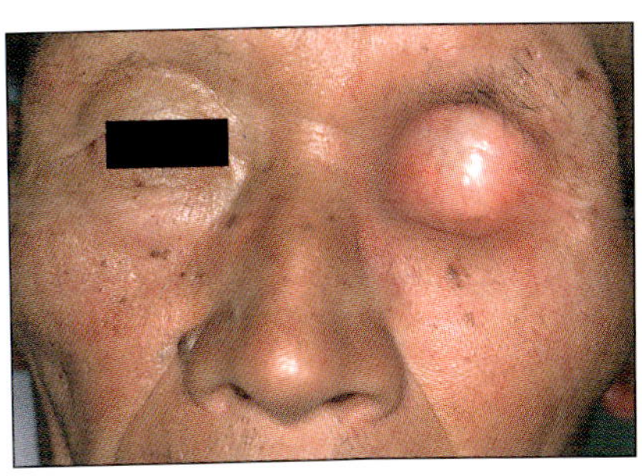

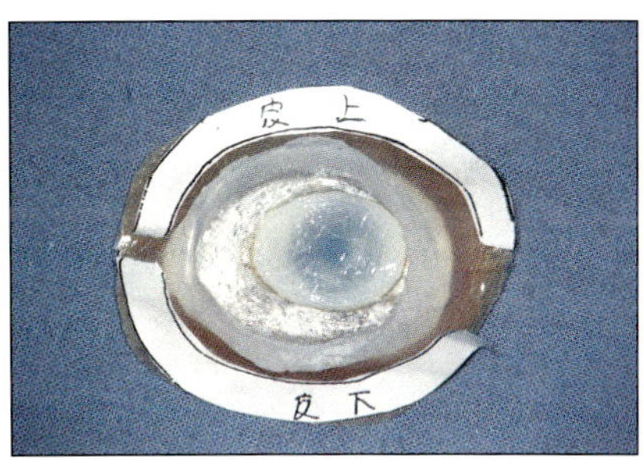

Fig. 17 *(left)* 68-year-old male with 32 × 28 mm skin defect including left orbital region. FC classification is F_1C_0.

Fig. 18 *(right)* Urethane tape was used as the base material for double-sided adhesive tape for the facial prosthesis. One side of the tape was coated with an adhesive agent for skin; the other side was for silicone. The double-sided tape was cut to conform to the shape of the margin of the facial prosthesis and the tape was adhered to the skin side (back side) of the prosthesis.

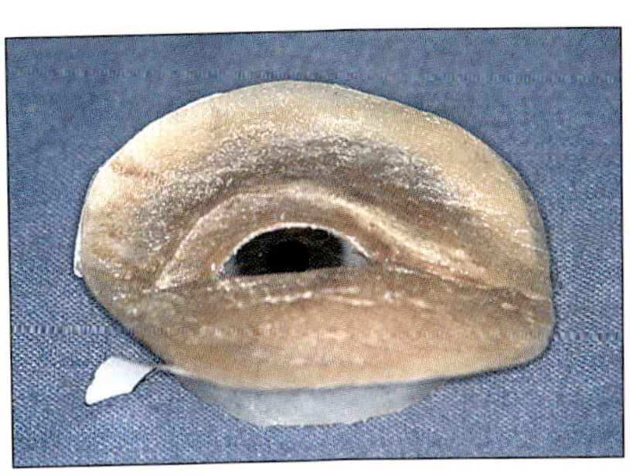

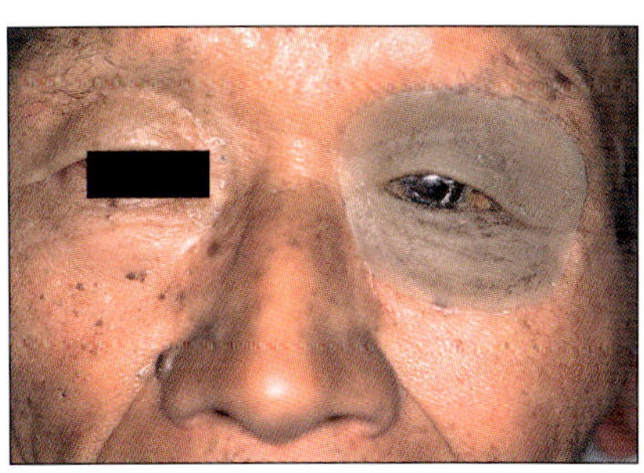

Fig. 19 *(left)* Surface of facial prosthesis.

Fig. 20 *(right)* View of facial prosthesis adhered.

Retention by adhesive tape (Case 2)

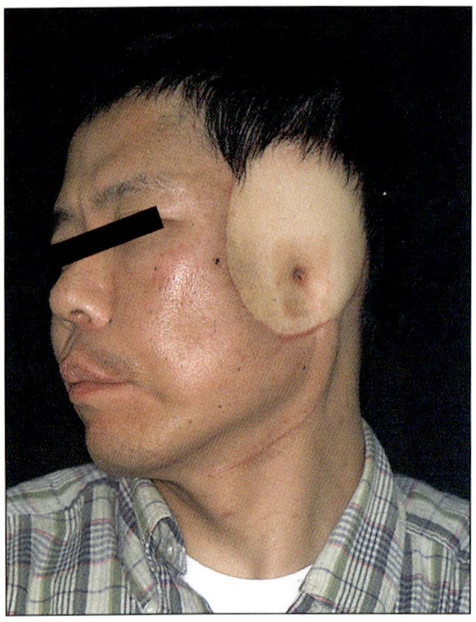

Fig. 21 39-year-old male with latissimus dorsi muscle skin flap reconstruction carried out over a wide area (95 x 115mm) of the temporal region, around the left ear.

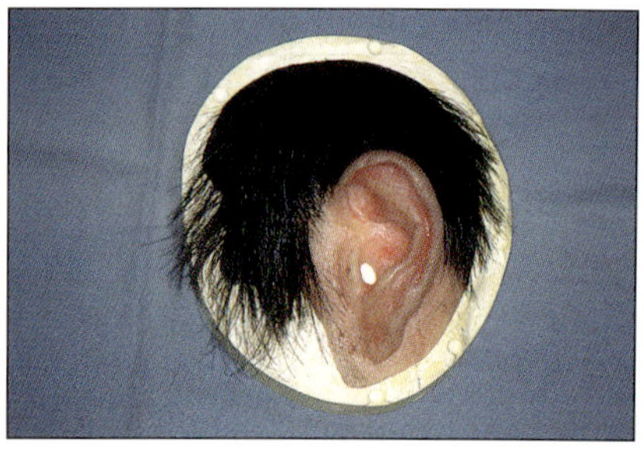

Fig. 22 A prosthesis for the temporal region, including auncle and hair, was produced to match the form of the reconstructed part, with reference to the auncle on the healthy side. Double-sided adhesive tape was used for retention.

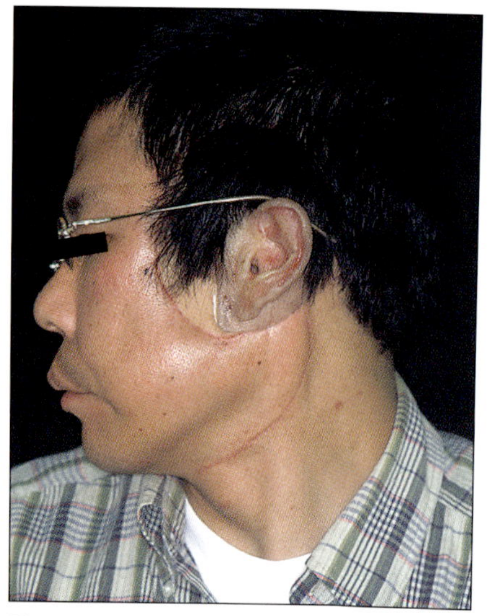

Fig. 23 The prosthesis was adhered to the defect region and eyeglasses were used as camouflage.

Retention by adhesive tape (Case 3)

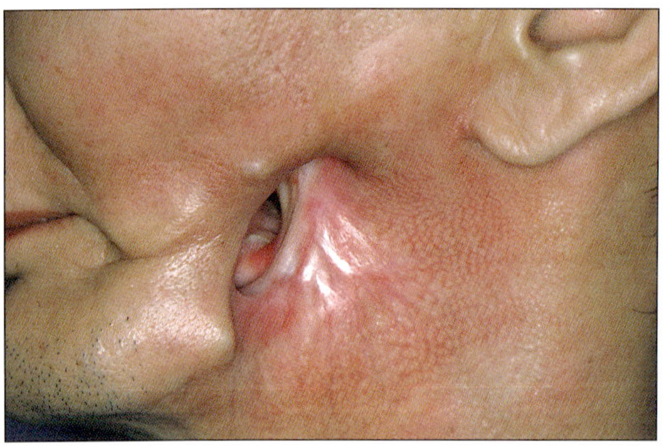

Fig. 24 46-year-old male, with skin defect 35 x 10mm in size on the left mandibular angle area. A dressing applied together with oilpaper in this region which has to be replaced 4 – 5 times every day. Leakage of saliva was the main problem.

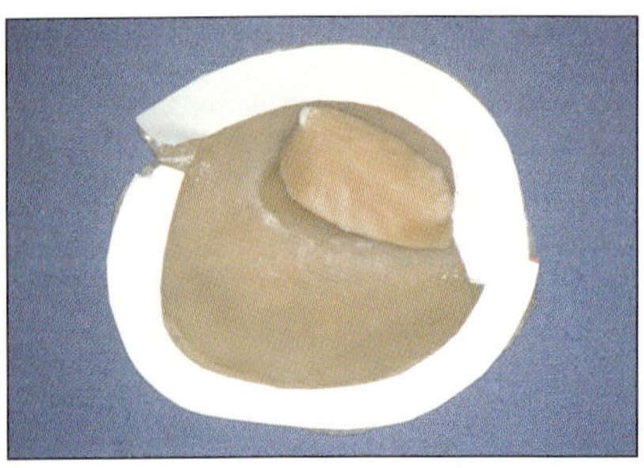

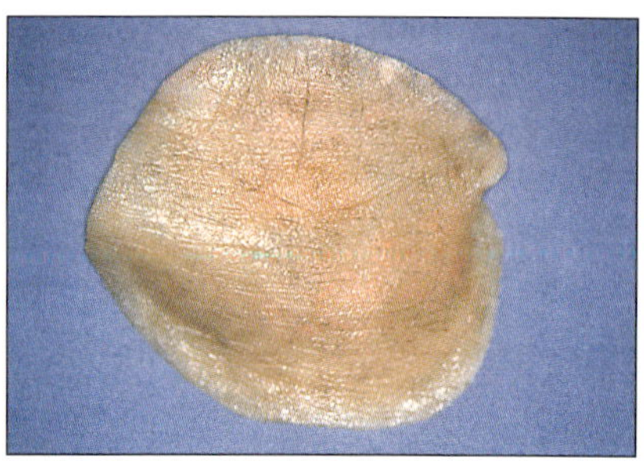

Figs. 25 and 26 The facial prosthesis was produced and double-sided tape retention was used. The left shows the skin (rear) of the prosthesis; The right shows the outer or surface side of the prosthesis. The use of double-sided tape was expected to result in interception of saliva leakage and retention of the prosthesis.

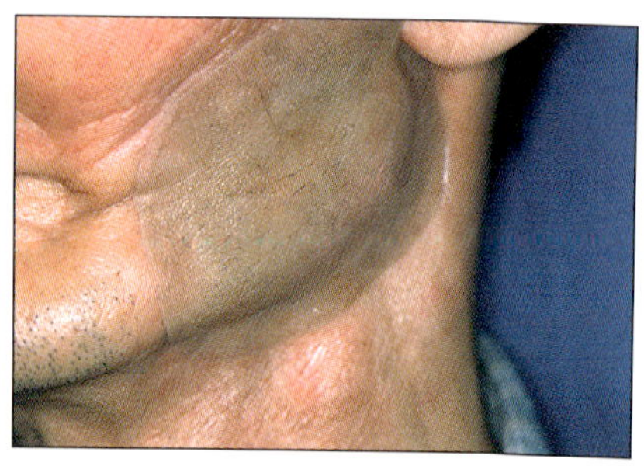

Fig. 27 View of facial prosthesis in place. Observation of the frequency of dressing replacement showed that the leakage of saliva was reduced to less than half of the previous amount.

Retention by adhesive tape (Case 4)

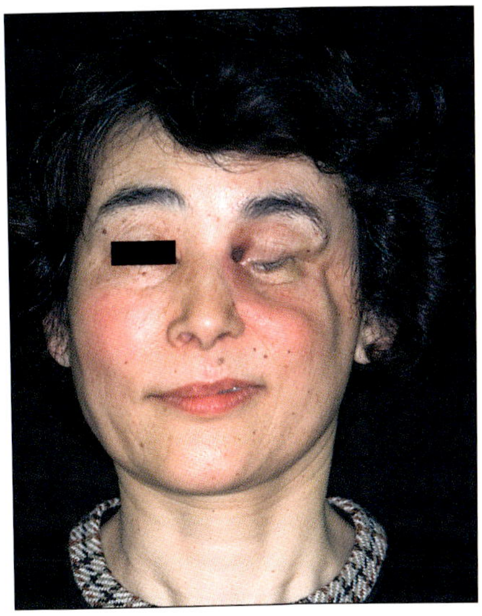

Fig. 28 54-year-old female with skin defect 10 × 10 mm in size on the left orbital region and concavities in the surrounding area. FC classification is F1C1234.

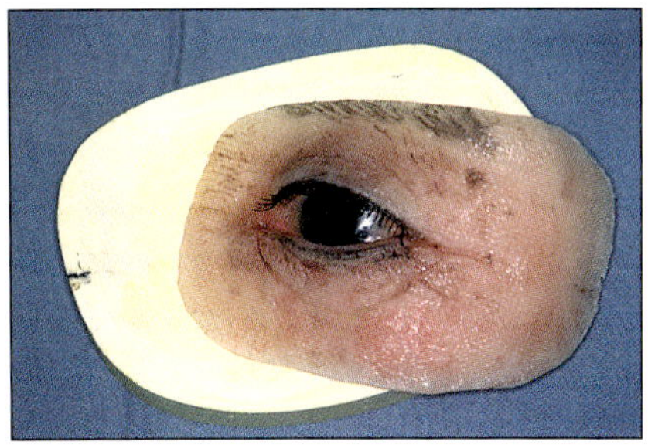

Fig. 29 The facial prosthesis is placed on the yellow plaster model used as the base for easy adhesion of the double-sided tape to the prosthesis.

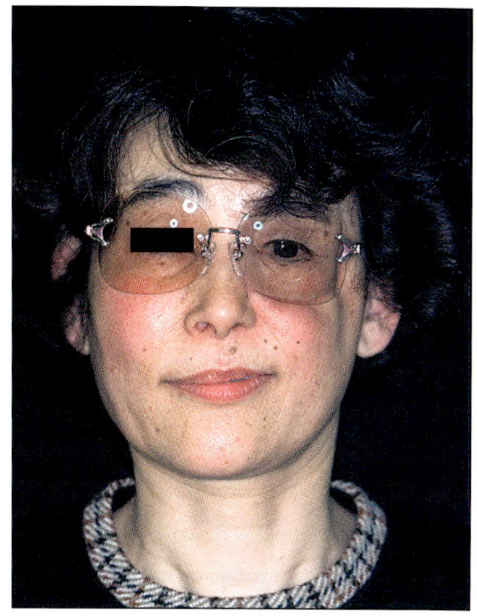

Fig. 30 View of facial prosthesis in place. Eyeglasses are used for camouflage.

Double-sided tape for facial prosthesis

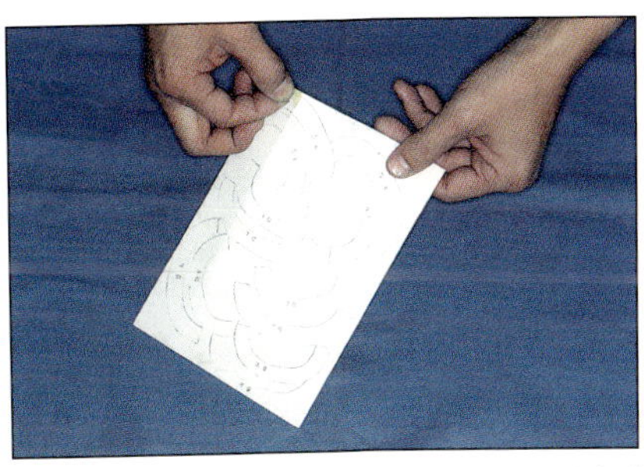

Fig. 31 The original sheet of double-sided tape for facial prosthesis use is A4 size (210 × 297mm). When the prosthesis is produced, make an exact copy of the shape of the surface to which the tape is to be adhered, then the form of this exact copy is transferred onto the tape sheet and cut out to shape.

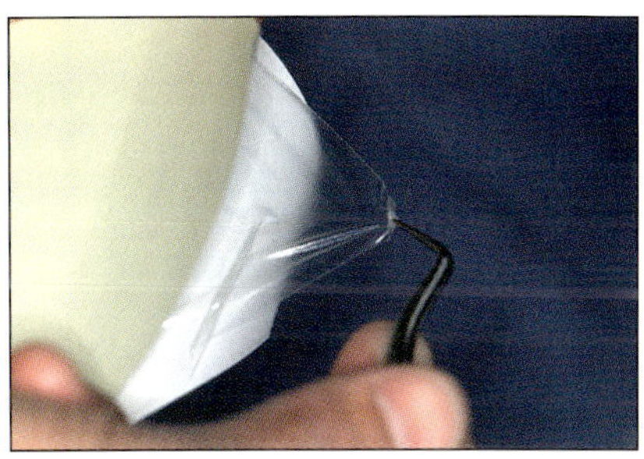

Fig. 32 When the release papers on the double-sided tape are peeled off, the urethane film which is the elastic base material of the tape can be seen. The adhesive agent for skin and for silicone are applied to the two surfaces of the film.

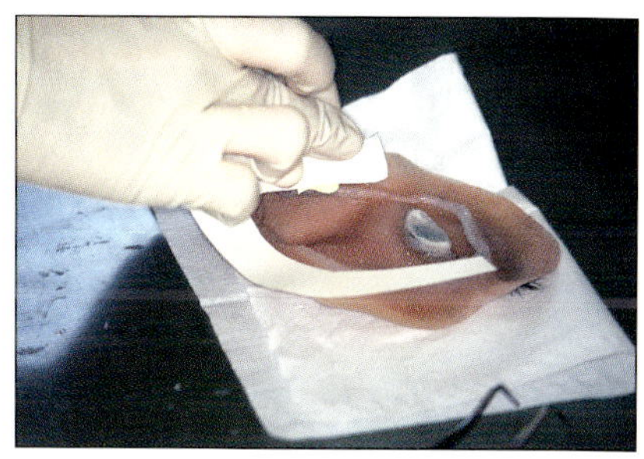

Fig. 33 The double-sided tape cut out is adhered to the prosthesis. The base for adhesion of the tape makes this easier to do.

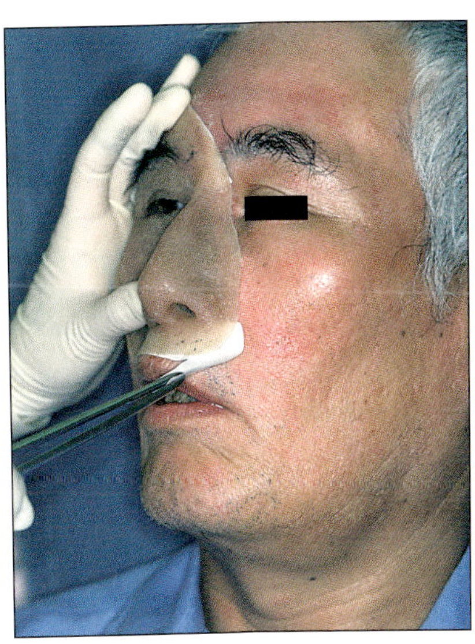

Fig. 34 The double-sided tape is adhered first to the prosthesis, then place the prosthesis in position, the release paper on the skin side is peeled off as if pulling it out, and the margin of the prosthesis is adhered to the position required. A relatively sound skin surface around the wounded part of the defect is used as the surface to which the double-sided tape is adhered; therefore the facial prosthesis can be placed in position less than 1 month after surgery.

CHAPTER 23

From installation of implants to placement of facial prostheses

1. Surgical simulation for facial prosthesis

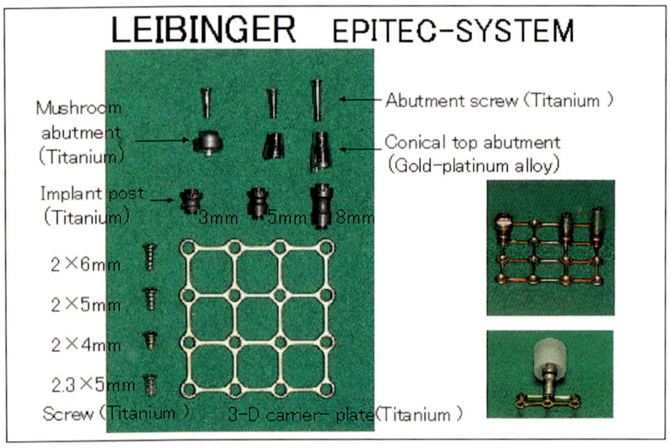

Fig. 1
EPITEC-SYSTEM is a type of implant used to maintain a facial prosthesis. In the EPITEC-SYSTEM a 3-D carrier plate made of titanium is fitted to a bone, the plate is fixed to the bone by screws made of titanium, the implant posts which are the skin-penetrating section are connected to the carrier plate, and mushroom abutments or conical-top abutments are connected to the implant post as the retainer for the facial prosthesis. Mushroom abutments are used in the same way as ball attachments. Conical-top abutments are used to attach an external crown, or bars are directly welded to the conical-top abutments.

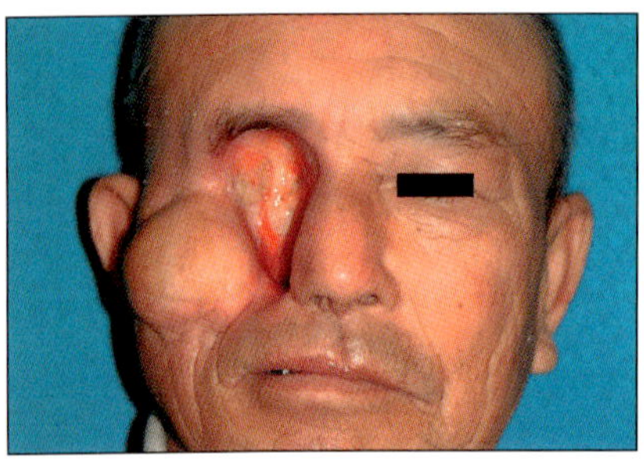

Fig. 2 In this case, part of the excised region was covered by a free musculocutaneous flap after excision of the right orbit malar bone and maxilla.

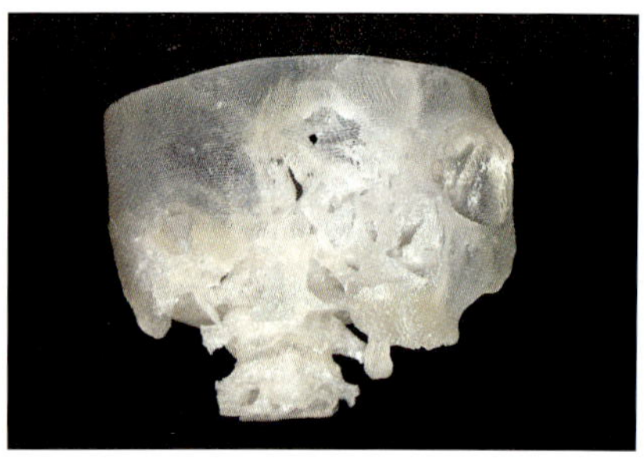

Fig. 3 Craniofacial skull model, based on the CT data, was fabricated by the stereo lithography technique and used for preoperative simulation.

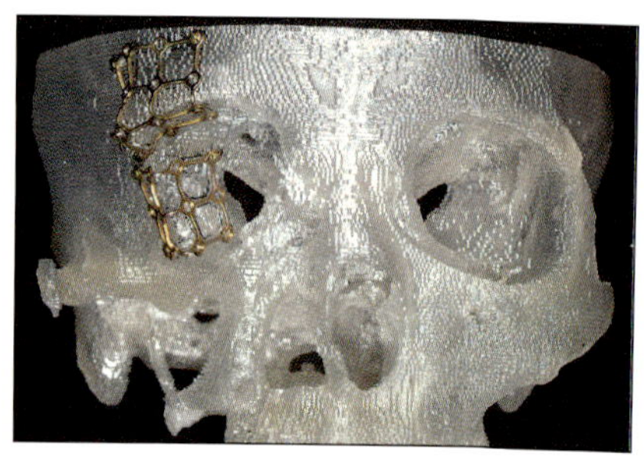

Fig. 4 A ready-made carrier plate (4 × 4 holes) was fitted to the craniofacial skull model. The position and angle of the retainer were inappropriate when the ready-made carrier plate was placed without simulation by a craniofacial skull model.

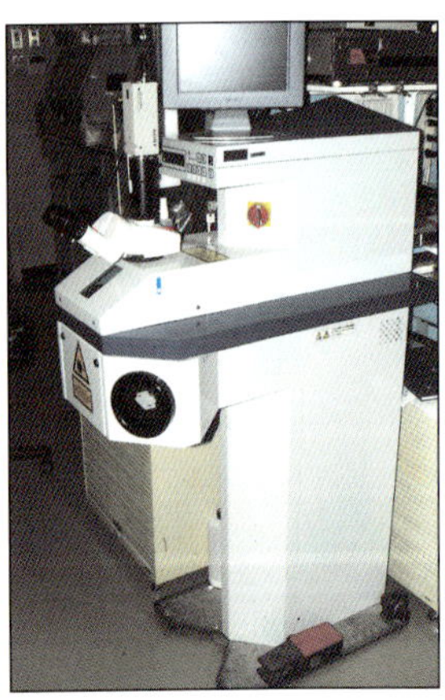

Fig. 5 Laser welding device used for weld-processing of carrier plate.

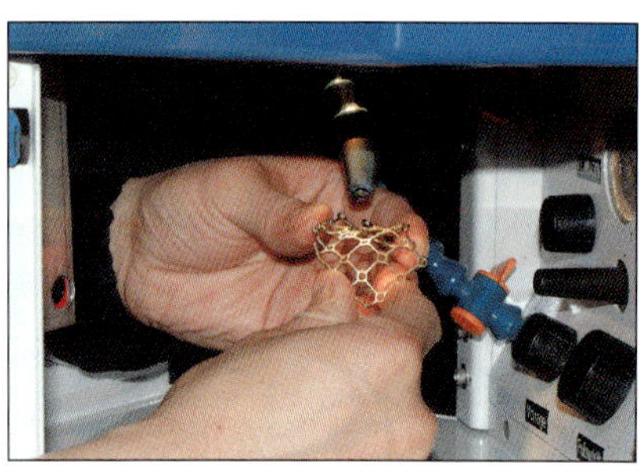

Fig. 6 Laser weld-processing was done to obtain the ideal form for the carrier plate.

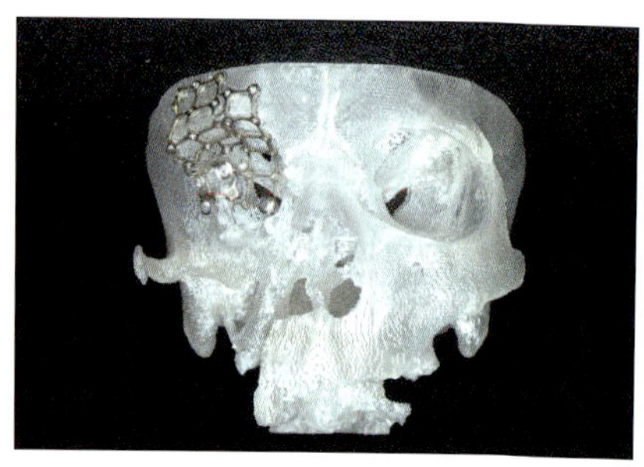

Fig. 7 Multiple carrier plates were processed by laser welding device to fit the plate to the model.

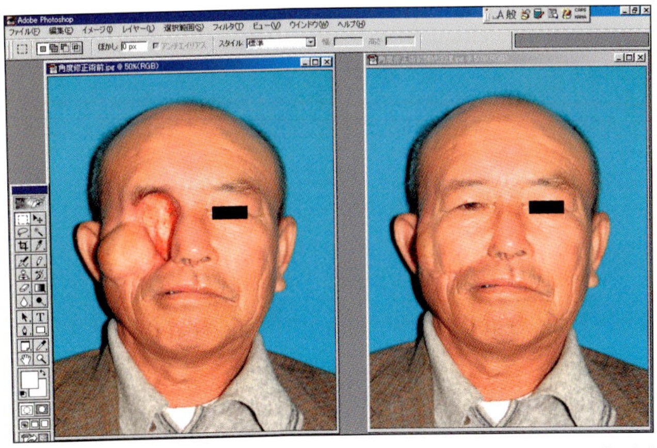

Fig. 8 Simulation for facial prosthesis by using patient's facial photographs and mirror image technique.

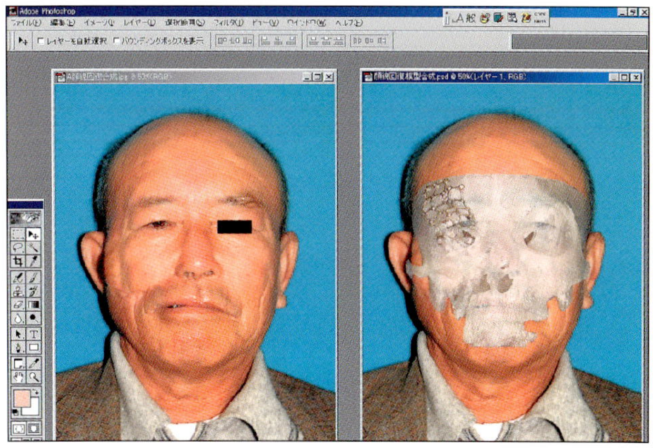

Fig. 9 The position of each abutment is determined by overlaying the picture image of the craniofacial skull model, on which the carrier plate has been fitted, over the facial photograph on the computer.

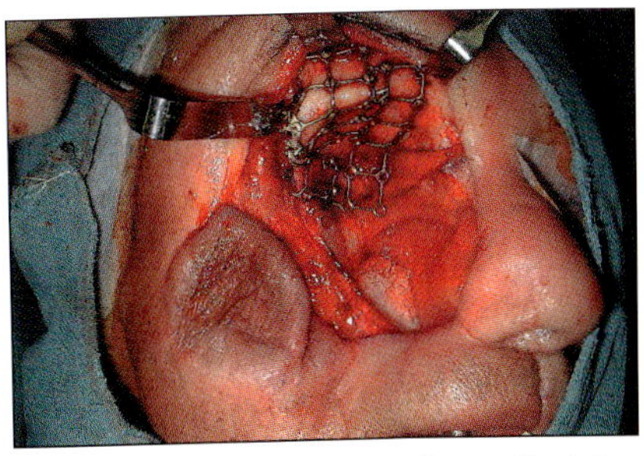

Fig. 10 There was no need to adjust the plate at the time of surgery, and fitting of the plate to the bone was good.

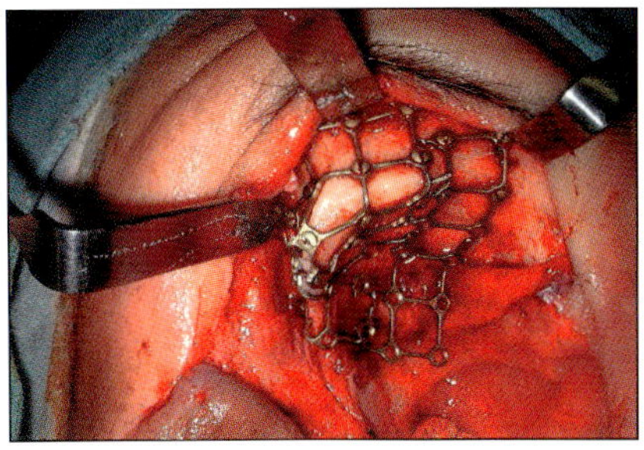

Fig. 11 Holes other than those in the region in which abutments will be placed in future are fixed in place by screws.

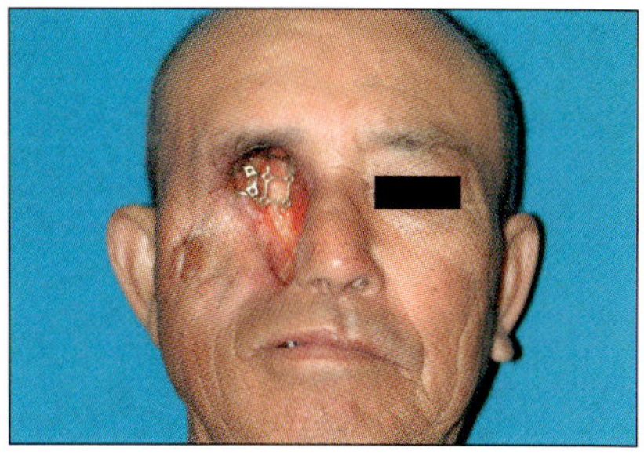

Fig. 12 Facial features after surgery, region has healed.

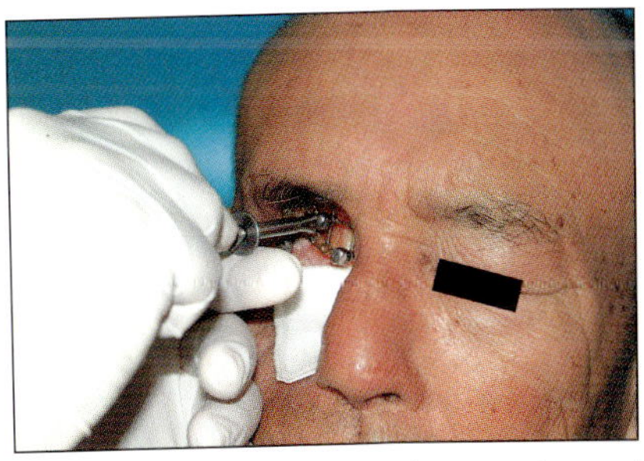

Fig. 13 Placement of implant posts and mushroom abutments.

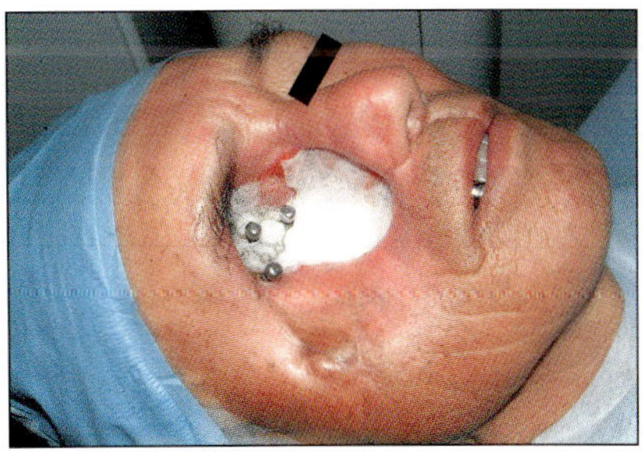

Fig. 14 Impression was taken after relief was done using gauze.

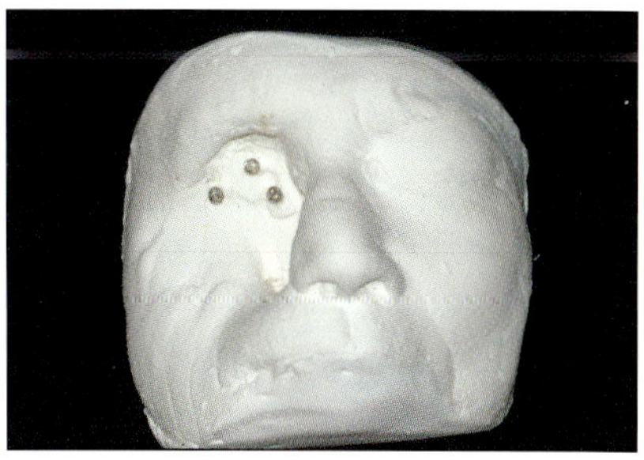

Fig. 15 Plaster model of face with abutments.

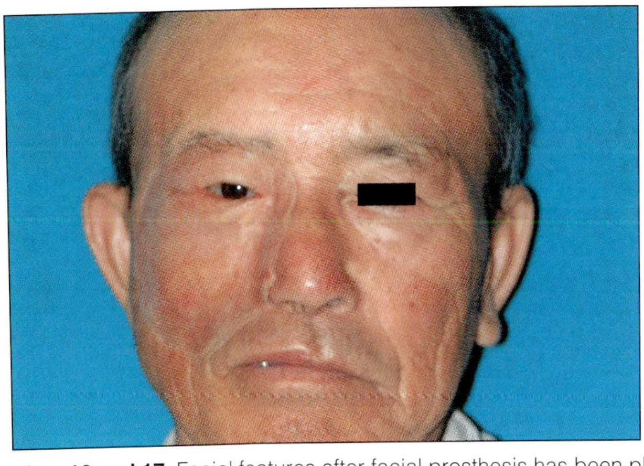

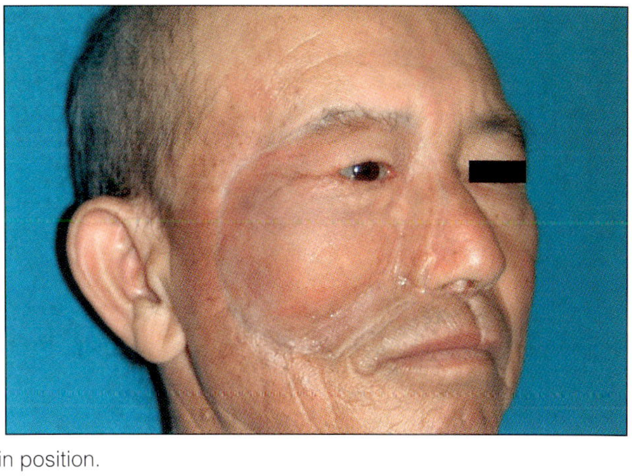

Figs. 16 and 17 Facial features after facial prosthesis has been placed in position.

2. Facial prosthesis

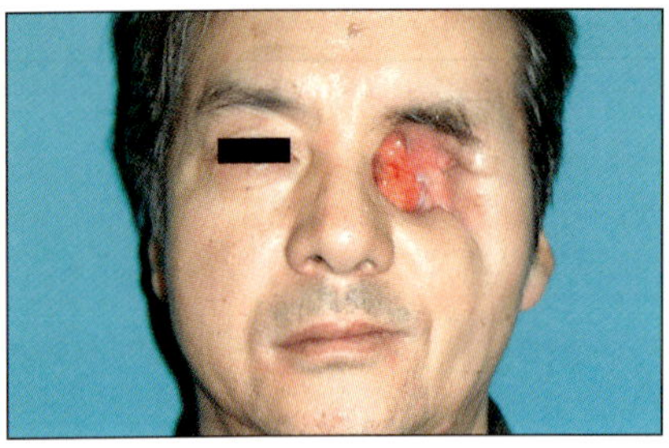

Fig. 18 Orbital defect case.

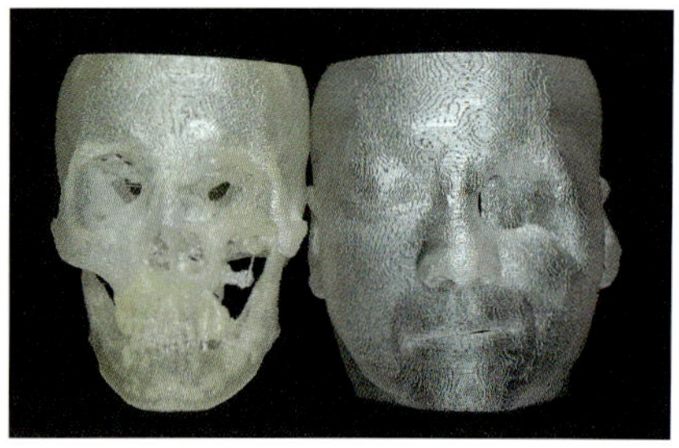

Fig. 19 Craniofacial skull model and facial soft tissue model produced by means of a stereolithography technique based on patient's CT data. These models are employed to provide understanding of the relationship between bone and soft tissue and to determine the position in which the implant is to be installed.

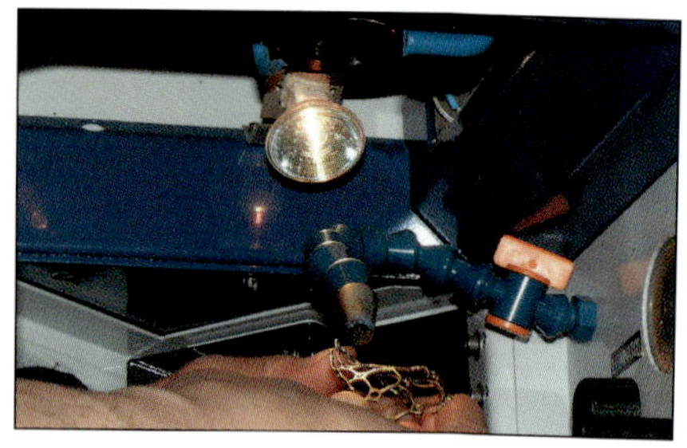

Fig. 20 Join the carrier plate to each other by laser welding so it matches the form of the bone.

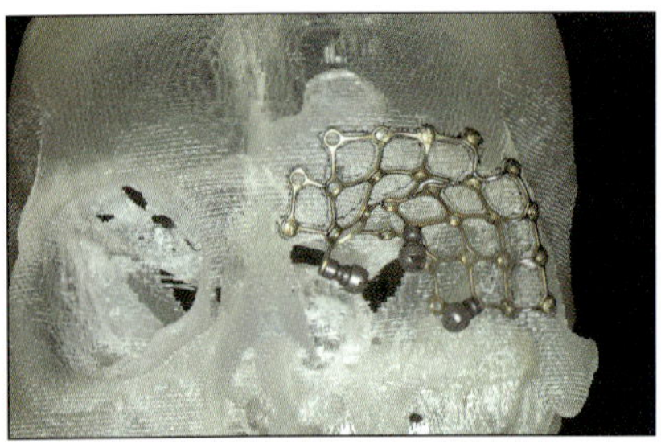

Fig. 21 Confirm that the laser-welded carrier plate fits the craniofacial skull model.

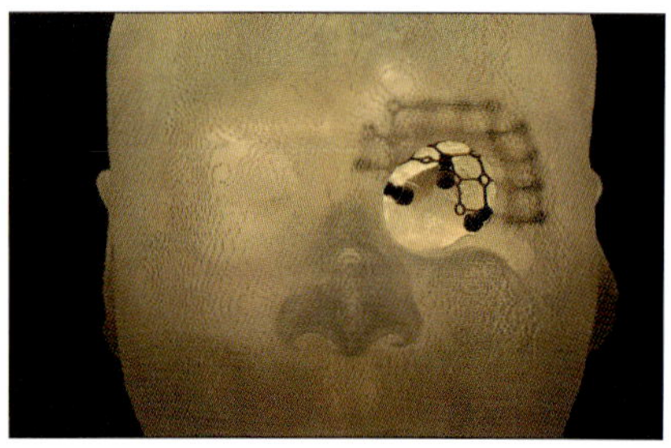

Fig. 22 Join the facial soft tissue model and craniofacial skull model together, and determine whether or not the position of mushroom abutments to retain the facial prosthesis is appropriate.

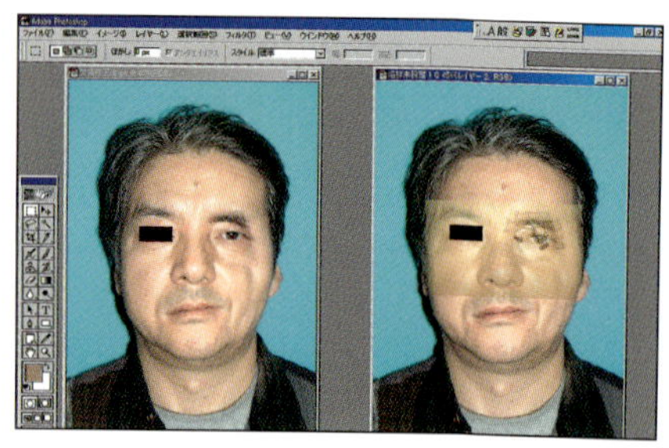

Fig. 23 After recovery of facial feature formed by mirror imaging has been done on the computer, the positional relationship between the facial prosthesis and abutment can be estimated when the photograph of the craniofacial skull model is overlaid on the recovered facial feature form.

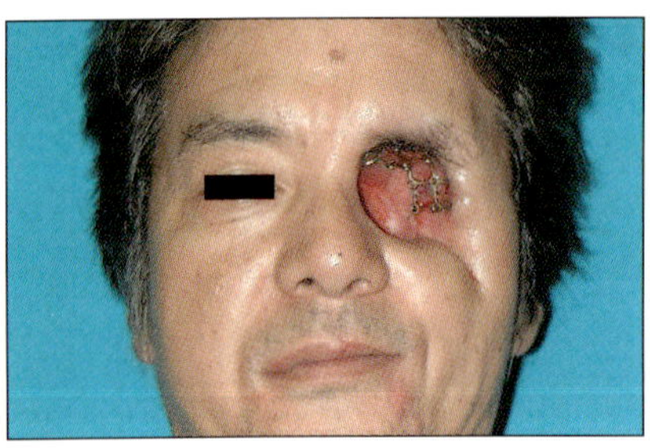

Fig. 24 After carrier plate placement operation has been done.

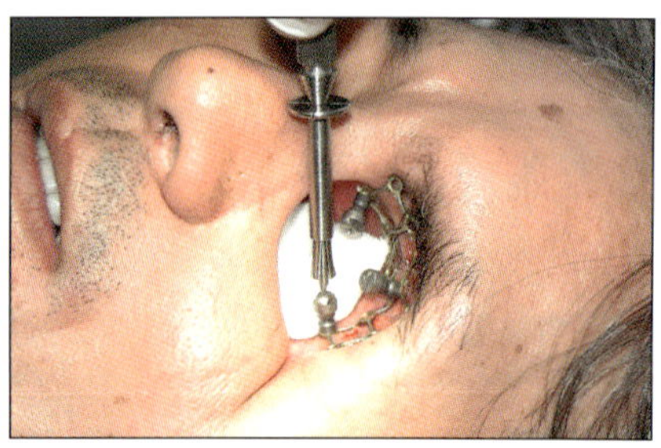

Fig. 25 Placing of mushroom abutments on carrier plates. At this time, fill the socket with gauze to keep the mushroom abutments from falling into the cavity.

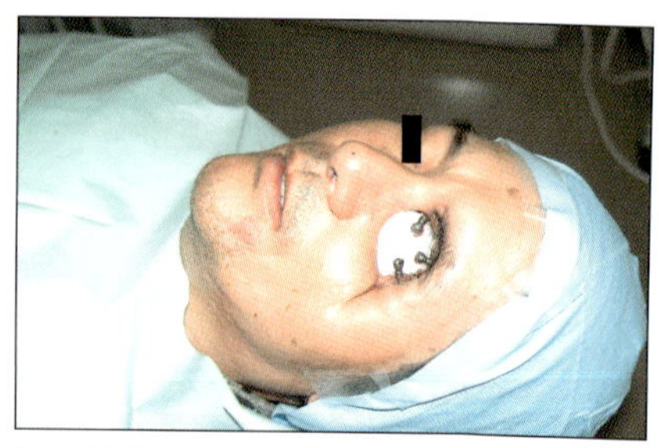

Fig. 26 Preparation for taking impression. Cover the entire head except for the face with a cap or other material, to avoid adhesion of impression material in the patient's hair. Also, position packs made of gauze to avoid the inflow of impression material into unnecessary regions.

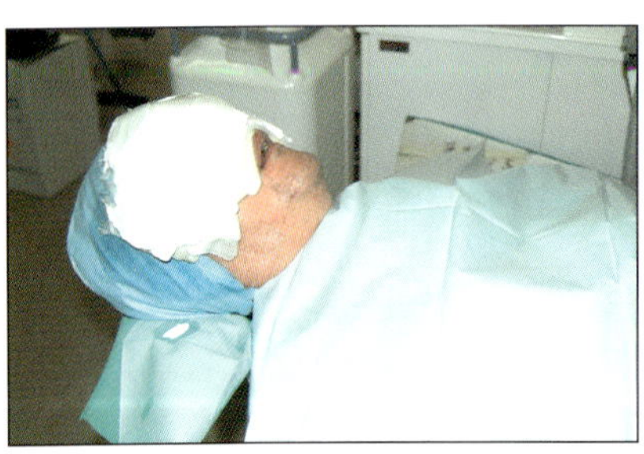

Fig. 27 Use alginate impression material to take the impression, and place gauze over the impression material before it cures. After the impression material has cured, cover the impression material with plaster to prevent deformation of the impression material when it is removed. The impression material and plaster are joined through the gauze.

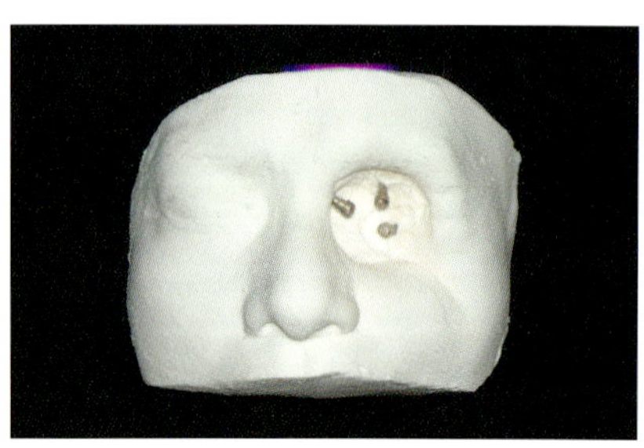

Fig. 28 Facial plaster model. Real abutments are invested in the model.

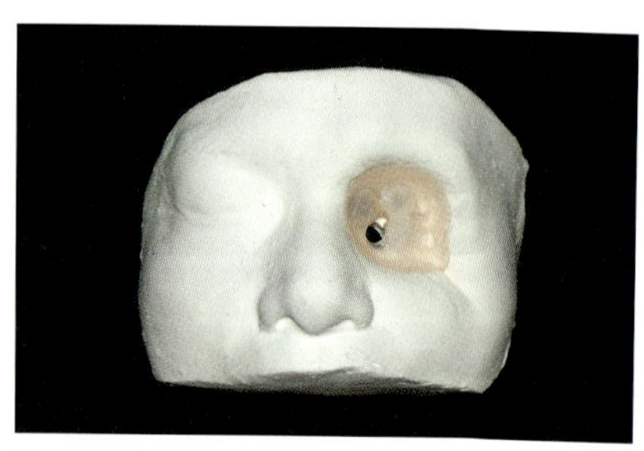

Fig. 29 Produce the resin frame that will be the base of the facial prosthesis.

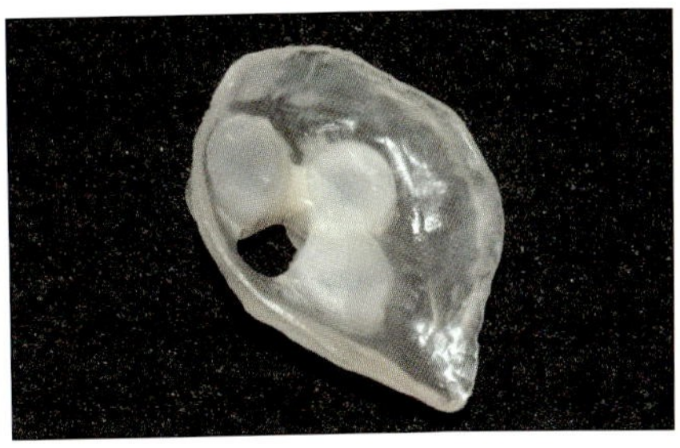

Fig. 30 Surface of resin frame.

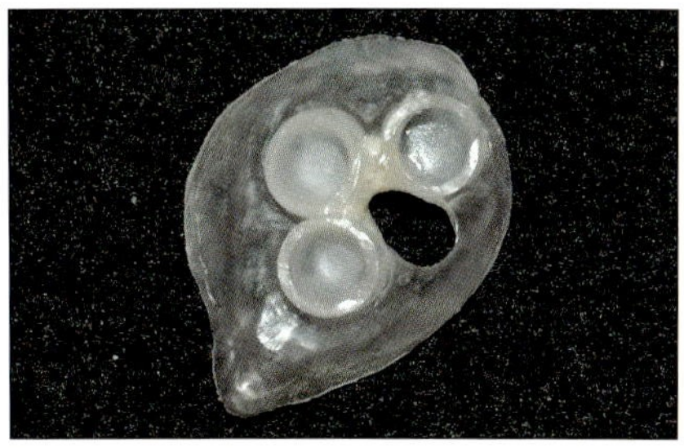

Fig. 31 Inner surface of resin frame. The resin frame and resin caps to receive the abutments are connected.

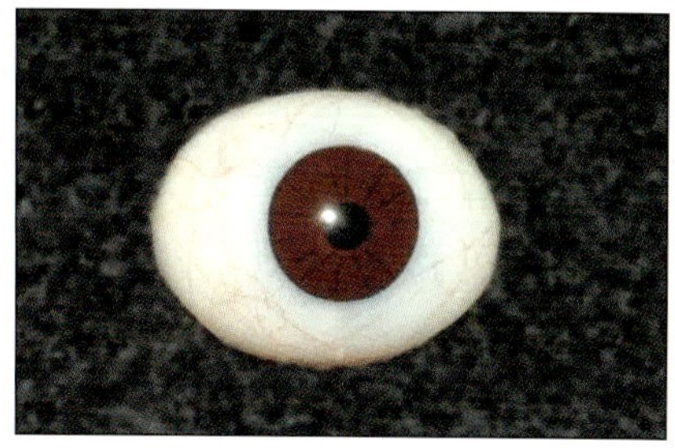

Fig. 32 Custom made artificial eye.

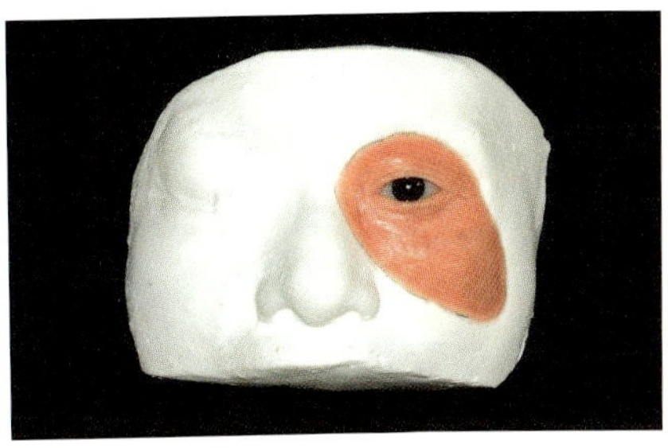

Fig. 33 A wax prosthesis is produced while referring to the picture image of recovered facial features on the computer. The wax used is prepared by adding pigment to achieve a color as close as possible to the patient's face color.

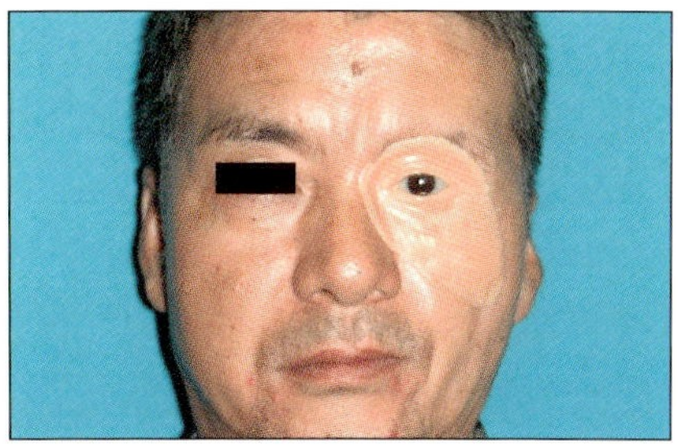

Fig. 34 Carry out trial fitting of the wax prosthesis to the patient's face, make adjustments, and complete the wax prosthesis.

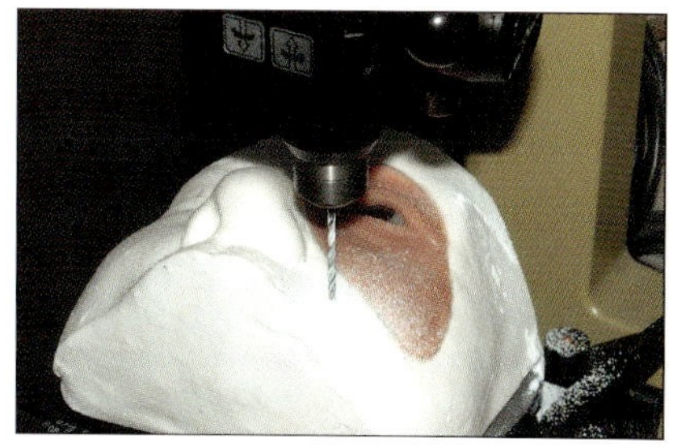

Fig. 35 Return the wax prosthesis to the facial plaster model, and make guide holes in 3 places to determine the position before the wax prosthesis is invested in plaster.

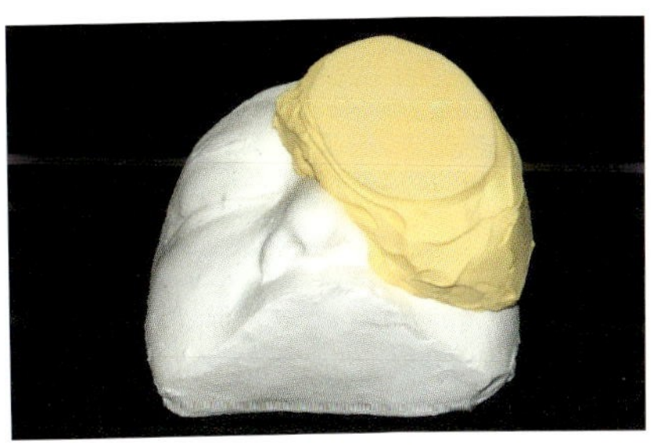

Fig. 36 Insert guide pins into the guide holes, do plaster investment, and prepare the core for silicon polymerization.

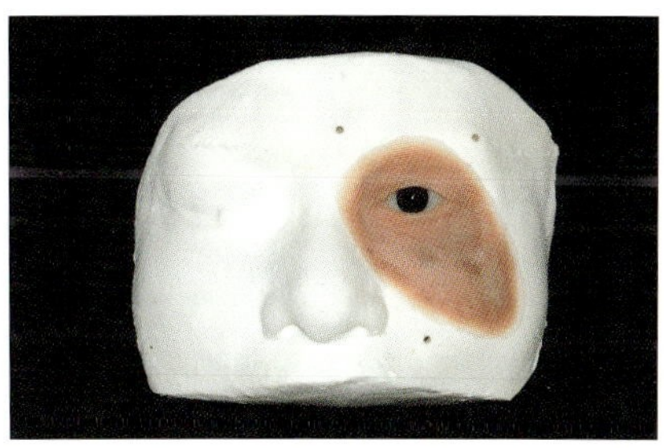

Fig. 37 After the plaster has cured, carry out dewaxing to complete the plaster core. Guide pins are attached to the plaster core, and the positional relationship between the plaster core and the patient's facial plaster model is accurately determined.

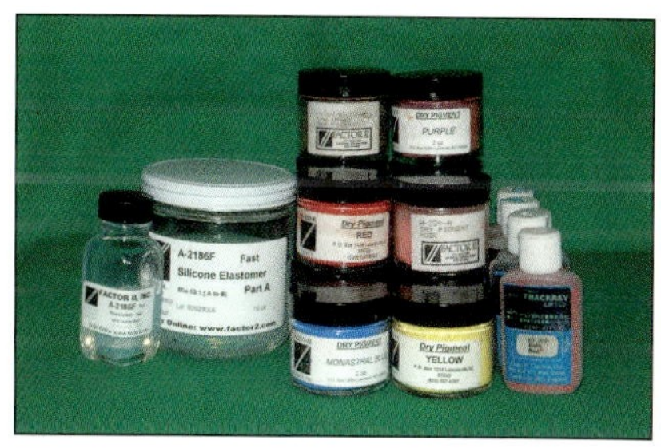

Fig. 38 Silicon and pigments (Factor II, INC. USA) used for facial prosthesis production.

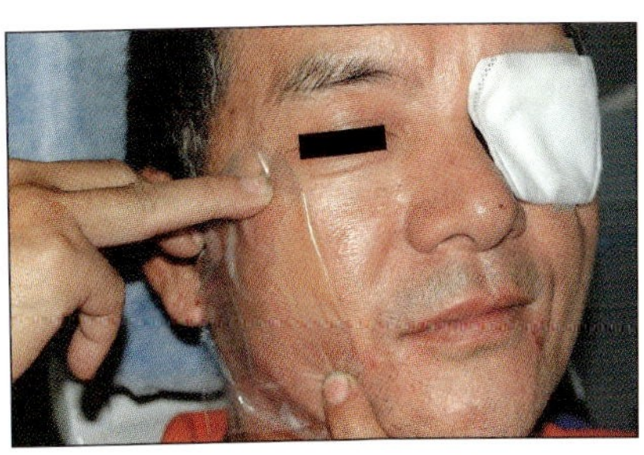

Fig. 39 Prepare the color of the base, matching it to the patient's face color by adding pigments to semi-transparent silicon.

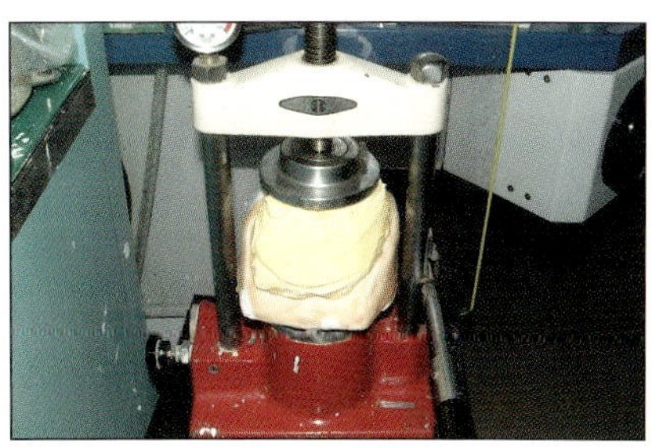

Fig. 40 Carry out the coloring in the plaster core, fill with the silicon base colored to match the patient's face color, and press it while it cures.

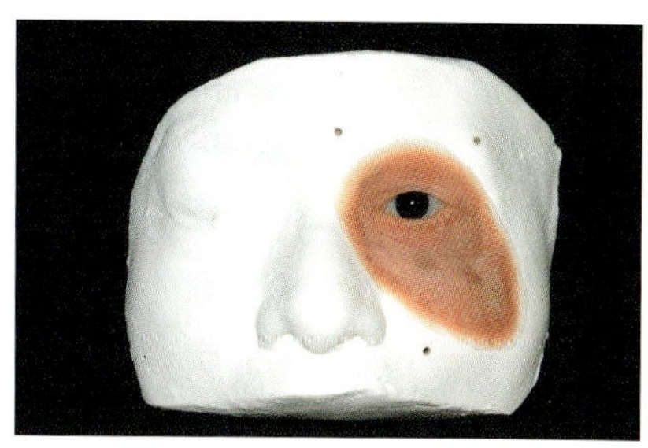

Fig. 41 Silicon after curing.

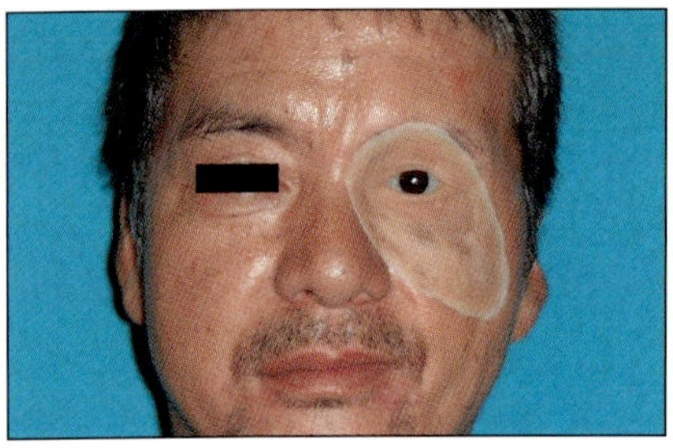

Fig. 42 Do trial fitting of the facial prosthesis to the patient's face, then color the outer surface of the facial prosthesis.

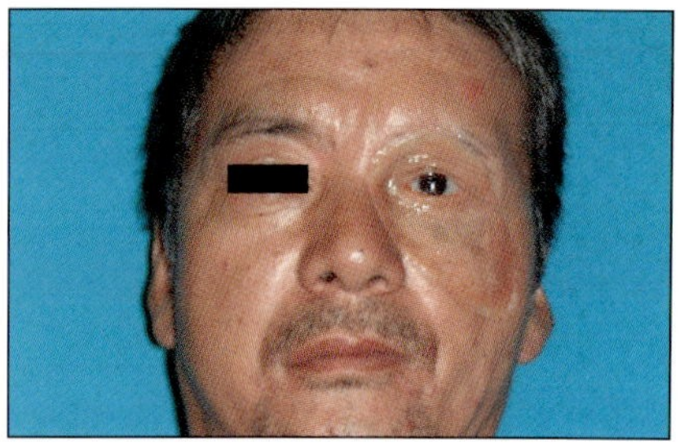

Fig. 43 Facial prosthesis after external coloring.

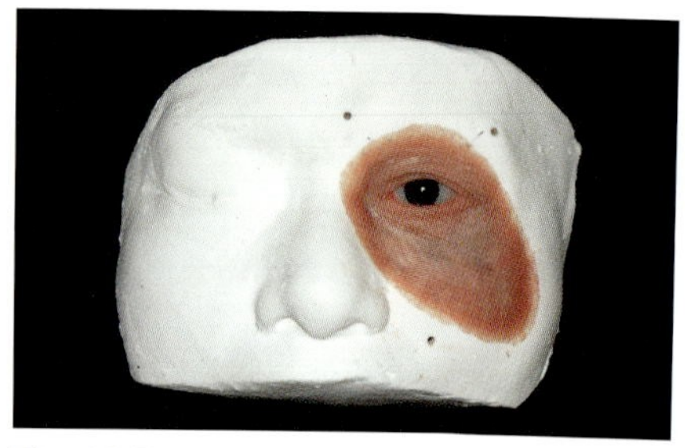

Fig. 44 Tapping the surface of prosthesis lightly with gauze before the external coloring on the prosthesis has completely cured reduces the luster on the surface of the facial prosthesis and produces more of a matte finish.

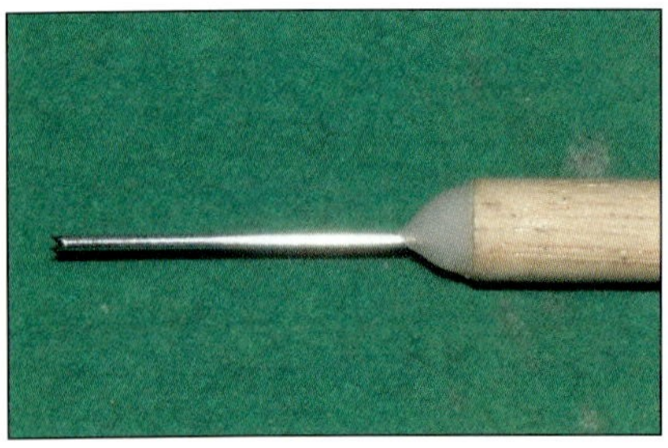

Fig. 45 For eyebrow implanting, use an instrument made of wire with a diameter of 0.7mm. The tip of the instrument has a V-shaped fork.

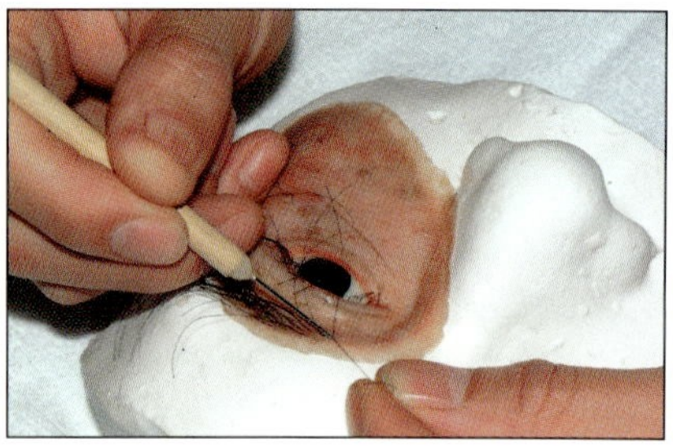

Fig. 46 Apply adhesive agent to the tip of the instrument and carry out eyebrow implantation.

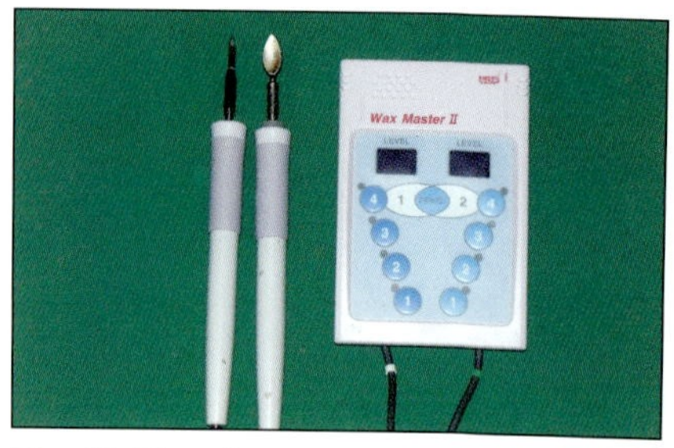

Fig. 47 Electric wax instrument used to curl the implanted artificial eyebrow.

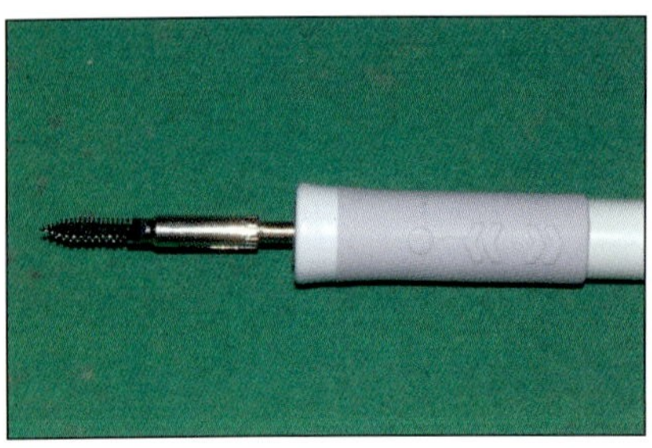

Fig. 48 Wax instrument with tip made comb-shaped by knurling.

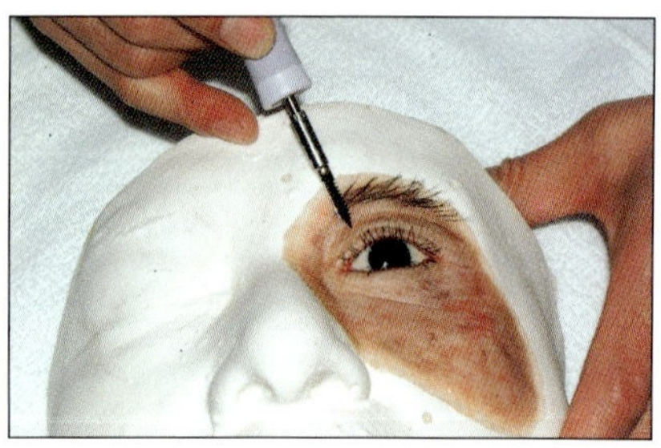

Fig. 49 Curling the artificial eyebrow.

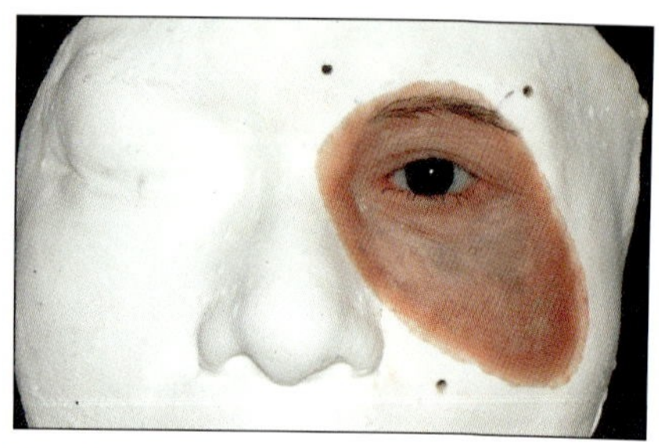

Fig. 50 Completed facial prosthesis.

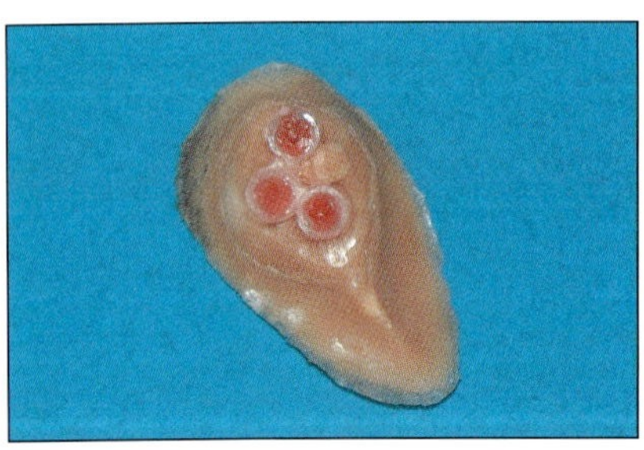

Fig. 51 Fill the resin caps on the inner surface of the facial prosthesis with silicon impression material, and impress the shape of abutments to make the attachment.

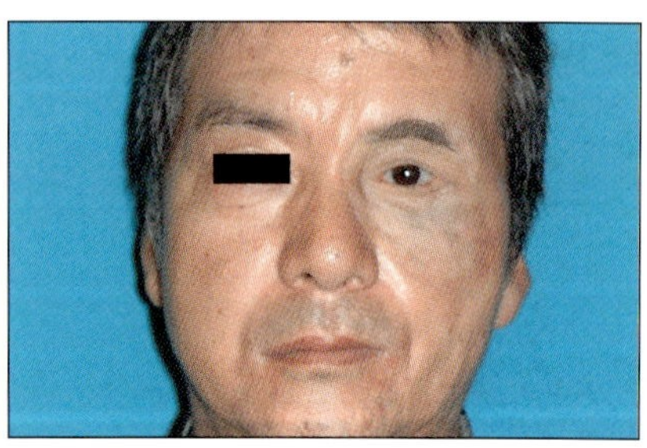

Fig. 52 Front view of patient with facial prosthesis in position. The facial prosthesis weighs 28g.

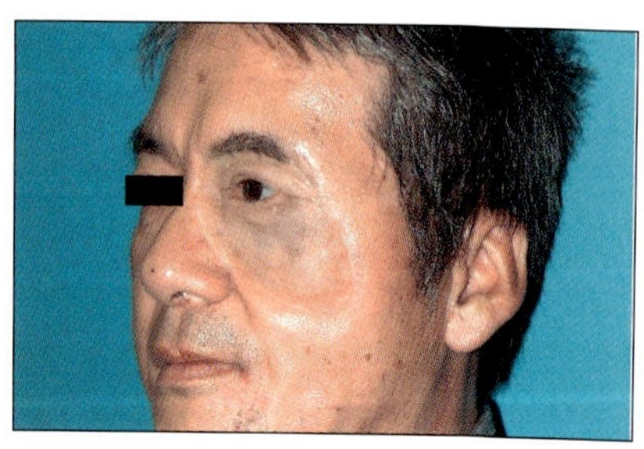

Fig. 53 Side view of patient with facial prosthesis in position.

CHAPTER 24

Camouflage of facial prostheses

It is not easy to prepare a facial prosthesis that is indistinguishable from surrounding structures, and many types of coloring methods and contrivances for the facial margin of the prosthesis have been presented. Also, no matter how good the facial prosthesis, there is also the problem of deterioration of the prosthesis over time. Various camouflage methods are used to make the margin of the prosthesis as unnoticeable as possible.

These various methods include the use of eyeglasses, hairstyles, wigs, cosmetics, hats, caps, scarves, etc., for camouflage to make prostheses less noticeable to other people's eyes.

Often it is not sufficient to use only one of these methods, so a combination of several kinds of methods should be considered.

Camouflage using eyeglasses and wig

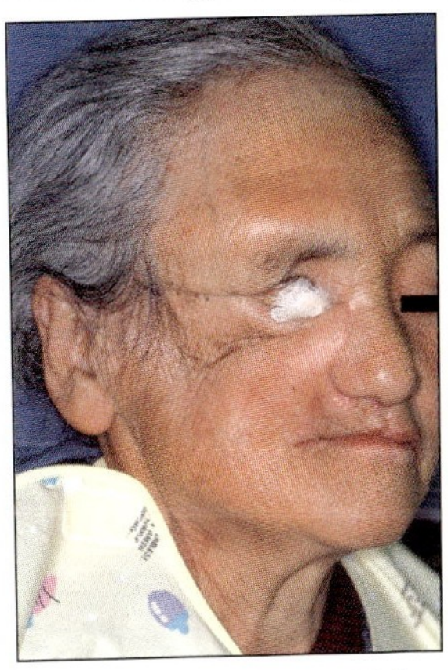

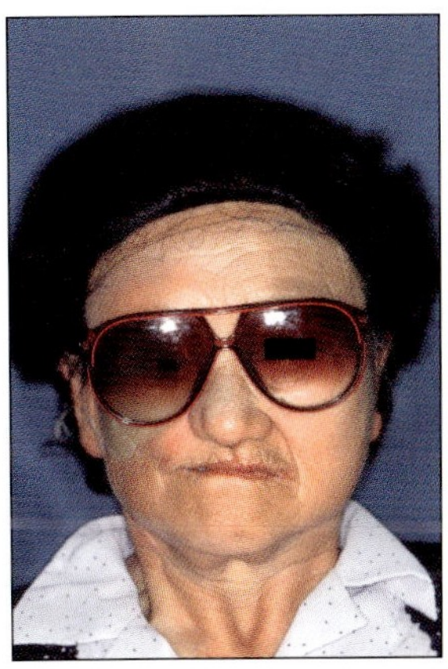

Fig. 1 *(left)* 66-year-old female with skin defect including right orbit region and depression of the periorbital area, infraorbital region, and zygomatic region.
Fig. 2 *(right)* The orbital prosthesis has been placed on the defect region and ready-made plastic framed sunglasses and a ready-made wig have been used for camouflage.

Camouflage using eyeglasses

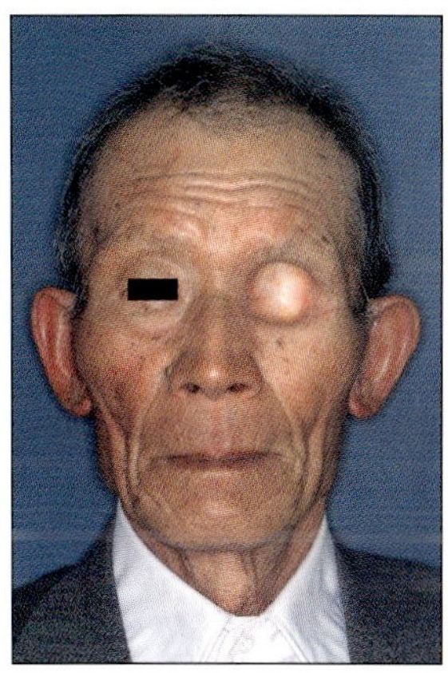

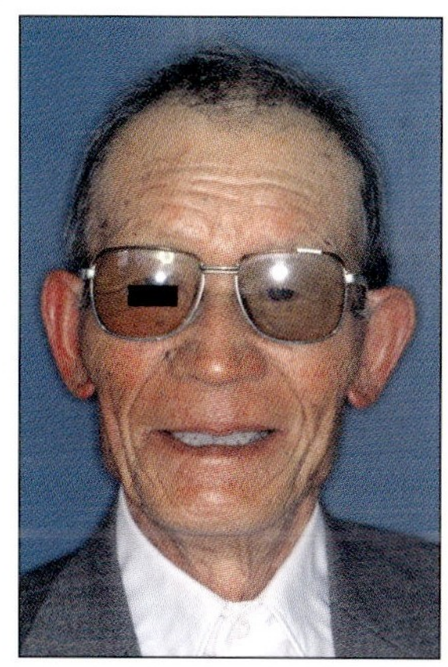

Fig. 3 *(left)* 68-year-old male fisherman with skin defect of orbital region, 32 × 28mm in size including left orbital content.
Fig. 4 *(right)* We selected a ready-made titanium eyeglass frame which matches the size and form of the defect, then set the margin of the facial prosthesis to match the frame, and prepared the facial prosthesis. We used maroon-color-based, dark lenses with light transmittance of 60%, as the patient desired. Under certain circumstances, such eyeglasses make the prosthesis more conspicuous and sometimes give the impression that the patient is visually handicapped.

Camouflage using eyeglasses and wig

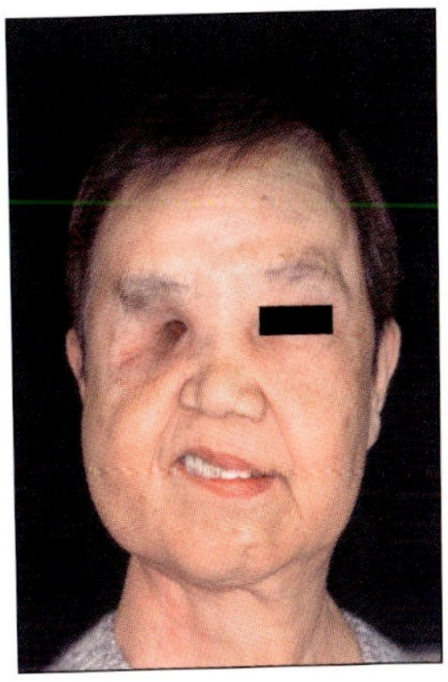

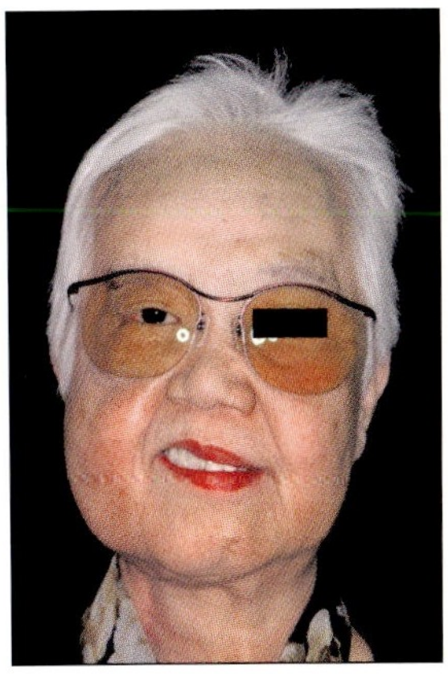

Fig. 5 *(left)* 66-year-old female with skin defect 16 × 7mm in size in the orbit and infraorbital region including right orbital content, and a depression 16 × 30 × 33mm in size including the zygomatic region surrounding the skin defect.
Facial prosthetics started while she was hospitalized following surgery.
Fig. 6 *(right)* As in the previous case, we asked an optician to adjust a ready-made titanium eyeglass frame and lenses to fit the size of the skin defect, and prepared the facial prosthesis to match the shape of the eyeglasses. Maroon-color lenses with light transmittance of 75% were prepared. Lenses with light transmittance of around 75% are considered to provide the most natural feeling. After leaving the hospital, she bleached her hair.

Camouflage using Covermark makeup, etc.

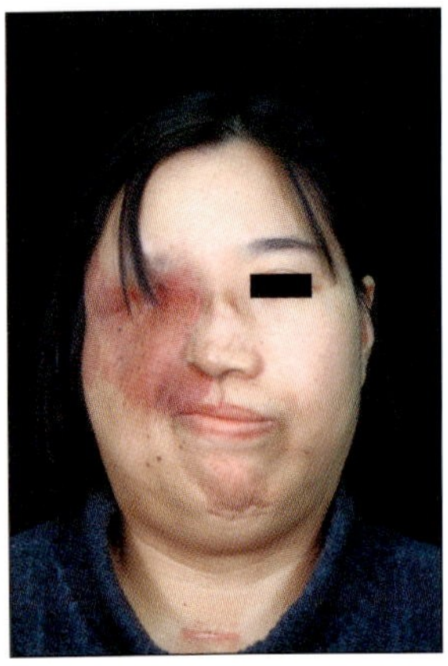

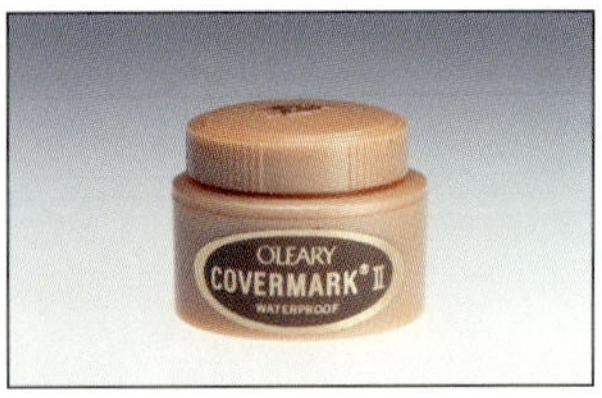

Fig. 7 *(left)* 42-year-old female: no skin defect because the skin of the eyelids was sutured together after extirpation of the orbital content, although there is a shallow depression in the orbit area centered around the surgical site and infraorbital region.
She was already using Covermark because of a red birthmark over a wide area on the right side of her face.
Fig. 8 *(right)* The photo shows a makeup foundation Covermark®, Grafa Laboratories Co.), which is most widely used for covering red or blue birthmarks.

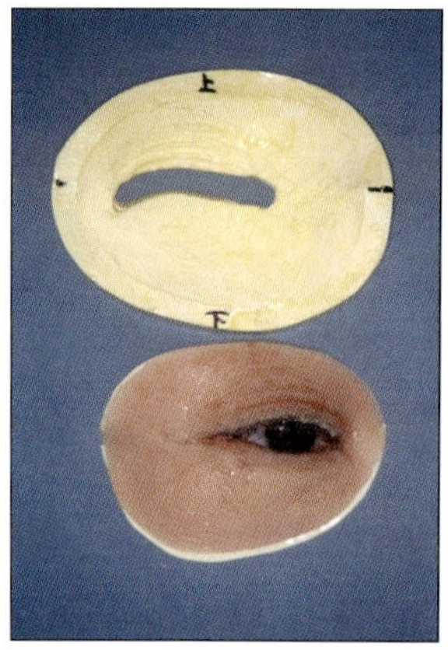

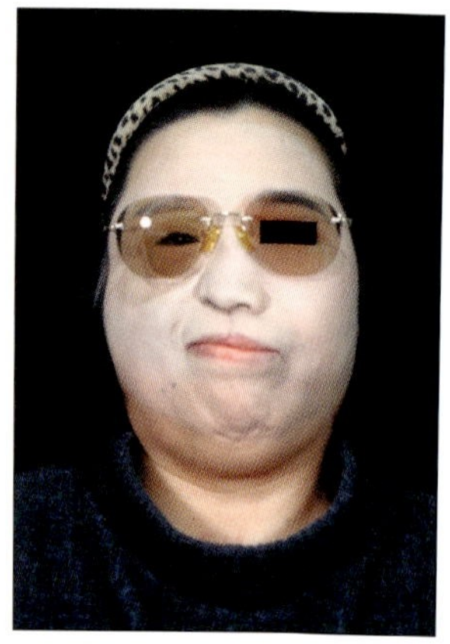

Fig. 9 *(left)* This photo shows the prosthesis produced.
Fig. 10 *(right)* As in the previous cases, an optician adjusted the eyeglass frame first and we set the external line of the prosthesis to fit the shape of the frame. In addition, she is using Covermark. The eyeglasses shown in this photo are for outdoor use during winter in snow country.

Camouflage using Covermark makeup, etc.

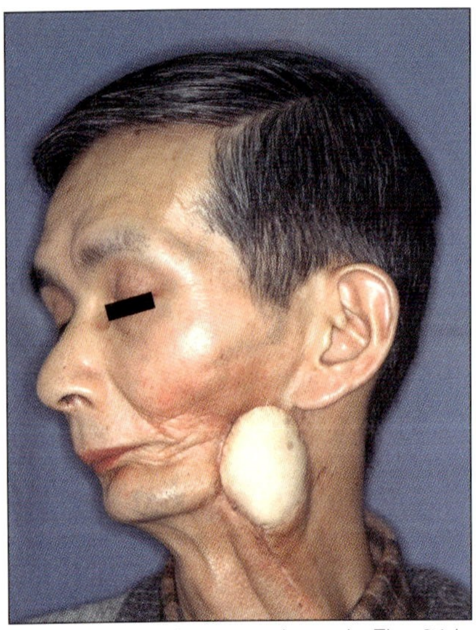

Fig. 11 This is the case shown in Fig. 24 in CHAPTER 22. The skin defect (35 × 10mm) of the left mandibular region was reconstructed using a pectralis major MC flap. Both the color and skin texture of flap greatly differ from those of the surrounding skin, and are conspicuous.

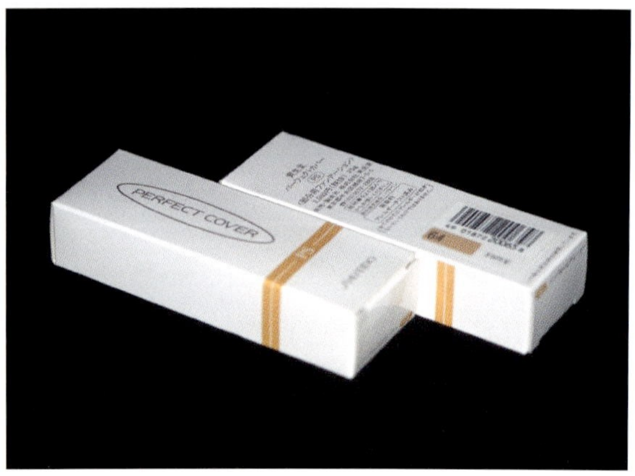

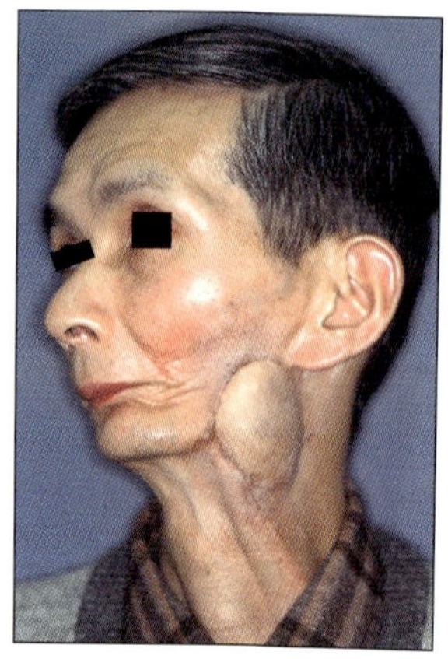

Figs. 12 and 13 The reconstructed region is camouflaged using greasepaint-based cosmetics (Perfect Cover®, Shiseido Co., Ltd.).

Camouflage by hairstyle and eyeglasses

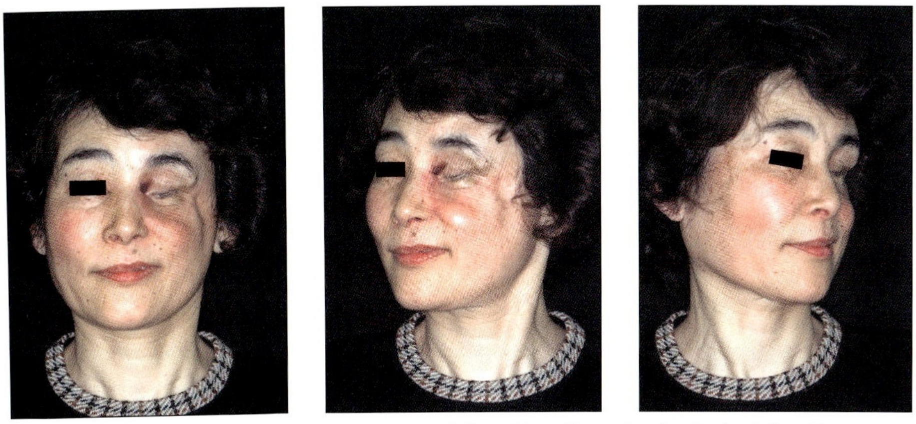

Figs. 14 to 16 54-year-old female with skin defect 10 × 10mm in size in the left orbital region with depression in the orbital, infraorbital and zygomatic regions. Production of the prosthesis was started following surgery, while she was still hospitalized. Together with the prosthesis, she has used eyeglasses and hairstyle for camouflage.

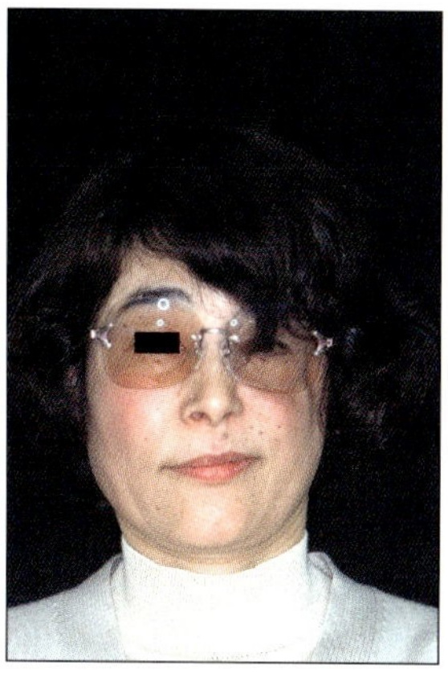

Fig. 17 Frontal view of patient's face 2 weeks after the prosthesis was placed. The eyeglasses are used as camouflage. She later tried various types of makeup and hairstyles.

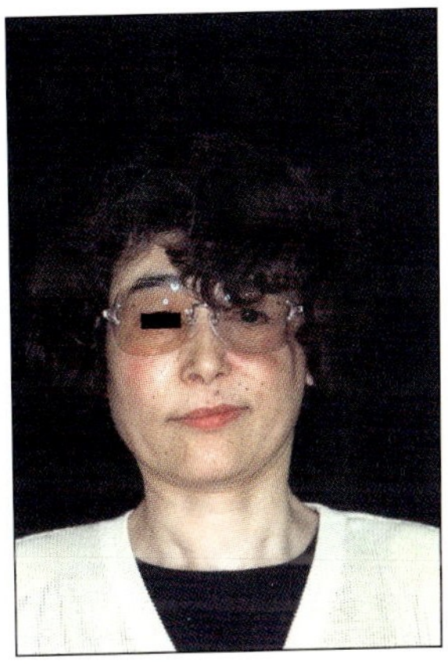

Fig. 18 Frontal view of patient's face 3 weeks after the prosthesis was placed.

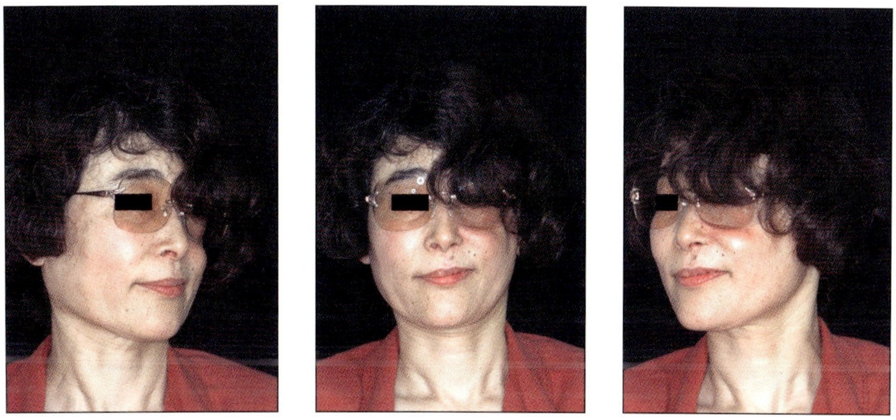

Figs. 19 to 21 Photos of patient's face 4 weeks after the prosthesis was placed.

SECTION 6

Radiation Stents

CHAPTER 25

Appliances for radiation therapy

Ancillary appliances for radiation therapy make radiotherapy more effective and prevent the aftereffects of radiation.

Their main functions are as follows:

① to contain and fix the radiation source in place, ② to exclude the surrounding normal tissue from the radiation field, ③ to seal the lead in and shield normal tissue, and ④ to protect normal tissue by creating distance between the normal tissue and the radiation source.

In practice, a single appliance often has multiple functions, or a combination of two appliances is generally used.

Principal types of ancillary appliances for radiation treatment

Spacer: an appliance for decreasing the radiation dosage of normal tissue by maintaining distance between the small radiation source and the normal tissue.

Mold: an appliance to contain and fix a small radiation source so that it is closely attached to the tumor site for radiation from the tumor surface.

Shield: an appliance to protect the surrounding normal tissue from radiation, using lead shielding.

Protector: an appliance that prevents exposure by mechanical exclusion, to keep the normal tissue adjacent to a tumor from entering the radiated field.

Spacers (Fig. 1)

These are used principally in interstitial radiation therapy for lingual cancer. It is more effective to make spacers as thick as possible to decrease the radiation dose directed toward the mandible (spacer thickness is equal to the distance between the tumor surface and the adjacent alveolar gingival surface). The spacer must be of a size that causes only minor pain when the interstitial radiation source is inserted. The spacer must be able to be used continuously during the treatment period. A minimum thickness of 8mm is necessary for the spacer; generally, a 10-12mm thickness is used.[1].

Materials for spacers :

For the spacer, usage of silicone, acrylic resins, modeling compounds, and gauzes are reported. The following conditions are required;

1) They must be biomaterials for medical use and of minimum irritation to the mucosa,

2) They must not degenerate or become deformed during the radiation period,

3) They must be readily available and easy to fabricate and adjust, and

4) Must be radiolucent and cause no problems related to transmissivity and radiation scatter. (Radiolucency is required because radiographs to calculate the dose are taken with the appliance in place.)

Production of spacers :

The essential conditions for the main units of spacers are ① accurate fit and excellent retention and stability, ② safety, sturdy design with no uncomfortable feeling when placed in the mouth, and ③ easy handling and a certain degree of control possible by patients themselves.

The author has obtained excellent results using a silicone resin for an orthodontic appliance, the "dynamic positioner" (Orthocon Light® : this is translucent, bland, innocuous, and radiolucent). Actual production procedures for devices used in the treatment of lingual cancer[2] are as follows.

1) Intraoral examination

The position and size of the primary tumor, and the area and depth of the internal aspect of the mandible, can be confirmed thoroughly by palpation to estimate the thickness and size for the spacer.

2) Impression-taking

The impression range for the spacer region is the maximum area from the oral floor to the internal aspect of the mandible.

The impression area for the spacer is outlined with an impression tray and utility wax, an impression of the entire device is taken with alginate impression material (Fig. 2).

The most effective way to take an adequate impression (Fig. 3) is first to instruct the patient to relax the head and shoulders, then slowly push down on the tray so it moves down deeply toward the oral floor, to the extent that it is not painful.

3) Registration of interocclusal relationship (bite-taking)

Registration of the interocclusal relationship should be conducted with the anterior teeth opened about 5mm in consideration of swelling of the tongue after insertion of the interstitial radiation source. When the jaw is edentulous or occlusion is unstable, occlusal

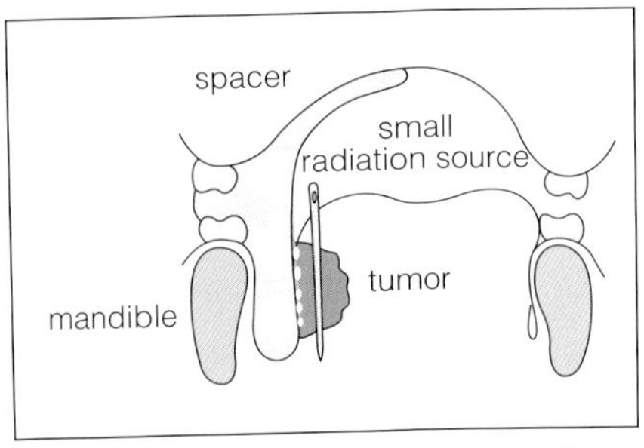

Fig. 1 Sectional view of spacer with interstitial radiation source, used in treatment of lingual cancer.

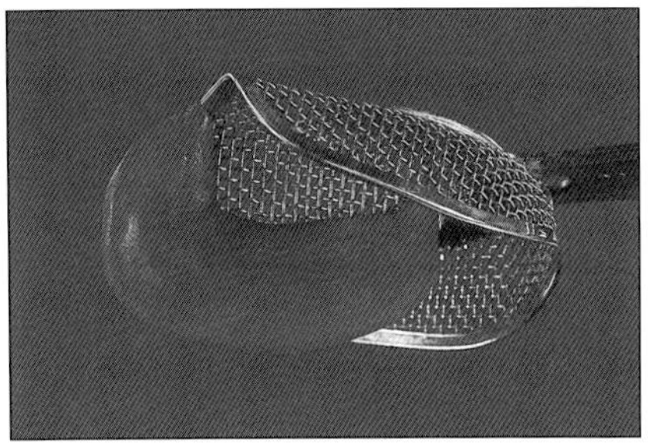

Fig. 2 Tray for impression. The tentative form of the spacer is pre-fabricated using a stock tray and utility wax.

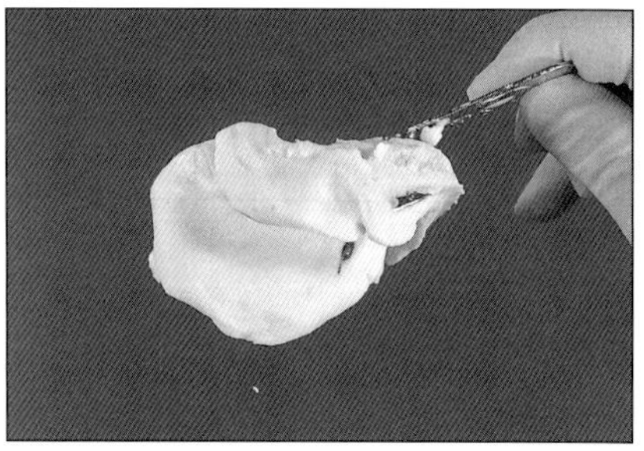

Fig. 3 Taking impression of spacer region. An impression is taken over a wide area from the mandibular inner surface to the deeper section of the oral floor.

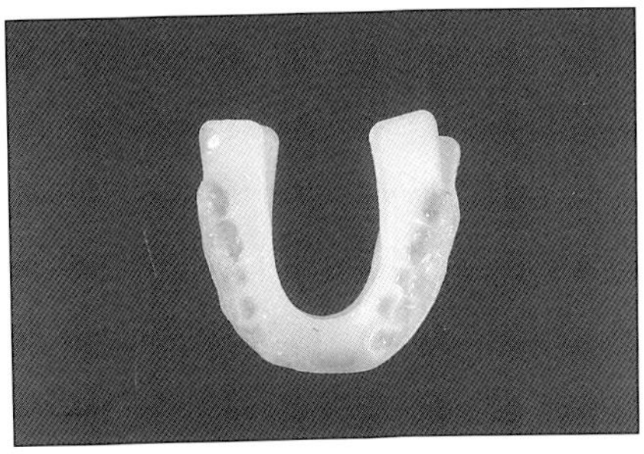

Fig. 4 Registration of interocclusal relationship (bite-taking) is done with the mouth slightly open, with upper and lower teeth separated by about 5mm.

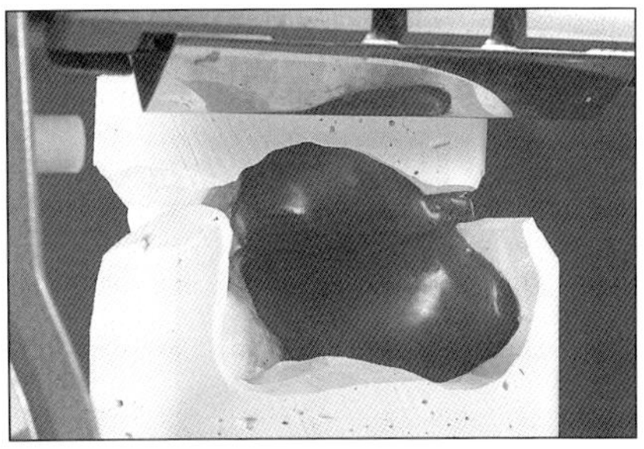

Fig. 5 Waxing-up of entire spacer. Waxing-up of upper-lower integrated mouthpiece type including palatal region.

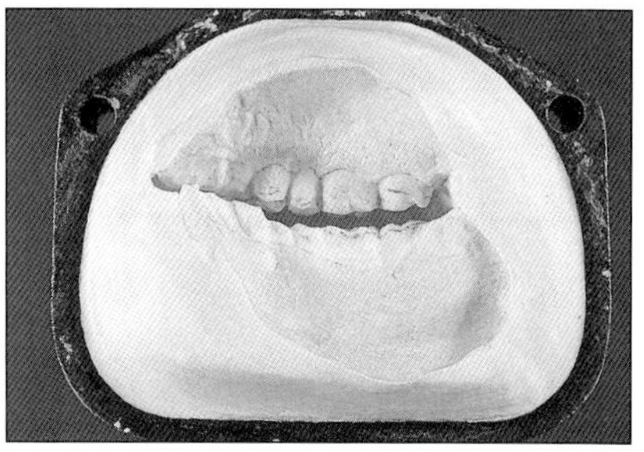

Fig. 6 Casting the spacer region mold after dewaxing. Orthocon® is compression-molded after dewaxing.

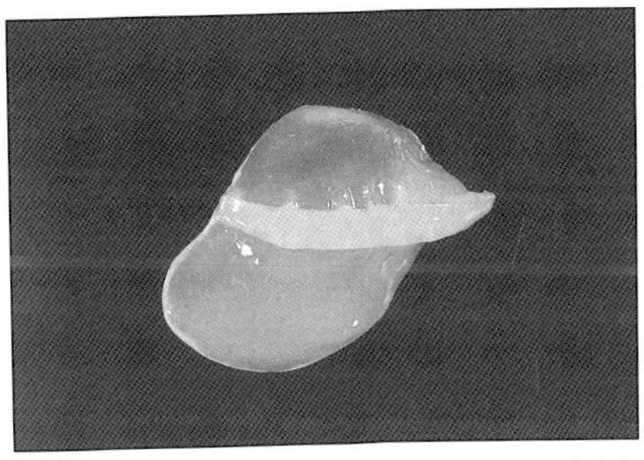

Fig. 7 Spacer (view from the outer side). The section below the center is the spacer section.

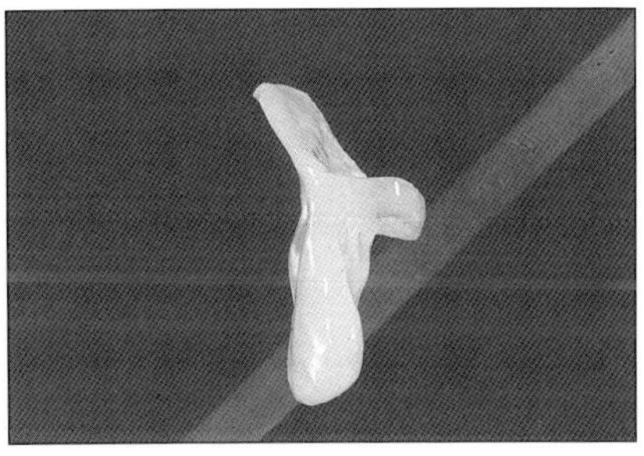

Fig. 8 Spacer (back view). Upper: palatal part. Center: occlusal part. Lower: spacer part.

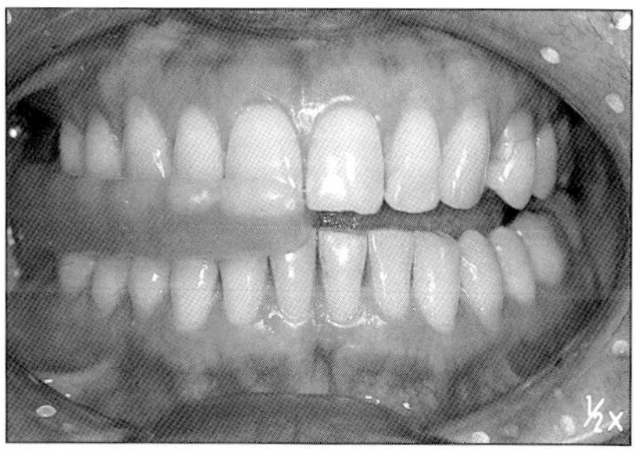

Fig. 9 Intraoral inserted view. Occlusal status after insertion of spacer.

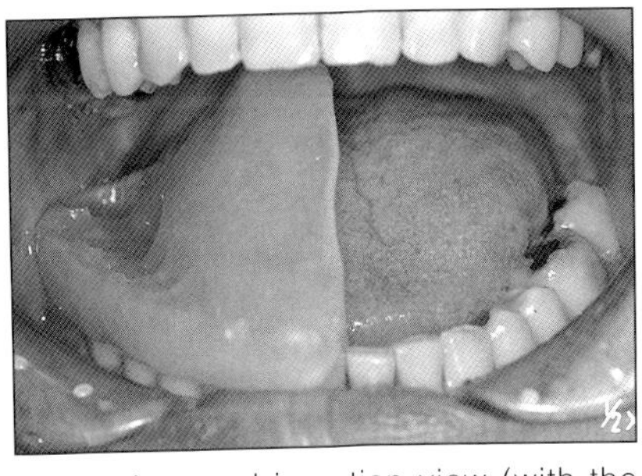

Fig. 10 Intraoral insertion view (with the mouth open). Even with the mouth open, the device never becomes displaced from the mandible.

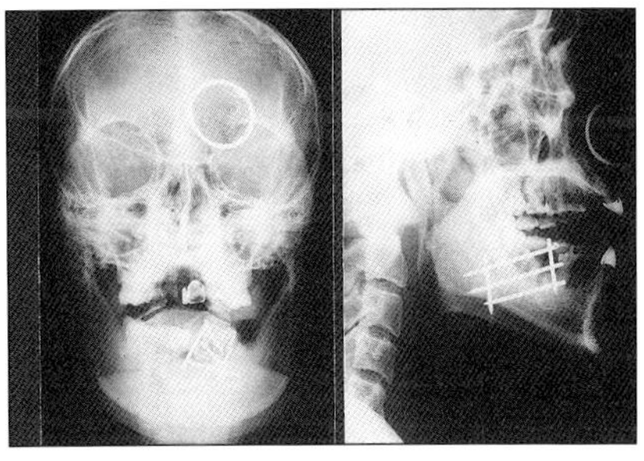

Fig. 11 Radiographic findings with spacer inserted. Because of its radiolucency, the taking of radiographs and calculation of dosage can be done with the spacer inserted.

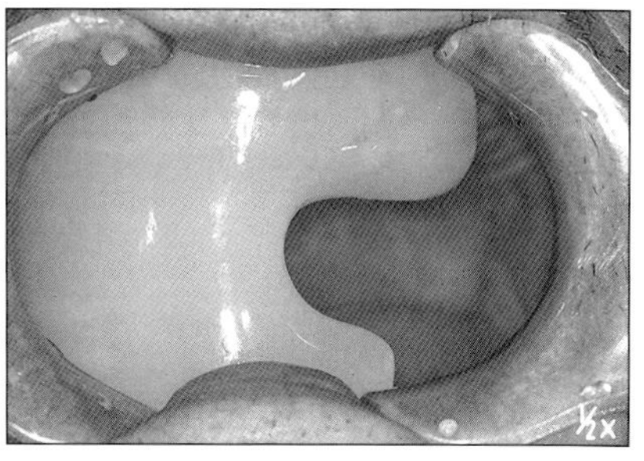

Fig. 12 Spacer for edentulous patient, inserted. Mouthpiece-type spacer combined with silicone resin.

plates should be formed first, before registration of the interocclusal relationship (Fig. 4).

4) With working casts mounted on an articulator, the entire appliance is waxed up.

The complete form of the appliance is the integrated mouthpiece type including the palatal region. Half-jaw size should be designed for a tumor close to the tongue root and 2/3-jaw size should be designed for a

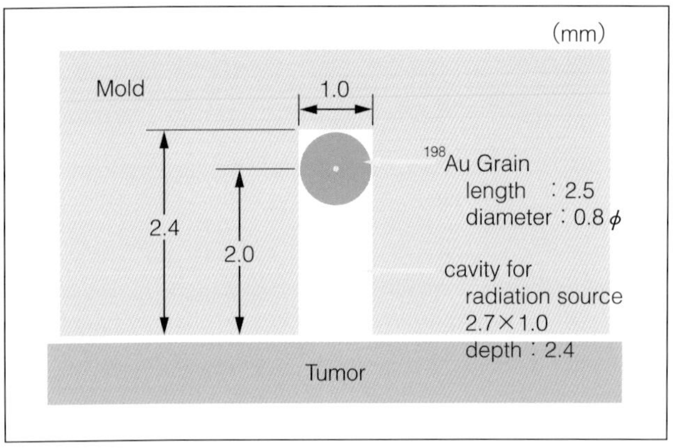

Fig. 13 Cross-sectional view of sealed cavity for small radiation source. The distance from the center of the radiation source to the tumor surface is designed to be 2mm.

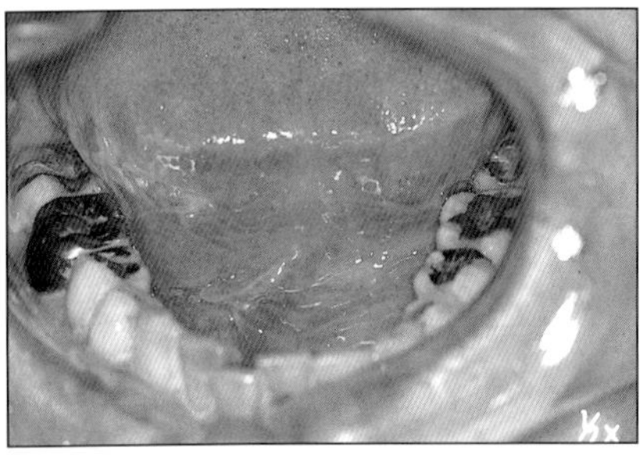

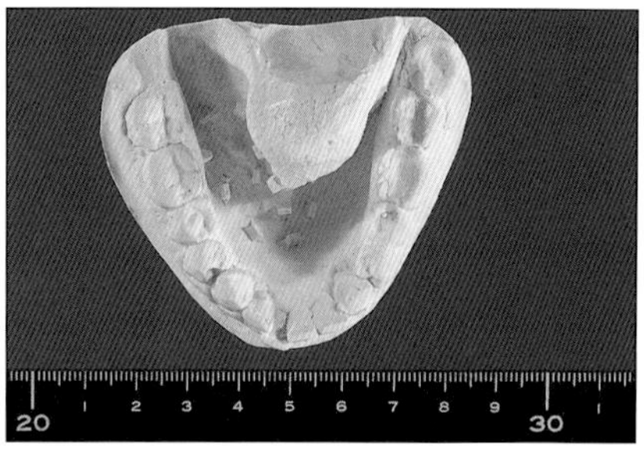

Fig. 14 *(left)* Oral-floor cancer. Pre-treatment view of the lesion for mold radiation therapy.
Fig. 15 *(right)* Position to which small radiation sources will be placed. A 1.0 × 2.7 × 2.4mm plastic block is attached to the cast (duplicate cast).

tumor close to the tongue apex.

Fixing the device in position in the oral cavity is achieved by inter-dental occlusion. In addition, retention must be achieved using the undercuts of lower teeth, to keep the device from floating off the mandible even when the mouth is partly open (Fig. 5).

5) After the working model is flasked, wax is removed and the Orthocon® is pressure-molded, then boiled for an hour for primary vulcanization (Fig. 6).

6) Following removal and polishing, a coating agent is applied, then drying by heating (second vulcanization) is done to complete the appliance (Figs. 7 and 8).

The completed spacer and the status of intraoral insertion are shown in Figs. 9 to 12.

Molds

Conditions for making molds :

Surface radiation means the method of irradiating a treatment surface by arranging small radiation sources according to certain specific standards and maintaining a fixed relationship to the surface to be treated.

Molds are devices for holding and fixing small radiation sources for a certain period of time to satisfy the requirements. Since even a slight error in the distance between the treatment surface and radiation sources will cause a large dosage error, it is important to take a precise impression of the radiation field and to do accurate positional fixation.

A sectional view of the cavity used to seal the small radiation source into the mold is shown here (Fig. 13).

Using ^{198}Au Grain (2.5mm in length, 0.8mm in diameter), the distance between the center of the radiation source and the tumor surface has been set at 2mm. These depths, intersource distances and arrangements are determined by the radiation planning required for radiation therapy itself.

Materials for molds :

Radiolucency is important to make it possible to calculate the radiation dose by taking radiographs after insertion of the radiation sources for interstitial radiation. For this, a dental base plate resin is normally used. When the use of a lead shield is required, the shield is often made separately from the mold.

Depending on the circumstances, materials for fixing molds may have to be specially designed. Clasps, mouthpiece types and/or bite block types can be used in combination with silicone resin.

Preparation and making of molds :

1) The position and area of the tumor and the status of the surrounding tissue should be thoroughly understood before making the mold, so that the radiation sources can be positioned effectively (Fig. 14).

2) A custom tray is prepared and a non-pressure impression is taken to avoid losing the form of the tumor and the surrounding tissue.

3) The position and direction of the radiation sources are marked on the working model.

4) Using an adhesive, small prefabricated plastic blocks, 1.0 × 2.7 × 2.4mm are attached vertically in the position of the radiation sources on the pre-marked cast (Fig. 15).

5) Polymerizing resin is then poured, followed by removal of the plastic blocks after setting. The cavities for indwelling of the small radiation sources are completed.

6) The completed mold is shown in Figs. 16 to 23.

Shields

The radiation dose of ^{198}Au Grain can be shielded by approximately 50% using a 4mm lead plate. The lead plate is fabricated by casting lead.

The lead plate is used by sealing it into the base plate resin. If the thickness of the resin is increased, this can also be used as a spacer.

A shield fabricated to protect the palatal region from exposure to the interstitial radiation therapy for cancer of the base of the tongue is shown in Figs. 24 and 25.

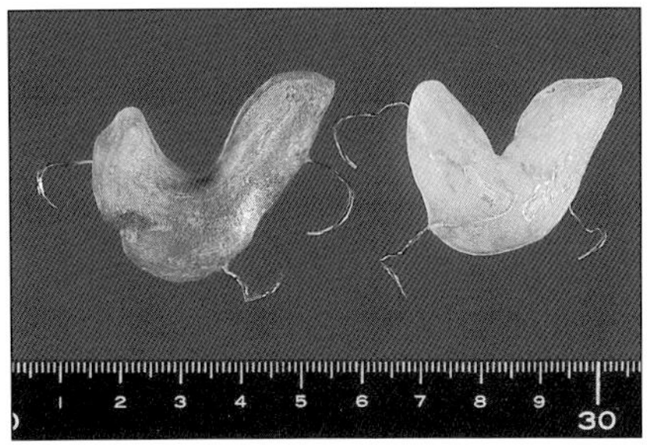

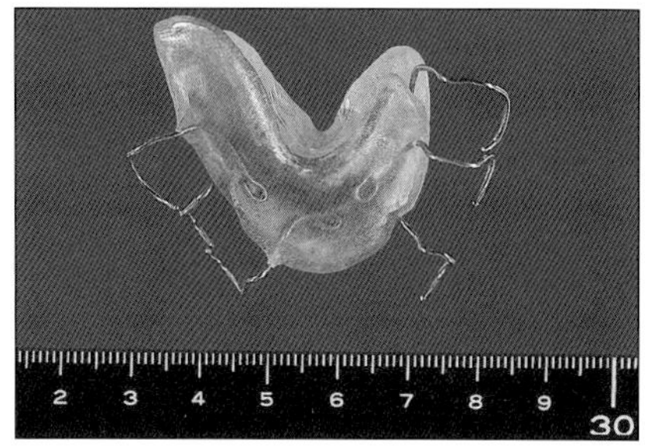

Fig. 16 *(left)* Left: shield. Right: mold The mold and shield are made as separate devices.
Fig. 17 *(right)* Mold and shield superimposed.

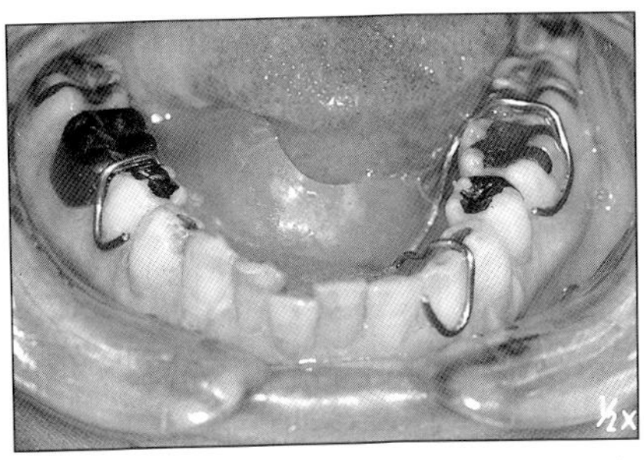

Fig. 18 Intraoral view when mold alone is inserted.

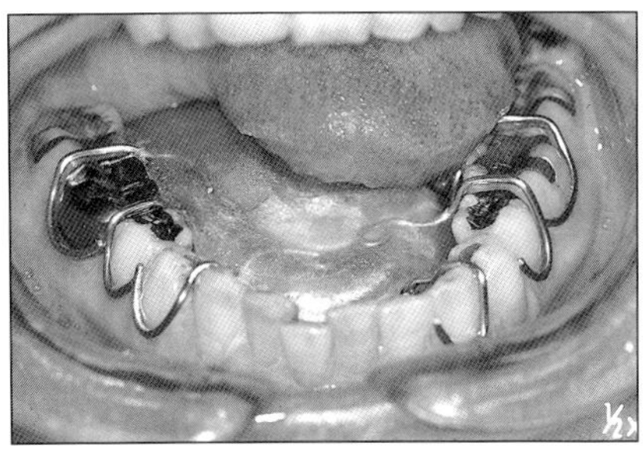

Fig. 19 Intraoral view when mold and shield are inserted.

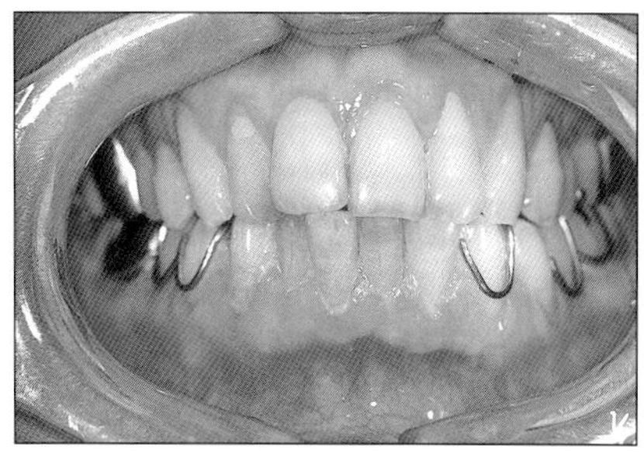

Fig. 20 Intraoral view when mold and shield are inserted. The patient can close his/her mouth even with the mold and shield inserted.

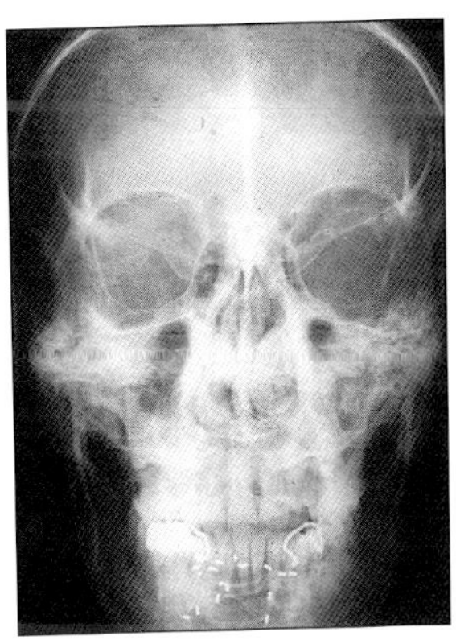

Fig. 21 Radiographic view with mold alone inserted (front view). Can be used for calculating dose.

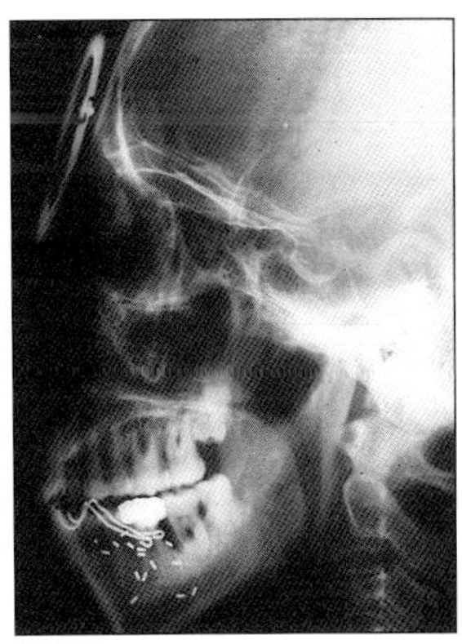

Fig. 22 Radiographic view with mold alone inserted (lateral view).

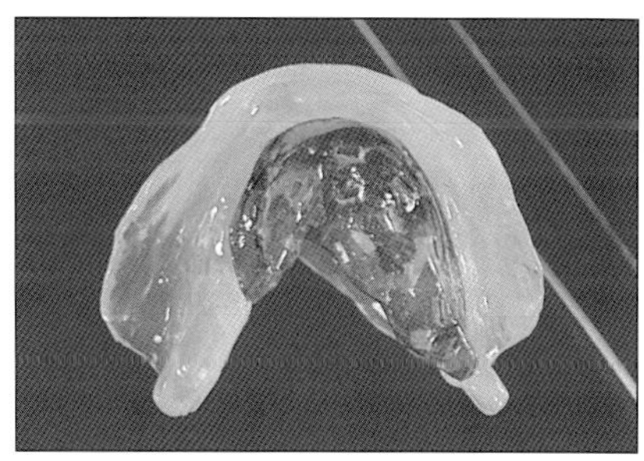

Fig. 23 Mold for edentulous patient. A bite-block type of mold made of silicone resin is attached to the resin mold to hold the appliance and fix it into the oral cavity.

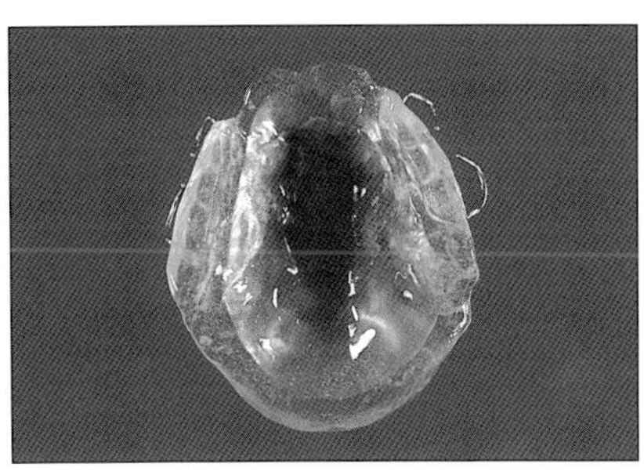

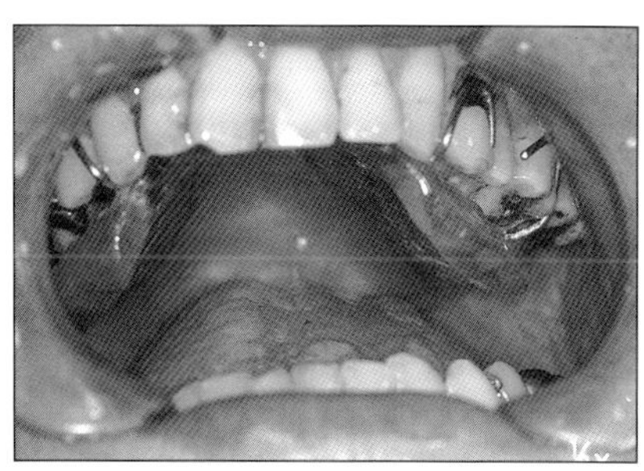

Fig. 24 *(left)* Shield for palatal region. Fabricated by sealing lead into a resin splint.
Fig. 25 *(right)* Shield for palatal region (intraoral insertion view). The appliance is fixed in position using clasps.

References

1) Koukichi Niwa, Kozo Morita, Hajime Kanazawa and Motoo Yokoi: Usefulness of a Radiolucent Spacer in Radiation Therapy for Cancer of the Tongue: Jap.J.Cancer Clin.,30(15): 1861 – 1865, 1984.

2) Motoo Yokoi, Yoshiyuki Ito, Nobukazu Fuwa, Eriko Kato, Takayuki Murao and Kozo Morita: Usefulness of a Radiolucent Spacer in Radiation Therapy for Cancer of the Tongue: Head and Neck Cancer. 19(2): 188 – 192, 1993.

Index